BF
2017

Ionizing Radiation Exposure of the Population of the United States

Recommendations of the
**NATIONAL COUNCIL ON RADIATION
PROTECTION AND MEASUREMENTS**

March 3, 2009

*WN
5
'N2775
2009
no.160*

National Council on Radiation Protection and Measurements
7910 Woodmont Avenue, Suite 400 / Bethesda, MD 20814-3095

LEGAL NOTICE

This Report was prepared by the National Council on Radiation Protection and Measurements (NCRP). The Council strives to provide accurate, complete and useful information in its documents. However, neither NCRP, the members of NCRP, other persons contributing to or assisting in the preparation of this Report, nor any person acting on the behalf of any of these parties: (a) makes any warranty or representation, express or implied, with respect to the accuracy, completeness or usefulness of the information contained in this Report, or that the use of any information, method or process disclosed in this Report may not infringe on privately owned rights; or (b) assumes any liability with respect to the use of, or for damages resulting from the use of any information, method or process disclosed in this Report, *under the Civil Rights Act of 1964, Section 701 et seq. as amended 42 U.S.C. Section 2000e et seq. (Title VII) or any other statutory or common law theory governing liability.*

Disclaimer

Any mention of commercial products within NCRP publications is for information only; it does not imply recommendation or endorsement by NCRP.

Library of Congress Cataloging-in-Publication Data

Ionizing radiation exposure of the population of the United States.
   p. ; cm. -- (NCRP report ; no. 160)
   Update of: NCRP report no. 93, Ionizing radiation exposure of the population of the United States, c1987.
   Includes bibliographical references and index.
   ISBN 978-0-929600-98-7
   1. Ionizing radiation--Dosage. 2. Ionizing radiation--Environmental aspects-- United States. 3. Health risk assessment--United States. I. National Council on Radiation Protection and Measurements. II. National Council on Radiation Protection and Measurements. Scientific Committee 6-2 on Radiation Exposure of the U.S. Population. III. National Council on Radiation Protection and Measurements. Ionizing radiation exposure of the population of the United States. IV. Series: NCRP report ; no. 160.
   [DNLM: 1. Environmental Exposure--United States--Statistics. 2. Radiation, Ionizing--United States--Statistics. 3. Radiation Dosage--United States--Statistics. WN 105 I58 2009]
   RA569.I66 2009
   363.17'990973--dc22

                                    2009005932

[For detailed information on the availability of NCRP publications see page 366.]

Preface

This Report was developed under the auspices of Program Area Committee 6 of the National Council on Radiation Protection and Measurements (NCRP), the Committee that provides oversight for radiation dosimetry and measurements. It is an update of NCRP Report No. 93, *Ionizing Radiation Exposure of the Population of the United States*, which was issued in September 1987. This Report evaluates the doses to the U.S. population from all sources of ionizing radiation for 2006, with particular attention to those sources that contribute the largest shares, and provides some information on doses that individuals may experience due to their specific circumstances. For example, patients undergoing specific medical procedures using ionizing radiation can in many cases obtain a nominal value of dose for a medical procedure (*e.g.*, an abdominal computed tomography examination) from data tabulated in this Report and a general idea of the total dose from multiple procedures by summing the values.

While the Report clearly describes the relative dose contributions to individuals and the population from the various radiation sources, it does not attempt to quantify the associated health risks nor specify the actions that should be taken in light of these latest data. The latter two subjects were outside the scope of the charge to the Committee.

NCRP has adopted the International System (SI) of Quantities and Units for its reports (NCRP Report No. 82, *SI Units in Radiation Protection and Measurements*) which includes gray, sievert and becquerel. However, some of the references cited in this Report originally used the previous system of quantities and units, namely rad, rem and curie, which have been converted to the SI system in this Report. For convenience, conversions between the SI system and the previous system are provided in Appendix A.

This Report was prepared by Scientific Committee 6-2 on Radiation Exposure of the U.S. Population, through the effort of five subcommittees, each of which addressed a specific category of radiation sources. Serving on the Committee (listed by category of radiation sources) were:

Joel E. Gray
DIQUAD, LLC
Steger, Illinois

Jill A. Lipoti
New Jersey Department of
Environmental Protection
Trenton, New Jersey

Mahadevappa Mahesh
Johns Hopkins University School
of Medicine
Baltimore, Maryland

John L. McCrohan
Center for Devices and
Radiological Health
Food and Drug Administration
Rockville, Maryland

Fred A. Mettler, Jr.
University of New Mexico
Albuquerque, New Mexico

Terry T. Yoshizumi
Duke University School of
Medicine
Durham, North Carolina

Consumer Products and Activities

Orhan H. Suleiman, *Subcommittee Chairman*
Center for Drug Evaluation and Research
Food and Drug Administration
Silver Spring, Maryland

Members

Jennifer Goodman
New Jersey Department of
Environmental Protection
Trenton, New Jersey

Raymond H. Johnson, Jr.
Dade Moeller and Associates
Gaithersburg, Maryland

Cheryl K. Rogers
Wisconsin Department of Health
Services
Madison, Wisconsin

Consultants

Paul W. Frame
Oak Ridge Associated
Universities
Oak Ridge, Tennessee

Ronald L. Kathren
Washington State University
Richland, Washington

Industrial, Security, Medical, Educational and Research Activities

Dennis M. Quinn, *Subcommittee Chairman*
Hopewell Junction, New York

Members

Ralph Andersen
Nuclear Energy Institute
Washington, D.C.

E. Scott Medling
San Onofre Nuclear Generating
 Station
San Clemente, California

Regis A. Greenwood
American Radiolabeled
 Chemicals, Inc.
Maryland Heights, Missouri

Carl J. Paperiello
Talisman International
Washington, D.C.

Cynthia G. Jones
U.S. Nuclear Regulatory
 Commission
Washington, D.C.

Linda M. Sewell
Diablo Canyon Power Plant
Avila Beach, California

Occupational Exposure

Kenneth L. Miller, *Subcommittee Chairman*
Penn State Hershey Medical Center
Hershey, Pennsylvania

Members

David J. Allard
Pennsylvania Department of
 Environmental Protection
Harrisburg, Pennsylvania

Kathleen L. Shingleton
Lawrence Livermore National
 Laboratory
Livermore, California

Kelly L. Classic
Mayo Clinic
Rochester, Minnesota

George J. Vargo
MJW Corporation, Inc.
Avondale, Pennsylvania

Michael A. Lewandowski
3M Company
St. Paul, Minnesota

NCRP Secretariat
Marvin Rosenstein, *Staff Consultant*
Cindy L. O'Brien, *Managing Editor*
David A. Schauer, *Executive Director*

The Council expresses its appreciation to the Committee members for the time and effort devoted to the preparation of this Report. NCRP also gratefully acknowledges financial support for this work provided by the U.S. Nuclear Regulatory Commission, the U.S. Environmental Protection Agency, and the Centers for Disease Control and Prevention.

Thomas S. Tenforde
President

Contents

1. Executive Summary

Detailed information on the exposure of the U.S. population to ionizing radiation, based on evaluations made in the early 1980s, was presented by the National Council on Radiation Protection and Measurements (NCRP) in Report No. 93, *Ionizing Radiation Exposure of the Population of the United States* (NCRP, 1987a). Since that time, the magnitude and distribution among the various sources of radiation exposure to the U.S. population have changed primarily due to increased utilization of ionizing radiation in diagnostic and interventional medical procedures. Documented in this Report are the contributions from all radiation sources in 2006. This Report neither quantifies the associated health risks nor specifies the radiation protection actions that should be taken in light of these latest data because these subjects are beyond the scope of this Report.

The radiation exposure to the U.S. population for 2006 is presented in five broad categories:

- exposure from ubiquitous background radiation, including radon in homes;
- exposure to patients from medical procedures;
- exposure from consumer products or activities involving radiation sources;
- exposure from industrial, security, medical, educational and research radiation sources; and
- exposure of workers that results from their occupations.

The dose assessments for the five categories and components within each category are derived from disparate types of information and variable methods of analysis. While not identical, these categories are closely aligned with those in NCRP (1987a).

The principal results are presented as annual values for:

- average effective dose to an individual in a group exposed to a specific source (E_{Exp}) (millisievert), which excludes individuals that are not subject to exposure from the specific source of radiation;

1

- collective effective dose (S) (person-sievert), which is the cumulative dose to a population of individuals exposed to a given radiation source or group of sources; and
- effective dose per individual in the U.S. population (E_{US}) (millisievert), computed by dividing S by the total number of individuals in the U.S. population (300 million in 2006) whether exposed to the specific source or not.

S and E_{US} provide useful indices for comparison among radiation sources and different time periods.

1.1 Ubiquitous Background Exposure

For purposes of analysis, this category was separated into four subcategories:

1. external exposure from space radiation (solar particles and cosmic rays);
2. external exposure from terrestrial radiation (primarily ^{40}K and the ^{238}U and ^{232}Th decay series);
3. internal exposure from inhalation of radon and thoron[1] and their progeny; and
4. internal exposure from radionuclides in the body.

An appendix to Subcategory 4 provides an independent assessment from domestic water supplies; however, the contribution from all food and water is already included in the evaluation for radionuclides in the body. Particular attention was given to evaluating the variability in these sources; arithmetic and geometric means and associated statistics for the effective dose distributions in each of the four subcategories were included. Estimates of effective dose for each subcategory were derived as follows:

1. *Space radiation*: A computer code was used for estimating outdoor ground level effective doses for 99 of the most populated U.S. urban areas and then adjusting for indoor levels and time spent outdoors and in dwellings.
2. *Terrestrial radiation*: Data from the National Uranium Resource Evaluation (NURE) Program for concentrations of uranium and thorium (parts per million by weight) and potassium (weight percent) in surface soil and rocks

---

[1]Radon is the common name for the radionuclide ^{222}Rn and thoron is the common name for the radionuclide ^{220}Rn. In this Report, the common names are generally used, and radon without qualification refers to ^{222}Rn.

at 10,650 locations across the continental United States were used to obtain activity concentrations for the principal radionuclides (^{238}U, ^{232}Th, and ^{40}K). The concentrations were then converted to air kerma and effective dose using age-dependent conversion coefficients, and adjusted for building attenuation for the time spent indoors.

3. *Radon and thoron and their progeny*: Radon concentrations (Bq m^{-3}) from the National Residential Radon Survey (NRRS) [conducted by the U.S. Environmental Protection Agency (EPA)], supplemented by data from the University of Pittsburgh and Lawrence Berkeley National Laboratory (LBNL), adjusted for equilibrium factors (Glossary) and fractions of time spent in various locations (indoors at home or away and outdoors) were used to obtain the potential alpha-energy exposure [in working level months (WLM)]. The dose conversion coefficient for radon and its progeny (millisievert effective dose per WLM) and its uncertainty are discussed.[2] Adjustments were made for estimated exposure to thoron and its progeny.

4. *Radionuclides in the body*: Age- and gender-dependent potassium measurements (gram of potassium per kilogram of body mass) from the U.S. Department of Energy's Hanford Site were used to derive activity concentrations for ^{40}K. Age- and gender-dependent dose conversion coefficients were obtained from the Radiation Dose Assessment Resource. For the ^{232}Th and ^{238}U series, effective dose estimates for the U.S. population were derived from reference values published by UNSCEAR (2000) and data for the United States. For the separate assessment of domestic water supplies, data for radium, uranium and radon concentrations in water supplies from the National Inorganic and Radionuclide Survey (NIRS) (public supplies) and the U.S. Geological Survey (USGS) (private wells), (adjusted for consumption rates), published dose conversion coefficients, and census data for number of individuals exposed were used.

---

[2]The dose conversion coefficient for radon and its progeny used in this Report is 10 mSv WLM^{-1} (Section 3.5.10). This value agrees with that obtained from a dosimetric analysis and is consistent with that used previously by NCRP (1987b). It is similar to that obtained in recent epidemiological analyses by Tomasek *et al.* (2008). The value of 10 mSv WLM^{-1} is greater than that used by UNSCEAR (2000), and more than twice that used by ICRP (1993) for exposure in homes based on a previous epidemiological analysis. Use of other dose conversion coefficients would result in a proportionate difference in S and E_{US}.

The results in 2006 for ubiquitous background radiation for S and E_{US} are 933,000 person-Sv and 3.1 mSv (arithmetic mean), respectively, compared with 690,000 person-Sv and 3 mSv in the early 1980s. The higher value for S reflects the 30 % increase in the U.S. population between the two time periods; the value for E_{US} is comparable with that for the early 1980s. The percent contribution to the total S and total E_{US} for this category from each of the four subcategories for 2006 is (in decreasing order):

- radon and thoron (73 %)
- space radiation (11 %)
- radionuclides in the body (9 %)
- terrestrial radiation (7 %)

The contribution to E_{US} from only ^{222}Rn (radon) for 2006 (2.1 mSv) (Table 3.14) is comparable with that for the early 1980s (2 mSv), given the uncertainty in derivation of the values. Since all members of the U.S. population are exposed to ubiquitous background radiation, E_{US} is also E_{Exp}. Values for total E_{Exp} and its components, including arithmetic means (AM), standard deviations (SD), geometric means (GM), geometric standard deviations (GSD), and 2.5 and 97.5 percentiles are given in Table 3.14 along with the factors affecting the variability of each component.

1.2 Medical Exposure of Patients

This category was separated into five subcategories for analysis grouped by medical modality:

1. computed tomography
2. conventional radiography and fluoroscopy
3. interventional fluoroscopy
4. nuclear medicine
5. external-beam radiotherapy

While a dose assessment was conducted for external-beam radiotherapy, the results are not included in the total for this category because of unique considerations, namely, E_{Exp} was 0.4 Sv, the population exposed is small (<3 % of the total U.S. population) and is a special group with life-threatening illness, and absorbed doses to some tissues or portions of tissues outside but nearby the treatment volume could approach and exceed 1 Sv. Thus the inclusion of this source in the assessment of dose to the U.S. population may not be applicable (Section 4.6).

The number of procedures for each modality for 2006 was derived mainly from several commercial market benchmark reports produced by IMV Medical Information Division [IMV (Des Plaines, Illinois)] that identify the universe of facilities providing the services. Supplemental sources of data that were available included: Medicare (administrative claims for fee-for-service enrollees), the U.S. Department of Veterans Affairs (VA) (administrative claims for VA health plan enrollees), a large national employer plan (LNEP) (administrative claims), and a commercial source for dental bitewing film packs. Effective doses for procedures were derived from the published literature as follows:

- *Computed tomography*: Based on data for dose length product and age and body region specific conversion coefficients.
- *Conventional radiography and fluoroscopy*: Based on data for effective dose.
- *Interventional fluoroscopy*: Based on data for kerma-area product (*KAP*) and protocol-specific dose conversion coefficients.
- *Nuclear medicine*: Based on data for dose conversion coefficients expressed as effective dose per unit administered activity.
- *External-beam radiotherapy*: Based on absorbed doses to organs and tissues located outside the treatment volume.

The available information on effective dose was not sufficient to permit an analysis of statistical measures of variability, nor was there sufficient information available to determine E_{Exp} for medical exposures.

The results for medical exposure of patients (excluding radiotherapy) for 2006, as contrasted with the early 1980s, show a marked increase in S (a factor of 7.3) and E_{US} (a factor of 5.7) during the intervening ~25 y. Some of the increase in S is due to the 30 % increase in the U.S. population during that time (230 million in 1980; 300 million in 2006). Since E_{US} is an effective dose per individual in the U.S. population, the effect of population growth is removed, and the increase is due primarily to increased utilization of CT, interventional fluoroscopy, and nuclear medicine. The percent contribution to the total S (899,000 person-Sv) and the total E_{US} (3 mSv) for medical exposure from each of the four modalities for 2006 is (in decreasing order):

- computed tomography (49 %)
- nuclear medicine (26 %)
- interventional fluoroscopy (14 %)
- conventional radiography and fluoroscopy (11 %)

1.3 Consumer Products and Activities

To analyze exposures in this category, it was divided into seven subcategories grouped by the origin of the source:

1. building materials
2. commercial air travel
3. cigarette smoking
4. mining and agriculture
5. combustion of fossil fuels
6. highway and road construction materials
7. glass and ceramics

The number of individuals exposed to a particular source was derived in various ways: updates of the values used by NCRP for the early 1980s to adjust for change in U.S. population (building materials, mining and agriculture, combustion of fossil fuels, and highway and road construction materials); numbers of passengers from the Bureau of Transportation Statistics (commercial air travel); the National Health Interview Survey (cigarette smoking); and assumptions for the small numbers of individuals involved (glass and ceramics). Estimates of effective dose for each subcategory were derived as follows:

- Subcategories 1, 4, 5 and 6. *Building materials, mining and agriculture, combustion of fossil fuels*, and *highway and road construction materials*: Based on the effective dose equivalent (H_E) (or updates of the values) used in deriving the estimates for the early 1980s.
- Subcategory 2. *Commercial air travel*: Based on effective doses calculated using the computer code CARI-6 for various flight segments and published by the U.S. Department of Transportation.
- Subcategory 3. *Cigarette smoking*: Based on published estimates for the effective dose from smoking one cigarette per day for a year, estimates from the Centers for Disease Control and Prevention on the average number of cigarettes smoked per day by an individual smoker, and the total number of smokers.
- Subcategory 7. *Glass and ceramics*: Based on published values from NRC expressed as H_E.

The available information on effective dose was not sufficient to permit an analysis of statistical measures of variability.

An extensive discussion of radiation exposure from consumer products is contained in NCRP Report No. 95 (NCRP, 1987d). Much of that information is still relevant. In this Report exposures from some of the more significant sources have been updated and information is included about some additional sources. The potential sources that are not discussed in any detail in this Report are noted as "other sources."

The results for consumer products or activities for 2006 for S and E_{US} are 39,000 person-Sv and 0.13 mSv, respectively, compared with 12,000 to 29,000 person-Sv and 0.05 to 0.13 mSv in the early 1980s [presented only in terms of ranges in NCRP (1987a)]. However, the collections of sources included in this category for 2006 and the early 1980s are dissimilar and no specific conclusions should be drawn from the S and E_{US} values other than that this category is a small contributor to U.S. population dose. The percent contribution to the total S and the total E_{US} for this category from each of the seven subcategories and the other sources for 2006 is (in decreasing order):

- cigarette smoking (35 %)
- building materials (27 %)
- commercial air travel (26 %)
- mining and agriculture (6 %)
- other sources (3 %)
- combustion of fossil fuels (2 %)
- highway and road construction materials (0.6 %)
- glass and ceramics (<0.03 %)

This category is characterized by sources that deliver small annual effective doses [*i.e.*, the range for E_{Exp} among the included subcategories is 1 to 300 μSv (Table 5.8)] to much of the U.S. population (Table 5.8).

1.4 Industrial, Security, Medical, Educational and Research Activities

This category was divided into six subcategories for analysis, grouped by the nature of the activity and associated type of source:

1. nuclear-power generation
2. DOE installations
3. decommissioning and radioactive waste
4. industrial, medical, educational and research activities
5. caregiving or other contact with nuclear-medicine patients
6. security inspection systems

The effective doses to members of the public (*i.e.*, not employees) and the number of individuals exposed for a particular source were derived as follows:

1. *Nuclear-power generation*: Based on H_E used by NCRP for the early 1980s adjusted for the current total power generation by nuclear reactors.
2. *DOE installations*: Based on DOE site environmental reports with doses expressed as H_E.
3. *Decommissioning and radioactive waste*: Based on various federal agency reports with doses expressed as H_E [or total effective dose equivalent (TEDE)].
4. *Industrial, medical, educational and research activities*: Based on projections to members of the public from the number of occupationally-exposed individuals and the effective doses for occupational exposures for similar facilities.
5. *Exposure from nuclear-medicine patients (as a result of caregiving or other contact)*: Based on projecting the annual number of procedures and the published effective dose per procedure (to a member of the public) in NCRP Report No. 124.
6. *Security inspection systems*: Based on assumptions for the small numbers of individuals receiving detectable exposure and the published literature data for dose equivalent from other than cabinet x-ray systems.

The available information on effective dose was not sufficient to permit an analysis of statistical measures of variability.

The estimates for industrial, security, medical, educational and research activities for 2006 for S and E_{US} are 1,000 person-Sv and 0.003 mSv, respectively, compared with 200 person-Sv and 0.001 mSv in the early 1980s. However, the collections of sources included in this category for 2006 and the early 1980s are dissimilar and no specific comparative conclusions should be drawn from the S and E_{US} values other than this category is a very small contributor to the U.S. population dose. The percent contribution to the total S and total E_{US} for this category from each of the six subcategories for 2006 is (in decreasing order):

- caregiving or other contact with nuclear-medicine patients (72 %)
- nuclear-power generation (15 %)
- industrial, medical, educational and research activities (13 %)

- DOE installations («1 %)
- decommissioning and radioactive waste («1 %)
- security inspection systems («1 %)

This category is characterized by sources that deliver very small annual effective doses to individuals who are in proximity to these activities (E_{Exp} for the included subcategories is 1 to 10 μSv).

1.5 Occupational Exposure

Six subcategories grouped by the nature of employment and associated type of source were used to analyze this category:

1. medical
2. aviation
3. commercial nuclear power
4. industry and commerce
5. education and research
6. government, DOE and military

Personal monitoring programs, accredited by either the National Voluntary Laboratory Accreditation Program or the DOE Laboratory Accreditation Program provided data for the numbers of workers monitored and doses for those with recordable dose (*i.e.*, doses greater than a minimum detectable level) in all the subcategories except aviation. Internal doses are included for those occupations where internal exposure is of concern. Since airline crews are not monitored, the numbers of airline crew were obtained from information published by the U.S. Department of Labor, and associated occupational doses were derived from calculations for space radiation based on altitude and latitude of typical flight routes. Effective doses were based on the following sources:

- Subcategories 1, 4 and 5. *Medical, industry and commerce, and education and research*: Personal monitoring data provided by Global Dosimetry Solutions, Inc. (Irvine, California) and Landauer, Inc. (Glenwood, Illinois), recorded as deep dose equivalent.
- Subcategory 2. *Aviation*: Effective dose estimates for various flight segments published by the U.S. Department of Transportation.
- Subcategory 3. *Commercial nuclear power*: Personal monitoring data provided by the U.S. Nuclear Regulatory Commission, recorded as TEDE.

- Subcategory 6. *Government, DOE and military*: Personal monitoring data provided by Global Dosimetry Solutions, Inc. and Landauer, Inc. for government agencies, by the military services for the Air Force, Army, Navy and Marines (all recorded as deep dose equivalent), and by DOE (recorded as TEDE).

For all subcategories except aviation, distributions of dose are presented for the monitored workers with recorded doses.

The results for occupational exposure for 2006 for S and E_{US} are 1,400 person-Sv and 0.005 mSv, respectively, compared with 2,000 person-Sv and 0.009 mSv in the early 1980s.

The percent contribution to the total S and the total E_{US} for this category from each of the six subcategories for 2006 is (in decreasing order):

- medical (39 %)
- aviation (38 %)
- commercial nuclear power (8 %)
- industry and commerce (8 %)
- education and research (4 %)
- government, DOE and military (3 %)

The estimate of E_{Exp} for 1.22 million workers (includes those with recordable doses and airline crew) is 1.1 mSv, and the variation in E_{Exp} among the included subcategories ranges from 0.6 mSv for government, DOE and military to 3.1 mSv for aviation. Distributions of annual effective dose for workers with recordable dose for each of the monitored subcategories (Figures 7.5, 7.7, 7.9, 7.10 and 7.11) indicate that the vast majority of individual dose values for those workers is <1 mSv.

1.6 Overall Results for 2006

The estimated totals from all sources for 2006 are 1,870,000 person-Sv for S and 6.2 mSv for E_{US}, based on a U.S. population of 300 million. Nearly all the S or E_{US} (98 %) results from ubiquitous background (50 %) and medical exposure of patients (48 %). Consumer products and activities account for 2 % and the remaining two categories (industrial, occupational) contribute very little (on the order of <0.1 % each). Figure 1.1 gives the percent contributions of various sources of exposure to the totals for S and E_{US}; the major sources are radon and thoron (37 %), CT (24 %), and nuclear medicine (12 %). Other background sources (external plus

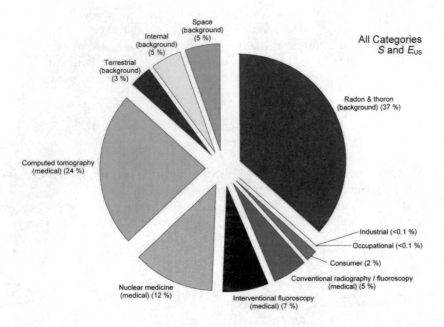

Fig. 1.1. Percent contribution of various sources of exposure to the total collective effective dose (1,870,000 person-Sv) and the total effective dose per individual in the U.S. population (6.2 mSv) for 2006. Percent values have been rounded to the nearest 1 %, except for those <1 % [see Table 1.1 for the values of S (person-sievert) and E_{US} (millisievert)].

internal) contribute 13 %, and other medical exposure (interventional fluoroscopy plus conventional radiography and fluoroscopy) contribute 12 %. The values for S (person-sievert), E_{US} (millisievert), and E_{Exp} (millisievert) for the five exposure categories and the main subcategories are provided in Table 1.1. In addition, thumbnail sketches are provided at the beginning of Sections 3 through 7 that provide a succinct overview of the results for each of the five exposure categories.

The value for S increased by a factor of 2.2 from the early 1980s to 2006. This includes an increase due to the change in number of individuals in the U.S. population between 1980 (230 million) and 2006 (300 million).The value for E_{US} increased by a factor of 1.7 from the early 1980s to 2006, primarily due to increased utilization of the medical modalities of computed tomography, nuclear medicine and interventional fluoroscopy. The values for S (person-sievert) and E_{US} (millisievert) for these comparisons are provided in Table 8.3.

TABLE 1.1—*Collective effective dose (S), effective dose per individual in the U.S. population (E_{US}), and average effective dose for the exposed group (E_{Exp}) for 2006.*[a]

Exposure Category	S (person-Sv)	E_{US} (mSv)	E_{Exp} (mSv)
Ubiquitous background	*933,000*	*3.11*	*3.11*
Internal, inhalation (radon and thoron)	684,000	2.28	2.28
External, space	99,000	0.33	0.33
Internal, ingestion	87,000	0.29	0.29
External, terrestrial	63,000	0.21	0.21
Medical	*899,000*	*3.00*	—[b]
CT	440,000	1.47	—[b]
Nuclear medicine	231,000	0.77	—[b]
Interventional fluoroscopy	128,000	0.43	—[b]
Conventional radiography and fluoroscopy	100,000	0.33	—[b]
Consumer	*39,000*	*0.13*	*0.001 – 0.3*[c]
Industrial, security, medical, educational and research	*1,000*	*0.003*	*0.001 – 0.01*[c]
Occupational	*1,400*	*0.005*	*1.1*
Medical	550		0.8
Aviation	530		3.1
Commercial nuclear power	110		1.9
Industry and commerce	110		0.8
Education and research	60		0.7
Government, DOE, military	40		0.6
Total	*1,870,000*[d]	*6.2*[d]	

[a]See Table 8.1 for more detail.

[b]Not determined for the medical category because the number of patients exposed is not known, only the number of procedures.

[c]The range of values for the various subcategories in this category.

[d]Rounded values.

Uncertainty in the 2006 estimates for effective dose (E), E_{Exp}, and S (and by extension E_{US}) are due to uncertainty in the underlying measurements from which these quantities are estimated, in the dosimetric models and their parameters, in the number of individuals exposed, and in the assumptions made in the absence of information. A detailed uncertainty analysis was possible only for E_{Exp} for ubiquitous background radiation (Table 3.14). In that case, the analysis applies also to S and E_{US} since all individuals in the United States are exposed and the number of individuals is relatively well known. The uncertainty in the estimates of E, E_{Exp}, and S for other exposure categories cannot be inferred from that analysis. For other exposure categories, at the present time, one is limited primarily to identification of the factors that contribute to uncertainty.

There are clearly two major contributors to the exposure of the U.S. population from ionizing radiation: exposure to ubiquitous background radiation and medical exposure of patients. As a word of caution in interpreting these results in terms of health detriment (*i.e.*, the stochastic health risks due to radiation exposure), it is important to recognize that the populations exposed to these two sources are not the same. Those exposed to ubiquitous background radiation represent the entire U.S. population in age, gender and health status. Groups of patients exposed to medical radiation often have distributions that are skewed in age to older individuals and in health status to sicker individuals. There also may be a skewed gender distribution. In addition the risk associated with the type of radiation encountered may differ from one source to another. The exposure to ubiquitous background radiation is generally to high-energy gamma rays and high-energy particles while the exposure from diagnostic medical procedures is generally to low-energy x rays. The radiation weighting factors $(w_{\text{R}}\text{s})$ used in the calculation of effective dose may not be the most appropriate in all cases for evaluation of radiation detriment for the type of radiation encountered. Therefore, the fact that S and E_{US} are approximately equal for the two populations does not convey that there is equal stochastic risk to the two populations. This caution, of course, applies to all sources of radiation exposure. Determination of radiation detriment was outside the scope of this Report.

2. Introduction

NCRP Report No. 93 (NCRP, 1987a) presented the exposure of the U.S. population to ionizing radiation as it was known in the early 1980s. NCRP (1987a) was supported by a series of five reports that detailed the population exposure from six specific source categories:

- NCRP Report No. 92, *Public Radiation Exposure from Nuclear Power Generation in the United States* (NCRP, 1987c);
- NCRP Report No. 94, *Exposure of the Population in the United States and Canada from Natural Background Radiation* (NCRP, 1987b);
- NCRP Report No. 95, *Radiation Exposure of the U.S. Population from Consumer Products and Miscellaneous Sources* (NCRP, 1987d);
- NCRP Report No. 100, *Exposure of the U.S. Population from Diagnostic Medical Radiation* (NCRP, 1989a); and
- NCRP Report No. 101, *Exposure of the U.S. Population from Occupational Radiation* (NCRP, 1989b).

Since that time, the magnitude of radiation exposure to the U.S. population and the distribution of that exposure among the various sources have changed because of changes in technology and use, primarily in medicine and industry, and changes in the assessment of radiation dose caused by radioactive material taken into the body, primarily radon gas and its particulate progeny. Consequently, a more current assessment of the radiation exposure of the U.S. population is required.

2.1 Present Report

The U.S. population is exposed to ionizing radiation from a variety of sources. The current Report categorizes those sources somewhat differently from NCRP (1987a), but it completely updates and replaces that report. However, some of the detailed discussions of the individual sources of exposure that are found in the original supporting documents are still applicable and are referred to in this Report.

This Report provides the available data and dose assessment for the radiation exposure to the U.S population for 2006 from five broad categories of sources. The dose assessments are derived from disparate types of information and varying methods of analysis. The sources included in each category, the resources from which the data regarding exposure were obtained, and to the extent possible the variability of doses to the U.S population from sources in that category are discussed in the following sections:

- Section 3: Ubiquitous background radiation;
- Section 4: Medical exposure of patients;
- Section 5: Consumer products and activities;
- Section 6: Industrial, security, medical, educational and research activities; and
- Section 7: Occupational exposure of workers.

Section 8 presents a summary and conclusions for the dose information.

2.2 Radiation Source Categories

2.2.1 *Ubiquitous Background Radiation*

Radiation exposure to ubiquitous background sources is covered in Section 3. Each subsection provides information on the data sources for the radiation source discussed in that subsection. The entire population is exposed to these sources, but the radiation dose received by any individual varies with that person's activities and place of residence. Consequently information is provided on the distribution of the sources and the variability in the radiation doses across the United States. Radiation is received from sources out- and inside the body and this is discussed in Section 3.3. Sources outside the body include radiation from space (solar particles and cosmic rays) and radiation emitted by radioactive elements in rocks and soil or their airborne decay products (terrestrial radiation). Radiation sources inside the body enter either by the ingestion of food and water (primarily radionuclides of potassium, uranium, radium and thorium) or the inhalation of air (primarily radon and its progeny).

2.2.2 *Patient Exposure from Medical Procedures*

Radiation exposure to patients is discussed in Section 4 and is divided into five groups of medical procedures because the radiation sources and the methods of determining radiation dose differ.

In each subsection the data sources are given for numbers of procedures performed and the radiation doses as follows:

- Section 4.2: Computed tomography;
- Section 4.3: Conventional radiography and fluoroscopy (including dental and chiropractic radiography, and bone densitometry);
- Section 4.4: Interventional fluoroscopy;
- Section 4.5: Nuclear medicine; and
- Section 4.6: External-beam radiotherapy.

2.2.3 *Consumer Products and Activities*

Certain consumer products and activities (somewhat arbitrarily classified) can expose the user or participant to radiation that is not considered ubiquitous background radiation. In almost all cases this added exposure is very small when compared with that from ubiquitous background radiation. The products and activities discussed in Section 5 are building materials, commercial air travel, cigarette smoking, mining and agriculture; combustion of fossil fuels, glass and ceramics. These and several other very minor sources are discussed in Sections 5.2 through 5.9. For all these sources except commercial air travel the radiation derives from naturally-occurring radioactive material (NORM) in the uranium and thorium decay series. Air travelers are exposed to additional radiation from cosmic and solar sources.

2.2.4 *Industrial, Security, Medical, Educational and Research Activities*

Many industrial operations, security inspection systems, medical facilities, and educational and research institutions use radiation sources or radioactive material. These are discussed in Section 6. Members of the public may be exposed to radiation when they are in proximity to such sources or material or when they are near a patient who has been administered a radiopharmaceutical. Each subsection discusses the radiation exposures that result from a particular activity or group of activities as follows:

- Section 6.2: Electricity generation using nuclear power;
- Section 6.3: Operation of DOE facilities;
- Section 6.4: Decommissioning of former sites where radioactive material was used and the disposal of radioactive waste;

- Section 6.5: Other industrial and commerce activities, medical facilities, and educational and research activities; and
- Section 6.6: Security inspection systems.

Exposure to members of the public from these various sources is minor compared with the exposure to ubiquitous background radiation.

2.2.5 *Occupational Exposure*

Individuals who are employed in medical facilities, as airline crew in commercial aviation, in certain industrial and commercial activities, in commercial nuclear power, in some educational and research activities, in the military, in certain government agencies, and in DOE facilities, may be exposed to radiation as part of their occupations. Almost all of these individuals (except airline crew) are regularly monitored for radiation exposure.[3] In 2006 this amounted to 3.86 million monitored workers, of which 1.04 million received doses above a minimum detectable level. In addition, 0.17 million airline crew members received occupational exposure. Section 7 includes detailed discussions of these radiation exposures.

2.3 Principal Radiation Dose Quantities in this Report

The International Commission on Radiological Protection (ICRP, 1991) and NCRP (1993a) reformulated the principal radiation dose quantities that were used in NCRP (1987a). To the extent possible this Report uses these reformulated quantities. Because of the way radiation dose has been reported in the literature, conversion to the reformulated dose quantities is not always possible and such cases are noted in this Report. The following dose quantities are the principal ones used in this Report and the rationale for each is discussed in Sections 2.3.1 through 2.3.4:

- effective dose (E);
- collective effective dose (S);
- average effective dose to an individual in a group exposed to a specific source (E_{Exp}); and
- effective dose per individual in the U.S. population whether exposed to the specific source or not (E_{US}).

---

[3]Exposures to individuals employed in some industries which utilize naturally-occurring radioactive materials (NORM) for manufacturing, or generate technologically-enhanced NORM (TENORM) as waste, may not be monitored and estimates of their doses have not been accounted for in this Report.

Therefore, effective dose is the primary quantity from which the other dose quantities listed above are derived for the purpose of comparisons among the radiation sources.

2.3.1 *Effective Dose*

Effective dose is used to normalize partial-body irradiations relative to whole-body irradiations to facilitate radiation protection activities (ICRP, 1991; NCRP, 1993a). The calculation of E requires knowledge of the mean absorbed dose to specific radiosensitive organs and tissues within the body (often obtained from Monte-Carlo transport calculations using anthropomorphic models). The unit for E in the International System (SI) of Quantities and Units is J kg^{-1}, with the special name sievert (Sv). A common magnitude reported is millisievert (*i.e.*, 10^{-3} Sv).

The formulation for E (ICRP, 1991; NCRP, 1993a) is:

$$E = \sum_T w_T H_T = \sum_T \left(w_T \sum_R w_R D_{T,R} \right), \tag{2.1}$$

where:

$D_{T,R}$ =   mean absorbed dose[4] in an organ or tissue T from radiation type R incident on the body

w_R =   radiation weighting factor that accounts for the biological effectiveness of the type of radiation in producing the stochastic health effect under consideration

w_T =   tissue weighting factor that accounts for the relative radiation detriment for the organ or tissue from the stochastic health effect

The sum of the products of $D_{T,R}$ and w_R gives the equivalent dose (H_T)[5] for the organ or tissue for all the radiation types involved. Multiplying H_T by the appropriate w_T (for each organ or tissue T) and summing the products for the specified organs and tissues gives E, which includes the effective dose from external sources and the committed effective dose (Glossary) from internal sources.

Values of w_T were developed from a reference population of equal numbers of males and females and a wide range of ages (ICRP, 1991). For this reason it is not appropriate to use values of E or

---

[4]The unit for absorbed dose in SI is also J kg^{-1}, but with the special name gray (Gy). A common magnitude reported is milligray (mGy) (*i.e.*, 10^{-3} Gy) (Glossary).

[5]The unit for equivalent dose in SI is also J kg^{-1}, with the special name sievert (Sv) (Glossary).

quantities derived from it (i.e., S, E_{Exp}, E_{US}) to assess the radiation detriment to an individual, or subsets of the U.S. population with an age and gender distribution significantly different from the reference population (ICRP, 2007a; 2007b).

The values for w_R relate to carcinogenesis in humans and were selected after consideration by ICRP and NCRP of the scientific literature on relative biological effectiveness (ICRP, 1991; NCRP, 1993a). The relative biological effectiveness values depend not only on the type and energy of radiation but also the test species, organ, and the particular biological effect in question. *This Report primarily applies the quantity E from ICRP (1991) and NCRP (1993a), which by definition assigns w_R a value of one for all exposures involving photons and electrons.* Recent publications indicate that the relative biological effectiveness values for carcinogenesis in humans for low-energy photons, such as used in medical imaging, may be as high as two or more based on chromosomal aberration data and on biophysical considerations (NAS/NRC, 2006). If such a change were adopted as a revised w_R for low-energy photons, the resulting values for such a redefined effective dose for low-energy photon sources would increase proportionally. To date, neither ICRP nor NCRP has revised the value of w_R for low-energy photons.

A previous formulation of E, named effective dose equivalent (H_E) (ICRP, 1977; NCRP, 1987e) is used occasionally in some of the dose assessments referenced in this Report, when other data are not available. Some values of w_T and w_R for H_E are different from those for E. Also, occupational exposure to radiation in the United States is currently reported by DOE and NRC as TEDE (DOE, 2006a; NRC, 2007a), a quantity close in formulation to H_E, and this Report utilizes data reported in that manner by DOE, NRC and others. ICRP (2007a) provided revised w_T and w_R values in its 2007 recommendations. This formulation (denoted E^*) is used in some instances in this Report when original calculations were made. (Note for all photon irradiation, w_R is assigned a value of one in the H_E, TEDE, and E^* formulations.) The reader should consult the noted references for the technical details of the definitions for these quantities including the respective values for w_T and w_R. *When data expressed as H_E, TEDE, or E^* are used in this Report, that fact is cited. However, when the data are compiled for comparison, the H_E, TEDE, and E^* values are included as though they were E (i.e., as surrogates for E). No attempt is made to adjust the H_E, TEDE and E^* values for the differences between their definitions and that of E.*

In this Report, E is often presented as an average or nominal value for a specified exposure situation that may or may not be consistent with the actual conditions experienced by a given individual.

Whenever possible, additional information is provided on the variability of the values of E for the exposure situation that would enable the reader to further refine an estimate for the circumstances that are actually encountered. As examples, the annual value of E for ubiquitous background radiation varies with location in the United States; E varies with the type of medical imaging procedure that is conducted, and the type of imaging equipment and technique factors used; and E varies depending on the radiation environment encountered in a particular occupational setting.

Effective dose is not and in fact cannot be determined directly, but rather through relationships with other radiation measurements or by calculation. Some examples are:

- exposure to ubiquitous background radiation from space and terrestrial sources reported as absorbed dose or kerma-in-air;
- exposure from radioactive material taken in as part of the diet reported as an average quantity of radionuclide consumed or deposited in the body;
- radon exposure reported as an average concentration of radon progeny in air;
- exposure to external sources for diagnostic medical applications reported as kerma-in-air or entrance skin exposure;
- exposure from CT procedures reported as the dose-length product (DLP);
- exposure from nuclear-medicine procedures reported as H_T to each organ exposed; and
- exposure from consumer products and industrial sources reported in various practical quantities.

However, many of these sources deliver very low doses (<0.01 mSv) annually to an individual and an attempt to derive precise values of E is usually unwarranted.

Various dose conversion coefficients are applied to obtain the quantity E from the reported quantities.

2.3.2 *Collective Effective Dose*

Collective effective dose is a measure of the cumulative dose to a population of individuals exposed to a given radiation source or group of sources. It is defined for purposes of this Report as:

$$S = \sum_j E_j N_j \qquad (2.2)$$

expressed in person-sievert, where:

E_j = average effective dose to population subgroup j

N_j = number of individuals in population subgroup j receiving E_j

The time period and the subgroups over which S is summed should be specified. In this Report, the S of interest is the annual value including committed effective dose.

Collective effective dose is used in this Report solely to provide a relative measure of the magnitude of population doses for general comparison among various radiation sources and to permit comparison with the collective dose results in NCRP Report No. 93 (NCRP, 1987a). No attempt is made to evaluate the radiation detriment associated with a given value of S, which is applicable only to stochastic health effects (*i.e.*, cancer and genetic effects). A thorough discussion of the concept of collective dose and NCRP recommendations concerning its use in radiation protection are given in NCRP Report No. 121 (NCRP, 1995a). For example, when comparing S values among different sources, one should take note of: (1) the known characteristics of the exposed population (*e.g.*, the age and gender distribution), and (2) the order of magnitude of the E values experienced by the exposed individuals. These two factors have implications with regard to the magnitude of radiation detriment (and its uncertainty) that the exposed population may experience.

2.3.3 *Average Effective Dose to an Individual in a Group Exposed to a Specific Source*

This quantity (E_{Exp}) is defined for purposes of this Report as:

$$E_{Exp} = \frac{S_{Exp}}{N_{Exp}} \qquad (2.3)$$

where:

S_{Exp} = collective effective dose for the N_{Exp} individuals who are considered to be in a defined exposed group

The exposed group excludes individuals who are not subject to exposure from that source of radiation.

The quantity E_{Exp} provides a measure of the magnitude of dose to individuals who are actually exposed, when such data are available. In this Report, the E_{Exp} of interest is the annual value. No attempt is made to evaluate the radiation detriment associated with a given value of E_{Exp}.

2.3.4 *Effective Dose per Individual in the U.S. Population*

The effective dose per individual in the U.S. population (E_{US}), whether exposed to the specific source or not, is defined for purposes of this Report as:

$$E_{US} = \frac{S_{Exp}}{N_{US}} \qquad (2.4)$$

where:

S_{Exp} = collective effective dose for the N_{Exp} individuals who are considered to be in a defined exposed group

N_{US} = total population of the United States (*e.g.*, 300 million in 2006)

In this Report, the E_{US} of interest is the annual value. The quantity E_{US} does not represent the actual dose received by any individual in the U.S. population, and it represents an average individual dose only in the case where all individuals are exposed to a given source (*e.g.*, ubiquitous background exposure). However, it is an index of the relative change in exposure between different time periods and is useful in comparisons with the results published in NCRP Report No. 93 (NCRP, 1987a) for the various radiation sources and from all sources. No attempt is made to evaluate the radiation detriment associated with a given value of E_{US}.

3. Ubiquitous Background Radiation

Thumbnail Sketch (for 2006) (rounded values):

- collective effective dose (S): 930,000 person-Sv[6]
- effective dose per individual in the U.S. population (E_{US}): 3.1 mSv (arithmetic mean)
  - percent of total S or E_{US} for the U.S. population (50 %)
- subcategories included (percent of total S and E_{US} for ubiquitous background radiation)
  - internal, inhalation (radon and thoron) (73 %)
  - external, space (11 %)
  - internal, ingestion (9 %)
  - external, terrestrial (7 %)
- mean effective dose for the exposed group (E_{Exp}): 3.1 mSv (arithmetic); 2.3 mSv (geometric)
  - statistics for E_{Exp}: 3.6 mSv (standard deviation); 2.0 (geometric standard deviation)
- group characteristics: all members of the population of the United States

3.1 Introduction

In 1975, NCRP presented a comprehensive report of exposure to natural background radiation in the United States as understood at that time (NCRP, 1975). The subsequent recognition of significant exposure from indoor radon decay products (NCRP, 1984a; 1984b) and additional data on exposure from other sources led to an updating of the report (NCRP, 1987b).

Useful summary reports on exposures to natural radiation are available from a number of sources. The most comprehensive are those prepared by the United Nations Scientific Committee on the Effects of Atomic Radiation (UNSCEAR, 1966; 1972; 1977; 1982; 1988; 1993; 2000). Oakley (1972) authored a report, *Natural*

---

[6]An independent assessment for domestic water supplies was ~34,000 person-Sv (Section B.3 in Appendix B); however, a contribution for ingestion of drinking water is deemed already included (from the assessment of radionuclides in the body) in the 930,000 person-Sv total.

Radiation Exposure in the United States, which dealt with external natural radiation. This was published by EPA and was used extensively in the preparation of NCRP Report No. 45 (NCRP, 1975). Also, the Committee on the Biological Effects of Ionizing Radiation of the National Academy of Sciences included data on natural background radiation in its 1972, 1980 and 2006 reports (NAS/NRC, 1972; 1980; 2006).

Since the 1987 publication of NCRP Report No. 93 and Report No. 94 (NCRP, 1987a; 1987b), which focused on average individual doses and exposures, increasing emphasis has been placed on variability and uncertainty of exposures and doses in a variety of settings. Exposure to ionizing radiation varies significantly with geographic location, diet, drinking water source, and building construction. Exposure varies somewhat with gender and age, primarily due to changes in body mass. The variability in most distributions of exposure and dose has been shown to be lognormal (Ott, 1995; UNSCEAR, 1977). Dose distributions inferred for populations are uncertain due to measurement uncertainty as well as uncertainty in dosimetric models and their parameters. Point estimates of dose inferred for any particular individual have an additional component of uncertainty introduced by that individual's position within the range of population doses, so that variability within a population becomes uncertainty for an individual. Additional uncertainty for individual doses occurs because individuals differ systematically from the average individual for whom model parameters are calculated.

3.2 Sources of Exposure

In this Report exposures to ubiquitous background radiation are divided into those from external sources and those from radionuclides in the body. The dose estimates for external source irradiation are based on direct measurements of dose rates, radionuclide concentrations, models, and calculations, while those for internal sources are calculated from a variety of radionuclide measurements. For exposures to ^{222}Rn (radon) and ^{220}Rn (thoron) and their short-lived decay products, doses are estimated from measurements and dosimetric and behavioral models. For intakes of other radionuclides by inhalation and ingestion, doses are estimated from limited analyses of radionuclide concentrations in individual organs, often from autopsy specimens.

3.2.1 *Naturally-Occurring Radionuclides*

Naturally-occurring radionuclides in the environment are of two general classes, cosmogenic and primordial.

Most cosmogenic radionuclides are beta-particle, gamma-ray, or x-ray emitters with low to intermediate atomic numbers, and are produced by interactions of cosmic nucleons with target atoms in the atmosphere or in the earth. While UNSCEAR (2000) lists 14 cosmogenic radionuclides, only ^{3}H, ^{7}Be, ^{14}C, and ^{22}Na occur with any significant abundance. Three of these, ^{3}H, ^{14}C, and ^{22}Na, are isotopes of major elements in the body. A number of other radionuclides are of scientific interest in tracing atmospheric and hydrological processes but are not of significance with respect to population doses.

Most primordial radionuclides are isotopes of the heavy elements of the three radioactive series headed by ^{238}U, ^{232}Th, and ^{235}U. The radiation emissions from the first two of these are significant contributors to the average effective dose to members of the population. The ^{232}Th decay series is shown in Figure 3.1, and the ^{238}U decay series is shown in Figure 3.2.

The major primordial radionuclides which decay directly to stable nuclides are ^{40}K and ^{87}Rb. The relatively constant isotopic abundance of ^{40}K in potassium is only 0.0117 %, but potassium is so widespread that ^{40}K contributes about one-third of both the external terrestrial and the internal whole-body dose arising from natural sources. The concentration of ^{87}Rb in soil is higher than that of ^{40}K, but ^{87}Rb is a pure beta-particle emitter and contributes essentially no external radiation dose. For internal exposure the average concentration of rubidium is about two orders of magnitude less than that of potassium. The dose conversion coefficient for ^{87}Rb is only one-tenth that of ^{40}K. Thus the contribution of ^{87}Rb to E or committed E from natural background is much lower than that of ^{40}K.

The primordial radioactive decay series headed by ^{232}Th, ^{235}U, and ^{238}U all transition through the element radon, in the form of ^{219}Rn (3.96 s), ^{220}Rn (55.6 s), and ^{222}Rn (3.82 d), respectively. In this Report, the radionuclide ^{220}Rn is called thoron, and radon without qualification refers to ^{222}Rn. Because of the rarity of its parent ^{235}U and its very short half-life, ^{219}Rn is inconsequential in terms of its airborne concentrations out- or indoors, and is not considered further. However, gaseous radon and thoron are found everywhere in out- and indoor air.

Outdoor radon concentration varies diurnally, temporally and geographically, depending on its emanation rate from upwind soil and its transport through the atmosphere (Section 3.5.7). For example, locations in Hawaii and some near the West Coast of the United States tend to have low outdoor concentrations in part because the prevailing winds are off the ocean, and radon emanation from the ocean is extremely low.

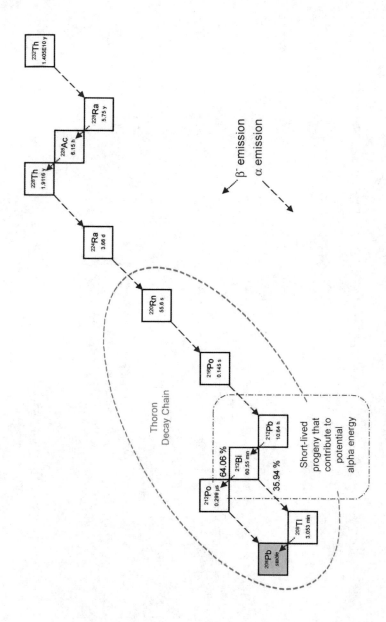

Fig. 3.1. The decay scheme of ^{232}Th that includes the ^{220}Rn decay chain. The time listed for each radionuclide is its half-life.

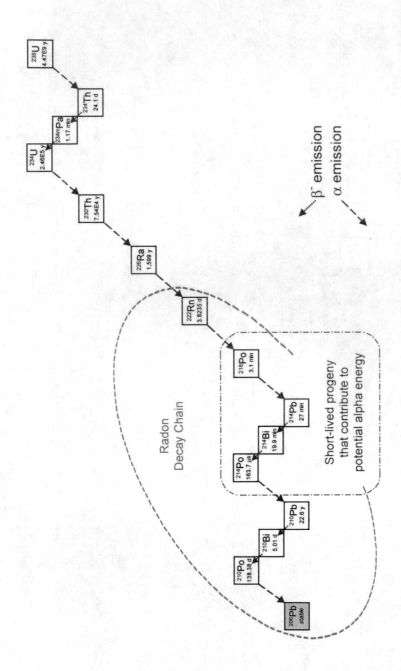

Fig. 3.2. The decay scheme of ^{238}U that includes the ^{222}Rn decay chain. The time listed for each radionuclide is its half-life.

Indoor concentrations of radon can be considerably higher than those found outdoors, primarily due to the buildup of radon emanating from soil underneath a building. In some cases, radon volatilized from water supplied to a building may be important (NAS/NRC, 1999a) (Appendix B.2). Building materials and natural gas may also be minor sources (Sections 5.8 and 5.9.3).

3.2.2 Anthropogenic Radionuclides

Human activities have resulted in the production and release of radioactive material to the environment. Over the years, such activities have included: atmospheric nuclear weapons testing; operations supporting the production of nuclear weapons such as reprocessing irradiated uranium to separate plutonium, uranium, and fission and activation products; the nuclear fuel cycle for electricity generation; the use of radionuclides in medicine, research and commerce; and accidents at nuclear reactors.

3.2.3 External Radiation

External radiation comes from two sources of approximately equal magnitude, the radiation from space and terrestrial gamma radiation from radionuclides in the environment, mainly the earth. The external radiation field consists of energetic penetrating radiations and may be considered, as a first approximation, to irradiate the whole body uniformly.

3.2.3.1 *Radiation from Space.* There are four kinds of space radiation incident on Earth's atmosphere:

1. solar energetic particles (associated with solar events);
2. anomalous cosmic rays (coming from interstellar space at the edge of the heliopause);
3. galactic cosmic rays (coming from outside the solar system); and
4. extragalatic cosmic rays (coming from beyond our galaxy).

These charged particles, primarily protons that are incident on Earth's atmosphere, have sufficiently high energies to generate secondary particles, mostly high-energy muons, electrons and photons, commonly referred to as the directly ionizing component, and a smaller number of neutrons. The neutrons are strongly absorbed in the atmosphere, so they contribute a relatively low effective dose at sea level but significant dose rates at higher altitudes.

3.2.3.2 *Terrestrial Radiation.* Naturally-occurring radionuclides of terrestrial origin are ubiquitous throughout the environment. Several of these have half-lives that are the same order of magnitude as the estimated age of Earth (~4.5 × 10^9 y) [*e.g.*, Figure 3.1 (^{232}Th) and Figure 3.2 (^{238}U)] and are often referred to as primordial radionuclides. They can be divided into "series radionuclides" that decay to a stable isotope of lead through a sequence of radionuclides with a wide range of half-lives and "non-series radionuclides" that decay into a stable nuclide.

These radionuclides occur in igneous and sedimentary rock, and ultimately in soil and the hydrosphere. A description of the geological processes that control migration and sedimentation of terrestrial radioactive material can be found in NCRP Report No. 45 and Report No. 94 (NCRP, 1975; 1987b).

The principal sources of external exposure are the penetrating gamma radiations emitted by ^{40}K and the series originating from ^{238}U and ^{232}Th. Most of the gamma radiation comes from the top 20 cm of soil, with a small contribution from airborne radon decay products. Soil concentrations of ^{40}K and the uranium and thorium series vary over a factor of 20 from place-to-place in the United States and Canada (Duval *et al.*, 2005, Grasty and LaMarre, 2004). USGS continuously acquires information from laboratory measurements of the concentrations of these radionuclides in soil or stream sediment samples, and maintains a database of soil concentration values inferred from airborne gamma surveys that began in the 1970s (Duval *et al.*, 2005). Maps of the 48 conterminous states, Alaska, and much of Canada showing concentrations of ^{40}K, ^{238}U and ^{232}Th using color scales are available at USGS (2005a; 2005b; 2005c; 2005d). Higher resolution maps can be found on the electronic version of the database (Duval *et al.*, 2005).

In a very few locations, gamma radiation from mine or mill tailings contributes to the exposure of local populations, but almost all areas have been remediated under the 1970 Formerly Utilized Sites Remedial Action Program (ACE, 2008), the Comprehensive Environmental Response, Compensation and Liability Act (CERCLA, 1980), or the Uranium Mill Tailings Radiation Control Act (UMTRCA, 1978).

Gamma radiation from global fallout from atmospheric weapons tests has been dramatically reduced by radioactive decay and weathering since major atmospheric testing ended in 1963. Gamma radiation from fallout from the reactor accident at Chernobyl in 1986 was not a significant source in North America (UNSCEAR, 2000).

3.2.4 *Internal Radiation (Radionuclides in the Body)*

The primordial radionuclides that are significant for human exposure by internal radiation include the isotopes of uranium, thorium, radium, radon, polonium, bismuth and lead of the ^{238}U and ^{232}Th series (Figures 3.1 and 3.2), and ^{40}K and ^{87}Rb. The only cosmogenic radionuclide of importance for human exposure by internal radiation is ^{14}C (UNSCEAR, 2000). These enter the body by ingestion of food, milk and water or by inhalation. The isotopes follow the normal chemical metabolism of the element and the long-lived radionuclides are usually maintained at an equilibrium concentration, but may change somewhat with age. The shorter-lived radionuclides disappear by decay, but concentrations in the body are continually renewed by additional intake. Ingestion intakes of decay series in secular equilibrium do not result in uniform tissue concentrations, because the fraction absorbed from the gastrointestinal (GI) tract depends strongly on the particular chemical element in question. Thus, for example, radium is much more readily absorbed than thorium, leading to vastly different tissue concentrations.

3.2.5 *Assessment of Sources of Exposure*

Sources of exposure may be distinct from routes of exposure, and distinct routes of exposure are treated separately here. External radiation exposure from ubiquitous background at any point on Earth is from naturally-occurring radionuclides in the earth and in building materials and radiation from space. Irradiation from internally-deposited naturally-occurring radionuclides occurs following inhalation of air or ingestion of food, milk and water.

Measurements can be used to estimate the total absorbed-dose rate from terrestrial and space radiation, but most instruments are not able to distinguish between these two sources. Calculations are usually needed to quantify each source separately.

3.3 Space Radiation

Because radiation from outer space is well characterized and well understood theoretically, a calculational approach is appropriate.

3.3.1 *Calculations*

A calculation of the effective dose to ground-level populations was executed using the code PLOTINUS which is fully described by O'Brien (2005). The only change was the replacement of the free-in-air neutron spectrum at ground level with ground-level neutron spectrum (Gordon *et al.*, 2004; JEDEC, 2006). The w_Rs in ICRP Publication 60 (ICRP, 1991) [or ICRP Publication 92 (ICRP, 2003)] and those in ICRP Publication 103 (ICRP, 2007a) were each used to determine an estimate of the effective dose. In the first case, the fluence-to-dose conversion coefficients of Ferrari *et al.* (1996; 1997a; 1997b; 1997c; 1997d; 1998), based on ICRP (1991), and Sato *et al.* (2003) transformation theory were used. In the second case, ICRP (1991) w_Rs were replaced by ICRP (2007a) w_Rs.

3.3.2 *Recent Results for U.S. Urban Areas*

Table 3.1 gives summary statistics for annual effective dose due to space radiation, using w_R (proton) = 2 (ICRP, 2007a)[7] and the fraction of time-spent data in Table 3.2. Had the earlier w_R for protons of five (ICRP, 1991) been used, these effective doses would have been 1.6 % higher at sea level, and almost 5 % higher at 1.8 km altitude.

In 99 of the most populated U.S. urban areas, the average annual effective dose outdoors from space radiation is 0.40 ± 0.08 mSv (for adults), with a range from 0.28 mSv in Honolulu to 0.82 mSv in Colorado Springs. Effective dose rates depend on geomagnetic latitude and elevation above sea level. These values were averaged over the 11 y solar cycle. A frequency distribution of outdoor values, which peaks sharply between 0.35 and 0.4, is shown in Figure 3.3. No account was taken for the age-dependence of dose. A factor of 0.8 was applied to compute indoor values, as in Volume I of *Sources and Effects of Ionizing Radiation* (UNSCEAR, 2000).

During the 2000 census, these urban areas comprised 168,067,825 people, just over half of the U.S population (USCB, 2008). Assuming this is representative of the entire U.S. population, the population-weighted average annual effective dose outdoors was 0.375 mSv. Using the age-dependent fractions of time spent out- and indoors given in Table 3.2, the age-dependent population-weighted average annual effective doses corrected for shielding and time spent indoors were 0.33, 0.34, and 0.33 mSv for age groups <4, 4 to 18, and >18 y, respectively. These values are 0.83, 0.85, and 0.83 times the respective outdoor values.

---

[7]O'Brien, K. (2006). Personal communication (Northern Arizona University, Flagstaff, Arizona).

TABLE 3.1—*Annual effective doses and associated statistical data for space radiation in 99 of the most populated U.S. urban areas, w_R (proton) = 2.*

Statistical Parameter	Outdoors	Indoors[a]	Weighted Averages[b]		
			Age <4 y	Age 4 – 18 y	Age >18 y
Average (arithmetic mean) (mSv)	0.397	0.318	0.330	0.338	0.330
SD (mSv)	0.077	0.062			
Coefficient of variation	0.195	0.195	0.25[c]	0.25[c]	0.25[c]
GM (mSv)	0.392	0.313			
GSD	1.17	1.17			
Minimum (mSv)	0.279	0.223			
Maximum (mSv)	0.818	0.654			
Maximum/minimum	2.93	2.93			

[a]Indoor values are 0.8 of outdoor values.
[b]Weighted averages use the fraction of time-spent data in Table 3.2.
[c]Larger coefficient of variation estimated based on variability of outdoor values, and uncertainty in indoor/outdoor time-use and building shielding.

TABLE 3.2—*Fractions of time spent outdoors and in dwellings used to obtain the weighted averages in Table 3.1.*

Age (y)	Fractions of Time Spent		
	Outdoors	Home	Work, School
<4	0.15	0.85	
4 – 18	0.25	0.6	0.15
>18	0.15	0.6	0.25

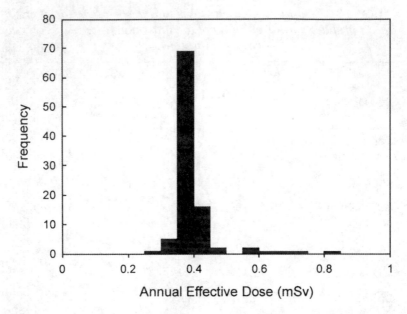

Fig. 3.3. Frequency distribution for average outdoor values of annual effective dose from space radiation in 99 of the most populated U.S. urban areas.

3.3.3 *Earlier Results*

Grasty and LaMarre (2004) reported calculations based on CARI-6 (FAA, 2004) of annual outdoor cosmic radiation doses at ground level throughout North America, including the contermi-nous United States and Alaska, ranging from 323 μSv at sea level to >1,000 μSv at high elevations. Figure 3.4 (Grasty and LaMarre, 2004) illustrates the great variability of annual cosmic radiation doses with geomagnetic latitude and elevation.

Culminating decades of measurements and analysis, Duval *et al.* (2005) published an extensive data set that includes outdoor cosmic radiation absorbed-dose rates (nGy h^{-1}) calculated using the methods of Boltneva *et al.* (1974), as well as dose rates due to ter-restrial radionuclides (Section 3.2.3.2). The cosmic radiation map from Duval *et al.* (2005) is available at USGS (2005e).

3.4 Terrestrial Gamma Radiation

The geographic distribution of sources of terrestrial gamma radiation is evaluated and estimates of age-dependent annual effective doses are presented in this section.

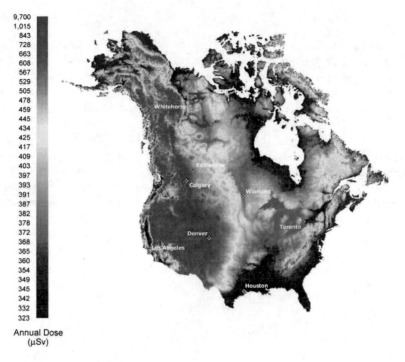

Fig. 3.4. False-color plot of CARI-6 calculations of annual cosmic radiation doses (microsievert) in North America (Grasty and LaMarre, 2004).

3.4.1 *Source Terms*

Previous assessments of exposure rates from terrestrial radiation were based on ground surveys as reported by Oakley (1972) and the aerial radiological measuring system program performed from 1958 to 1963 (Doyle, 1972). The aerial surveys were conducted over 25 areas within the continental United States and each covered ~24,000 km².

The NURE Program was initiated by the U.S. Atomic Energy Commission in 1973 with a primary goal of identifying uranium resources in the United States. When the U.S. Atomic Energy Commission was abolished in 1974, the NURE Program was transferred to the newly created Energy Research and Development Administration, and subsequently to DOE. The NURE Program effectively ended about 1983 when funding was terminated, but USGS continues to perform aerial surveys and to acquire and analyze soil and stream sediment samples.

3.4.2 *Methodology*

To obtain the population-weighted effective dose from external terrestrial radiation, the NURE data presented in a 25 by 25 km grid across the continental United States were used (Darnley *et al.*, 2003; Duval and Riggle, 1999). The data set consists of fractional mass concentrations $[(C_m)_{i,x,y}]$ in parts per million by weight (mg kg^{-1}) for uranium and thorium and in weight percent for potassium. The subscript i denotes the radionuclide (^{238}U, ^{232}Th, ^{40}K); the subscript x represents the longitude in degrees, minutes; and the subscript y represents the latitude in degrees, minutes. There are ~10,650 locations for each radionuclide. These data were converted to an activity concentration $(C_{i,x,y})$ (Bq kg^{-1}) for the primary radionuclide using:

$$C_{i,x,y} = 10^{-6}(C_m)_{i,x,y}\frac{\lambda\, N_A\, f\,(^{232}\text{Th or }^{238}\text{U})}{M_{el}} ,$$

for ^{232}Th and ^{238}U, and

$$C_{i,x,y} = 10^{-2}(C_m)_{i,x,y}\frac{\lambda\, N_A\, f\,(^{40}\text{K})}{M_{el}} , \tag{3.1}$$

for ^{40}K, where:
λ = radioactive transformation (decay) constant (s^{-1})
N_A = Avogadro constant (mol^{-1})
M_{el} = atomic mass of the element (kg mol^{-1})
$f\,(^{232}$Th or ^{238}U) and $f\,(^{40}$K)
  = mass fractional abundances of ^{232}Th, ^{238}U, or ^{40}K, respectively

The boundaries for each state in terms of longitude and latitude were used to select data and obtain average concentrations according to the following expression:

$$C_{S,i} = \frac{\sum\limits_{x,y}^{S} C_{i,x,y}}{n_{S,i}} \tag{3.2}$$

where:
S = a given state
$n_{S,i}$ = number of data points for radionuclide i in the state
$C_{S,i}$ = average concentration in the soil (Bq kg^{-1}) for radionuclide i in the state

The air-kerma rate at 1 m height per nuclear transformation of the parent radionuclide was determined using results of computations assuming equilibrium of all progeny and uniform distribution in the ground.

$$\dot{K}_{S,i} = k_i C_{S,i} \tag{3.3}$$

where:

k_i = air-kerma conversion coefficient [nGy h^{-1} (Bq kg^{-1})$^{-1}$]

$\dot{K}_{S,i}$ = average value of air-kerma rate in state S from parent radionuclide i (nGy h^{-1})

Alternatively, effective dose rate coefficients [tabulated as Sv h^{-1} (Bq kg^{-1})$^{-1}$] from contaminated soil can be used (Eckerman and Ryman, 1993; Eckerman and Sjoreen, 2006).

The annual effective dose based on the average concentration of radionuclide in state S (E_S) was obtained from the following expression:

$$E_S = \sum_i \sum_a f_{S,a} \sum_t f_{a,t} \sum_H f_H L_H d_{i,a} \dot{K}_{S,i} \tag{3.4}$$

where:

$d_{i,a}$ = age-dependent conversion coefficient from air-kerma rate outdoors to annual effective dose [mSv (mGy h^{-1})$^{-1}$] (due to anthropomorphic differences) for each parent radionuclide i; a represents the age category

$f_{S,a}$ = fraction of the population in state S in age category a

$f_{a,t}$ = fraction of time (t) persons in age category a are outdoors or inside buildings

H = type of buildings including housing and work-related structures

f_H = fraction of housing or buildings in this category

L_H = attenuation of exposure for this type of buildings

The annual effective dose for the conterminous 48 states based on the geographical-weighted average state radionuclide concentrations (E_G) is:

$$E_G = \frac{\sum_S E_S}{48} \tag{3.5}$$

The population-weighted effective dose (E_{US}) (millisievert) for the conterminous 48 states is:

$$E_{US} = \frac{\sum\limits_{S} N_S E_S}{\sum\limits_{S} N_S} \qquad (3.6)$$

where:

N_S = population for state S

3.4.3 Data

The air-kerma conversion coefficients (k_i) are listed in Table 3.3 (Saito and Jacob, 1995). These are similar to those given for the assessment of exposure to the U.S. population in Table 5.1 of NCRP Report No. 94 (NCRP, 1987b).

Figures 3.5, 3.6, and 3.7 show the frequency distribution of the data for uranium, thorium and potassium for all points in the NURE data set (Darnley *et al.*, 2003; Duval and Riggle, 1999). The data are summarized in Table 3.4.

The age-dependent kerma-to-effective dose conversion coefficients are shown in Figure 3.8 (Saito *et al.*, 1998). These coefficients reflect the effect of body size and use w_Ts recommended in ICRP Publication 60 (ICRP, 1991).

Although the dose distribution from penetrating gamma rays is not uniform throughout the body, no single organ receives the dominant contribution to absorbed dose. Variations in estimates of w_Ts should not significantly alter the coefficients shown in Figure 3.8.

Population data by state were obtained from USCB (2007a). The index a was used to indicate three age groups: infants and toddlers (<4 y), children and adolescents (4 to 14 y), and adults (>14 y). The fraction of the population in each state ($f_{S,a}$) was obtained from census pyramids (CS, 2007). The distribution of housing by type in each state (f_H) was obtained from USCB (2007b).

TABLE 3.3—*Conversion coefficients from activity concentrations in the ground to kerma-in-air above the ground (Saito and Jacob, 1995).*

Radionuclides	Air-Kerma Conversion Coefficient (k_i) [nGy h^{-1} (Bq kg^{-1})$^{-1}$]
^{238}U series	0.463
^{232}Th series	0.604
^{40}K	0.0417

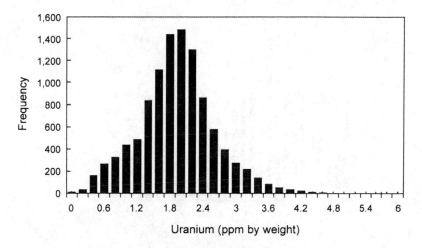

Fig. 3.5. Histogram showing the variability of uranium concentrations (parts per million by weight) in U.S. soils based on the NURE data (Darnley *et al.*, 2003; Duval and Riggle, 1999).

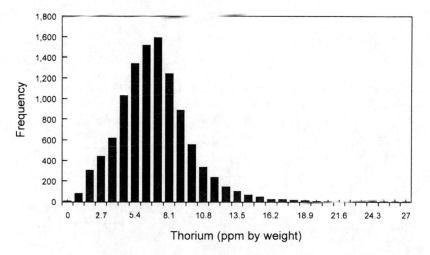

Fig. 3.6. Histogram showing the variability of thorium concentrations (parts per million by weight) in U.S. soils based on the NURE data (Darnley *et al.*, 2003; Duval and Riggle, 1999).

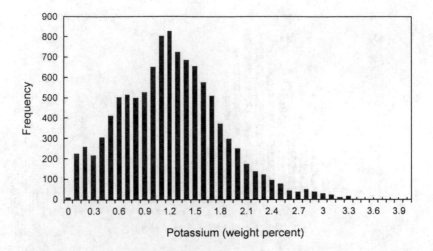

Fig. 3.7. Histogram showing the variability of potassium concentrations (weight percent) in U.S. soils based on the NURE data (Darnley *et al.*, 2003; Duval and Riggle, 1999).

TABLE 3.4—*Summary of soil concentration data for uranium, thorium and potassium from USGS (based on the NURE data) (Darnley et al., 2003; Duval and Riggle, 1999).*

Element	Mean	Median	Standard Deviation	5th Percentile	95th Percentile
Uranium (ppm[a] by weight)	1.84	1.81	0.7	0.63	3.1
Thorium (ppm by weight)	6.45	6.30	2.8	2.2	11
Potassium (weight percent)	1.16	1.14	0.6	0.22	2.2

[a]Parts per million.

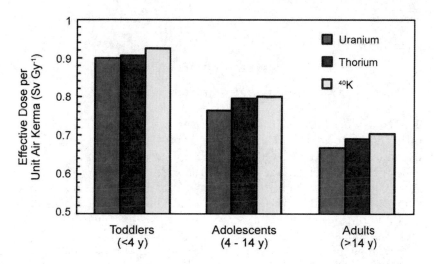

Fig. 3.8. Age-dependent conversion coefficients for effective dose per unit air kerma (Sv Gy^{-1}) for the two primordial radionuclide chains (uranium and thorium) and ^{40}K (Saito *et al.*, 1998). The conversion coefficients from Saito *et al.* (1998) for baby (eight weeks), child (7 y), and adult were applied to three age groups designated by the index a representing infants and toddlers (<4 y), adolescents (4 to 14 y) and adults (>14 y), respectively.

Exposure to terrestrial radiation indoors is modified by construction materials as well as by the location of the room with respect to the ground. The first compilation of natural background radiation in the United States recommended a "housing factor" of 80 % (*i.e.*, a 20 % reduction of outdoor exposure rates) (NCRP, 1975). Another factor of 0.8 was applied to outdoor exposure rates to serve as a self-shielding factor to estimate the dose rate to the gonads and blood forming organs. In the second compilation of exposure of the population in the United States from background radiation, the average indoor exposure was assumed to be equal to the outdoor exposure (NCRP, 1987b). This was based on the consideration that attenuation of photons originating outdoors is compensated indoors by photons originating from building materials.

Miller (1992) made an estimate of building attenuation from measurements in dwellings in several regions of the country. There is evidence that building materials may contribute to indoor exposures, and in some parts of the world dose rates are higher indoors (Arvela *et al.*, 1995; Miller, 1992). Miller (1992) found that for wood frame (including brick veneer) houses, which represented 85 % of the type encountered in his survey, the absorbed-dose rate indoors ($\dot{D}_{in}$) was given by:

$$\dot{D}_{in} = 8 + 0.59\, \dot{D}_{out} \qquad (3.7)$$

where:

$\dot{D}_{in}$ = absorbed-dose rate indoors (nGy h^{-1})

$\dot{D}_{out}$ = absorbed-dose rate outdoors (nGy h^{-1})

The 8 nGy h^{-1} ($\pm$20 %) constant represents the contribution from building materials, and 0.59 ($\pm$6 %) represents the average building shielding factor for outdoor radiation.

For this Report, L_H for indoor categories are shown in Table 3.5. A procedure to incorporate Equation 3.7 for estimating L_H in Equation 3.4 was used in the computations. The results for the state- and population-weighted effective-dose rates were essentially the same as those using the values listed in Table 3.5.

Since people spend a small fraction of their time outdoors (EPA, 1997), outdoor dose rates should be corrected for fraction of time spent indoors. This correction factor is not generally known for the United States, and has been taken as 0.8 in past publications (NCRP, 1987b; UNSCEAR, 2000). The fraction of time spent indoors is difficult to estimate and highly variable. It is age dependent and seasonal in nature. Table 3.2 shows the nominal values used in this Report.

3.4.4 Results

Figure 3.9 shows USGS data (Duval et al., 2005) presented as the absorbed-dose rate ranging from <6 to >83 nGy h^{-1}. The white areas indicate no measurement. The data show a significant geographical variation.

TABLE 3.5—*Building attenuation factors (L_H) used in this Report.*

Building Category	L_H
Single-family detached	0.9
Single-family attached	0.9
Apartments 2 to 4 units	0.85
Apartments >5 units	0.7
Mobile home	1.0
Other: recreational vehicle, boat	1.0
School, work	0.9

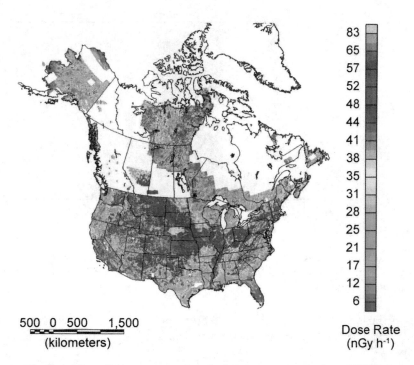

83
65
57
52
48
44
41
38
35
31
28
25
21
17
12
6

500 0 500 1,500
(kilometers)

Dose Rate
(nGy h⁻¹)

Fig. 3.9. Plot of gamma-ray absorbed-dose rate in air from USGS data, with blue being the lowest (<6 nGy h^{-1}) and lavender the highest (>83 nGy h^{-1}) (Duval *et al.*, 2005).

The average outdoor annual gamma-ray effective dose in the conterminous 48 states derived from airborne radiation measurements done under the NURE Program (Grasty, 2002; Grasty and LaMarre, 2004) is 0.26 mSv, with a fifth percentile value of 0.07 mSv and a 95th percentile value of 0.47 mSv. The annual effective dose on the Atlantic and Gulf Coastal Plain is lowest, while that in the mountainous regions in the west is highest.

The frequency distribution of average annual effective dose compiled for 49 states (the 48 conterminous states and Alaska) is shown in Figure 3.10. The values are weighted according to age, housing distributions, and fraction of time indoors. The annual value for this geographical distribution weighted by state is 0.23 ± 0.06 mSv. The population-weighted annual effective dose is 0.21 mSv.

A Monte-Carlo procedure was developed to estimate the influence of uncertainties and variability in the determination of effective dose rate by analyzing variations in the equations and coefficients used to transform the NURE data. Figure 3.11 shows the results of this analysis in terms of the distribution of the

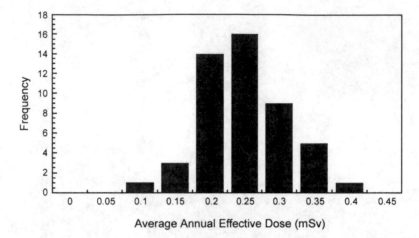

Fig. 3.10. Histogram showing the variability of terrestrial average annual effective dose (millisievert) in 49 states (the 48 conterminous states and Alaska).

population-weighted annual effective dose. The 95 % confidence interval for the estimate of population-weighted annual effective dose is 0.15 to 0.29 mSv.

3.5 Radon and Thoron and Their Short-Lived Decay Products

Radon is an inert gas and most of that inhaled is rapidly exhaled without being retained in the body. Although a small fraction of inhaled radon passes into the bloodstream, very little radiation dose results because nearly all radon recirculates to the lung and is exhaled before radioactive decay. Much more important is the alpha-particle dose to the lung produced by the decay of inhaled short-lived radon decay products, referred to as radon "progeny" or historically as radon "daughters" (Figure 3.2 for decay chain). The progeny are produced as positively-charged atomic ions in the air, where they quickly form complexes with water vapor and attach to ambient aerosol particles. The inhaled progeny, whether or not they are "attached," deposit on airways of the respiratory tract, including the extrathoracic region, and are retained long enough to irradiate sensitive cells in the bronchial epithelium.

The alpha-particle dose to sensitive cells in the lung cannot be measured, but it can be estimated using lung dosimetry models and information regarding the radon progeny exposure. Doses to tissues outside the respiratory tract from inhaled radon progeny are relatively small compared with the dose received by the lung

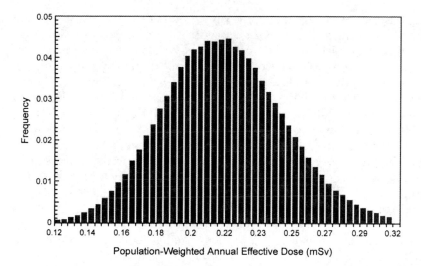

Fig. 3.11. Results of Monte-Carlo simulation demonstrating uncertainty in the population-weighted annual effective dose (terrestrial gamma radiation) due to parameter uncertainty. The integral is normalized to one.

(Harley and Robbins, 1992; Jacobi and Eisfeld, 1980; Kendall and Smith, 2002).

3.5.1 *Radon Quantities and Units*

Traditionally, radon progeny concentration is expressed as potential alpha energy per unit volume of air that can be released by short-lived radon decay products. The potential alpha-energy concentration $[c_p \ (\text{J m}^{-3})]$ is commonly expressed as the working level (WL), now defined[8] to be exactly 1.30×10^5 MeV L^{-1} ($\sim 2.08 \times 10^{-5}$ J m^{-3}). WL can be related to equilibrium equivalent radon concentration, that is, the concentration of radon in secular equilibrium with its short-lived progeny. This relationship depends on the best estimates of the half-lives and branching ratios of the short-lived progeny, and the energies and abundances of their alpha-particle emissions. The equilibrium equivalent concentration

[8]A working level (WL) was originally defined as the potential alpha-energy concentration associated with the radon progeny in equilibrium with 100 pCi L^{-1} (3,700 Bq L^{-1}) of radon, a concentration that was $\sim 1.30 \times 10^5$ MeV L^{-1} (Evans, 1980), but the precise value depended on the estimates of potential alpha energy per disintegration. WL is now defined as a concentration of potential alpha energy of exactly 1.30×10^5 MeV L^{-1} (ICRP, 1993).

[c_{eq} (Bq m^{-3})] of any nonequilibrium mixture of short-lived radon progeny in air is the activity concentration of radon in radioactive equilibrium with its short-lived progeny that has the same potential alpha-energy concentration as the actual nonequilibrium mixture. WL as now defined corresponds to c_{eq} = 3,739 ± 11 Bq m^{-3} (rounded to 3,740) based on averages of data from ICRP (Eckerman and Sjoreen, 2004), the National Nuclear Data Center (NNDC, 2008a), and the *Chart of the Nuclides and Isotopes* (LMC, 2003).

The time-integral of exposure to radon progeny is called potential alpha-energy exposure [ε_p (J h m^{-3})], commonly expressed as the working level month (WLM). Defined originally for occupational exposures, 1 WLM is the exposure to 1 WL for 170 h, a conventional definition of an occupational month (ICRP, 1993; NAS/NRC, 1999a; 1999b).

In most situations, radon progeny are not in secular equilibrium with radon gas. The equilibrium factor (F) is defined to be the ratio of potential alpha energy present in the form of short-lived progeny divided by what would be present at secular equilibrium. Thus:

$$c_p = \frac{c_{eq}}{3,740} = F \frac{C}{3,740} , \qquad (3.8)$$

where:

c_p	=	potential alpha-energy concentration (WL)
c_{eq}	=	equilibrium equivalent concentration of radon gas (Bq m^{-3})
C	=	observed concentration of radon gas (Bq m^{-3})

Knowledge of the equilibrium factor thus allows one to infer potential alpha-energy concentration from measurements of radon gas and to infer radon progeny exposure from a time-integrated determination of radon-gas exposure.

Measurements of radon gas are simpler and less expensive than those of radon progeny; moreover, there have been several national radon testing proficiency programs since the mid-1980s to standardize radon-gas measurements (EPA, 2008). Consequently, radon progeny are rarely monitored outside the occupational or research settings.

3.5.2 *Residential Exposure*

Many studies of radon levels in U.S. homes have been conducted, but the most definitive, by far, is NRRS carried out by EPA. NRRS, completed in 1991, measured radon-gas concentrations in a representative sample of 5,694 U.S. homes (EPA, 1992; Marcinowski *et al.*, 1994). The survey covered single-family detached homes, multi-unit structures, and mobile homes. Year-long measurements were carried out with alpha-particle track detectors placed on each living level of the house.

The results of NRRS for the United States are summarized in Table 3.6 and Figure 3.12. The radon concentration for each home was taken to be the arithmetic mean of the measured annual average concentrations for each living level. The frequency distribution of radon concentration was approximately lognormal with a median of 24.8 Bq m^{-3} and a GSD of 3.11. The mean concentration was 46.3 ± 4.4 Bq m^{-3} (one standard error of the mean). There is significant variability even among averaging areas as large as EPA regions. For example, EPA Region VIII (Montana, North Dakota, South Dakota, Wyoming, Utah, and Colorado) had an arithmetic mean concentration of 95.8 Bq m^{-3}, 4.54 times higher than the value of 21.1 Bq m^{-3} for EPA Region X (Alaska, Washington, Oregon and Idaho).

There is likely some error introduced by assigning equal weight to each living level of the home. As part of NRRS, a questionnaire was administered to residents in which they were asked how much time they spent on each level of the house. When the radon concentration for each house was obtained by weighting the radon reading on each floor by reported occupancy on that floor, the national mean radon concentration was computed to be 43.3 ± 4.3 Bq m^{-3} (one standard error of the mean), slightly lower than obtained from a simple arithmetic average of the concentrations on each level. However, since it appeared likely that the questionnaire, administered primarily in the summer, was a poor reflection of year-round occupancy habits, the simple arithmetic average was adopted by EPA (Marcinowski *et al.*, 1994).

Two other major nationwide collections have been assembled of measurements made during the 1980s. While they are not carefully designed to give accurate averages, these serve to show geographic variability. These studies involved primarily short-term measurements, which may be a poor reflection of the yearly average radon level; many measurements were made only in the lowest level of the house or the lowest living area.

The University of Pittsburgh data set represents hundreds of thousands of measurements (usually lasting one week) using diffusion barrier charcoal adsorbers in 1,601 counties in 47 states and Washington, D.C., but does not include data for Arizona, California, or Florida[9] (Cohen 1992; 1996).

---

[9]Arizona, California and Florida were omitted because they have a high proportion of retirees who presumably received their radon exposures elsewhere.

TABLE 3.6—*Results of NRRS (Marcinowski et al., 1994) by EPA region.*

EPA Region[a]	Observations	Arithmetic Mean $(Bq\ m^{-3})$	Median $(Bq\ m^{-3})$	Geometric Standard Deviation
I	355	43.7	25.5	2.96
II	632	31.8	13.0	4.66
III	810	50.7	25.2	2.76
IV	801	42.2	24.4	2.62
V	1,504	62.5	39.2	2.91
VI	419	30.0	16.7	3.00
VII	314	87.3	57.7	2.44
VIII	279	95.8	60.7	2.91
IX	390	29.6	21.8	2.71
X	190	21.1	13.3	2.54
Overall	5,694	46.3	24.8	3.11

[a]EPA regions were:

I	Maine, Vermont, New Hampshire, Massachusetts, Connecticut, and Rhode Island
II	New York and New Jersey
III	Pennsylvania, Delaware, Maryland, Virginia, and West Virginia
IV	Kentucky, Tennessee, North Carolina, South Carolina, Mississippi, Alabama, Georgia, and Florida
V	Minnesota, Wisconsin, Michigan, Illinois, Indiana and Ohio
VI	New Mexico, Texas, Oklahoma, Arkansas, and Louisiana
VII	Nebraska, Iowa, Kansas and Missouri
VIII	Montana, North Dakota, South Dakota, Wyoming, Utah, and Colorado
IX	California, Nevada, Arizona and Hawaii
X	Alaska, Washington, Oregon and Idaho

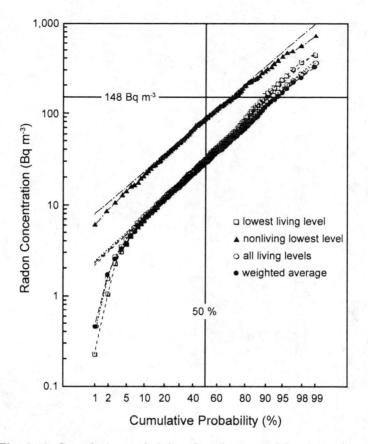

Fig. 3.12. Cumulative probability distributions of the observed radon parameters in single-family housing units: (square) radon concentration on the lowest level of living space, (triangle) radon concentration on the lowest level in housing units where the lowest level was not living space, (open circle) average radon concentration over all levels used as living space, and (solid circle) weighted average of radon concentrations over all levels. The dashed straight lines represent lognormal distributions. The solid horizontal line represents EPA recommended action level for mitigation (148 Bq m^{-3}) (Marcinowski *et al.*, 1994).

The LBNL data set (Price *et al.*, 2007) contains summaries for 3,079 counties.

A comparison of summary statistics for the data from the three sources is given in Table 3.7. Because the University of Pittsburgh and LBNL data are averages for counties or states, the largest values for these averages are less than the maximum values in individual residences. Indeed, the maximum concentration of decay

TABLE 3.7—*Comparison of radon concentration measurement results from the University of Pittsburgh (Cohen, 1992; 1996), LBNL (Price et al., 2007), and NRRS (Marcinowski et al., 1994).*

	University of Pittsburgh		LBNL			EPA
	(states)	(counties)	(states)	(counties)	(regions)	(residences)
Average (arithmetic mean) (Bq m^{-3})	59.8	65.5	56.6	59.1	49.5	46.3
SD (Bq m^{-3})	25.4	37.8	31.6	39.4	25.2	
Standard error of the mean (Bq m^{-3})						4.4
Coefficient of variation	0.42	0.58	0.56	0.67	0.51	
GM (Bq m^{-3})	55.0	56.0	49.5	47.3	44.3	24.8
GSD	1.50	1.76	1.68	1.98	1.63	3.11
Minimum (Bq m^{-3})	22.1	9.7	13.1	6.3	21.1	
Maximum (Bq m^{-3})	116	237	141	266	95.8	
Maximum/minimum	5.2	24.5	10.8	42.2	4.54	
Number[a] used for average and SD	46	1,601	49	3,079	10	5,694

[a]Number of states, counties, regions or residences.

products of radon, 13 WL, was found in the Reading Prong Region of Pennsylvania and is equivalent to 96,200 Bq m^{-3} of radon gas (Gerusky, 1996). Measured in 1984, the 96,200 Bq m^{-3} value brought indoor radon to national attention. If radon concentrations were truly distributed lognormally, this value would be 7.28 SDs above the median of NRRS, an event with a probability of 1.6 × 10^{-13}. Suffice it to say that a few Americans are exposed to far higher concentrations than the average values would suggest. Indoor radon concentrations are far more variable than any other component of ubiquitous background radiation.

For the calculations of indoor exposure below, an average concentration in U.S. residences of 46.3 Bq m^{-3} is assumed.

The data for NRRS were collected in 1989 to 1990. It is known that there are sizable year-to-year fluctuations in radon concentrations within houses (Darby et al., 2006; Harley and Terilli, 1990; Hopke et al., 1995), due to changes in weather patterns and other factors such as changes in living habits. Unless U.S. weather patterns during the year in which the data were collected were highly abnormal, the estimated mean and median should not be perturbed appreciably. However, the effect of the variations is to broaden the distribution over what one would obtain over a much longer term set of measurements. Errors in the annual measurements would also cause a broadening, but these errors were relatively small for homes with elevated radon concentrations.

3.5.3 Changes in Exposure to Radon and Thoron Decay Products Since 1987

Since NRRS, substantial efforts have been made by EPA and by state governments to reduce elevated radon levels in existing homes and to encourage construction of new homes that are "radon resistant" (i.e., that have been built mitigation-ready by including passive mitigation systems that can be easily activated through the addition of a radon vent fan, if necessary). Altogether, EPA estimates that, as of 2005, ~632,000 homes had an operating fan-powered radon mitigation system. Even though such systems significantly reduce the radon concentrations in dwellings in which they are operating, the impact of operating fan-powered mitigation systems on average U.S. indoor radon exposure is likely small.

Of the tens of millions of new homes constructed since NRRS, the National Association of Home Builders reports ~1.4 million have been built "radon resistant," an estimated 60 % of these in areas with high potential for having an elevated radon level indoors.[10] There is evidence that the passive features, properly installed in radon-resistant new construction, may in themselves reduce indoor radon concentration by up to 40 % in some cases, but data are sketchy (NAS/NRC, 1999b). This suggests that a substantial reduction in average radon exposure might be achieved over the long term by wide adoption of radon-resistant new home construction techniques.

Another limitation of NRRS is that it simply measured radon gas, with no attempt to assess the equilibrium factor or other factors, such as aerosol characteristics, that influence lung dose. These kinds of parameters have been measured in only a limited number of homes, not necessarily a representative sample.

Since 1987, it has become apparent that thoron may interfere with some kinds of radon measurements (Section 3.5.13).

3.5.4 Exposure Characteristics of Radon and Radon Decay Products

NAS/NRC (1999b) estimated an average value of 40 % for the equilibrium factor. This estimate was primarily based on 565 measurements in just six homes (Hopke *et al.*, 1995; NAS/NRC, 1999b). Large temporal variability was found within houses, and the overall range of "instantaneous" measurements encompassed values from <10 to 99 % (Hopke *et al.*, 1995). The equilibrium factor was found to be higher, on average, in homes of nonsmokers than in homes of smokers (GM = 0.469 versus GM = 0.346). However, there was little difference in the calculated lung dose for a given radon-gas exposure once differences in the attachment fractions and particle size distributions were taken into account.

George and Breslin (1980) made measurements in 21 houses from which EPA (2003a) derived a central estimate of 50 % for the equilibrium factor. A survey of 200 houses conducted by the state of New Jersey reported a mean equilibrium factor of 45 % (NJDEP, 1989). An earlier study of 20 houses in Butte, Montana, yielded a mean of 32.9 % for the equilibrium factor (Israeli, 1985). Based on the available information, a nominal central estimate of 40 % for the equilibrium factor has been assigned in this Report, with an uncertainty range of 30 to 50 %.

---

[10]Jalbert, P.P. (2006). Personal communication (U.S. Environmental Protection Agency, Washington).

3.5.5 *Time-Use and Radon Exposure*

Airborne radon and its progeny are present everywhere, so exposure occurs not just in residences but also outdoors, indoors at work or school, or in vehicles. Americans spend, on average, ~70 % of their time indoors at home, ~10 % outdoors or in transit, and the rest indoors at other locations (EPA, 1997). A more detailed break-down by age and gender is shown in Table 3.8. Some studies have attempted to account for differences in breathing rate during different activities (Rogers *et al.*, 1990), but this is not attempted here.

TABLE 3.8—*Recommended values for physical activity factors (EPA, 1997).*

Location of Physical Activity	Value (h d^{-1})	Key Studies
Indoor	*Children (ages 3 – 11 y)* 19 h d^{-1} (weekdays) 17 h d^{-1} (weekends) *Adults (ages ≥12 y)* 21 h d^{-1}	 Timmer *et al.* (1985) Timmer *et al.* (1985) Robinson and Thomas (1991)
Outdoor	*Children* 5 h d^{-1} (weekdays) 7 h d^{-1} (weekends) *Adults* 1.5 h d^{-1}	 Timmer *et al.* (1985) Timmer *et al.* (1985) Robinson and Thomas (1991)
Vehicle	*Adults* 1.3 h d^{-1} 1.6 h d^{-1} (mean)	 Robinson and Thomas (1991) Tsang and Klepeis (1996)
Indoors at work	6.6 h d^{-1} (mean) 7.3 h d^{-1} (median)	Tsang and Klepeis (1996)
Residential indoors	16.4 h d^{-1} (median) 16.7 mean: 17.5 (female); 15.8 (male)	Tsang and Klepeis (1996)

3.5.6   *Variability in the Geographic Distribution of Radon*

Radon levels vary widely across the United States. Elevated levels are most commonly found in the Appalachians, the upper Midwest, and the Rocky Mountain states. A geographic plot of the LBNL data (Price *et al.*, 2007) shows clusters of high concentrations (Figure 3.13).

Figure 3.14 shows a map that assigns each U.S. county to a zone of "radon potential" (EPA, 2007a). Zone 1 includes those counties where the average screening measurement for radon in the lowest livable level of the house would be predicted to exceed the EPA action level of 148 Bq m^{-3}, Zone 2 includes counties where the predicted screening level is 74 to 148 Bq m^{-3}, and Zone 3 includes those counties where the predicted screening level is <74 Bq m^{-3}. The estimated radon potential was based on: indoor radon measurements, geology, aerial radiation mapping, soil permeability, and foundation types of homes. The maps in Figures 3.13 and 3.14 are not strictly comparable because the first is based on short-term measurements, while the second is based on an evaluation of potential radon concentrations.

The radon potential map is useful in guiding efforts to reduce radon through mitigation of existing homes or through construction of radon resistant new homes. Nevertheless, it should be noted

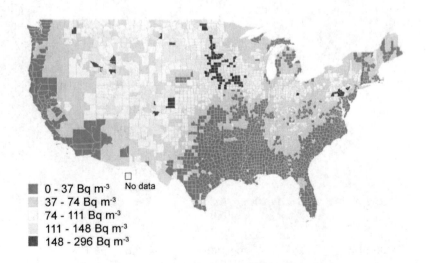

□ No data
■ 0 - 37 Bq m^{-3}
   37 - 74 Bq m^{-3}
   74 - 111 Bq m^{-3}
   111 - 148 Bq m^{-3}
■ 148 - 296 Bq m^{-3}

Fig. 3.13. Map of the United States with LBNL predicted long-term average radon concentrations in living areas (Price *et al.*, 2007).

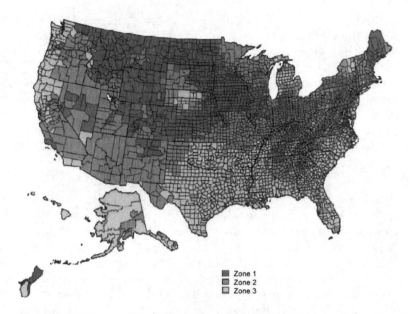

Fig. 3.14. EPA map of radon zones (EPA, 2007a). The map was developed using five factors to determine radon potential: indoor radon measurements, geology, aerial radiation mapping, soil permeability, and foundation type. Radon potential assessment is based on geologic provinces, which were adapted to county boundaries for this map. Each of the 3,141 counties in the United States was assigned to one of three zones based on radon potential (*i.e.*, the predicted average indoor radon screening level). Zone 1 counties (red) are >148 Bq m^{-3}; Zone 2 counties (orange) are between 74 and 148 Bq m^{-3}; and Zone 3 counties (yellow) are <74 Bq m^{-3}.

that radon levels also vary widely from house to house within counties, depending on factors such as outcroppings of uranium rich granite, soil permeability, and building characteristics.

3.5.7 *Outdoor (Ambient) Radon*

Data on outdoor levels of radon have been obtained by EPA through E-Perm® (Rad Elec, Inc., Frederick, Maryland) determinations of annual average concentrations at one location in each U.S. state (Hopper *et al.*, 1991). The results varied from 5.92 to 21.1 Bq m^{-3}, with a mean concentration of 15.1 ± 0.5 Bq m^{-3}. Primarily based on this study, a National Research Council committee concluded that the most probable value for the ambient radon concentration is 15 Bq m^{-3}; they also characterized the uncertainty as being uniformly distributed over the range 14 to 16 Bq m^{-3}

(NAS/NRC, 1999a). Results from other measurements made around the world tend to be lower than this, and UNSCEAR (1993; 2000) estimated the worldwide average radon-gas concentration to be 10 Bq m^{-3}.

The equilibrium factor outdoors is generally somewhat higher than indoors, typically between 50 and 70 % (UNSCEAR, 2000), although a much wider range (20 to 100 %) can be found, depending on conditions. UNSCEAR (2000) estimated an average value of 60 % for the equilibrium factor outdoors.

3.5.8 *Other Indoor Exposure*

Radon concentrations in schools and offices appear to be substantially lower than in residences. Based on EPA long-term measurements, the mean concentration in ground-contact schoolrooms is 29.6 Bq m^{-3} (EPA, 1993a).

As part of its Building Assessment and Evaluation Study, EPA has also conducted short-term radon measurements using charcoal canisters in a random sample of 100 public and commercial office buildings (EPA, 2006). For the 291 measurements taken in occupied areas, the average radon concentration was only 14.8 Bq m^{-3}, similar to the outdoor average. Due to plate-out of radon progeny in the ventilation system, however, the equilibrium factor in large buildings would be considerably lower, typically, than that found outdoors (~0.6) and possibly lower than in the average residence (~0.4).

3.5.9 *Estimate of Population Exposure*

An individual's time-averaged potential alpha-energy concentration [c_p (WL)] can be written as a weighted sum of the exposure rates where the person spends time:

$$c_p = \frac{\sum_i C_i F_i f_i}{3{,}740} \qquad (3.9)$$

Each term in the expression on the right is the product of the radon-gas concentration (C_i) in Bq m^{-3}, the equilibrium factor (F_i) and the fraction of time (f_i) spent in each location i. As an approximation, it is assumed, on average, that 70 % of the time is spent indoors at home, 20 % indoors away from home, and 10 % outside. Based on material discussed above, average radon concentrations in these locations are 46.3, 14.8, and 15 Bq m^{-3}, and average equilibrium factors are 0.4, 0.4, and 0.6, respectively. Based on these values, the time-weighted average potential alpha-energy concentration is:

$$c_p = \frac{(46.3)(0.4)(0.7) + (14.8)(0.4)(0.2) + (15)(0.6)(0.1)}{3,740 \ (\text{Bq m}^{-3}) \ \text{WL}^{-1}}$$

$$= 4.02 \times 10^{-3} \ \text{WL}$$

The average annual potential alpha-energy exposure (ε_p) is then estimated to be:

$$\varepsilon_p = c_p t = \frac{(4.02 \times 10^{-3} \ \text{WL})(24 \ \text{h d}^{-1})(365 \ \text{d y}^{-1})}{170 \ \text{WL h WLM}^{-1}} = 0.207 \ \text{WLM} \ .$$

Given the lognormal variability in residential exposure (a GSD of 3.11 in NRRS), this potential alpha-energy exposure is consistent with a lognormal distribution whose GM is 0.109 WLM, and whose SD is 0.336 WLM. As an extreme value, using the peak indoor radon exposure in Pennsylvania of 96,200 Bq m^{-3} in results in a value of ε_p equal to 372 WLM.

3.5.10 *Average Dose from Radon Progeny*

The most important uncertainty in the estimate of average dose from inhaled radon progeny is the uncertainty in the dose conversion coefficient. The dose conversion coefficient depends on assumptions made about the radon decay product aerosol (including whether cigarette smoke is present), and properties of the human respiratory tract including dissolution rates for radon decay products deposited there and whether the person is a smoker.

The alpha-particle dose to target cells in the lung from exposure to radon progeny is estimated from calculations based on models, which may use different modeling techniques. Some models use biological parameters, measured bronchial airway dimensions, mucociliary clearance rates, particle deposition, and target cell depths, while others compute total deposition in a few selected regions. The deposition of inhaled progeny in the airways is dependent on physical parameters such as: the activity-weighted particle size distribution of the ambient aerosol; the fractions of radon progeny in the "unattached" mode (0.5 to 2 nm) or "nucleation" mode (2 to 30 nm), which contribute disproportionately to the dose because of their high rates of diffusional deposition (Altshuler *et al.*, 1964; Harley and Pasternack, 1972; 1982; James *et al.*, 2004; Knutson and George, 1992; NAS/NRC, 1999b; NCRP, 1984b); and the relative amounts of the individual radon decay products. The dose depends also on biological parameters such as breathing rate, details of the lung anatomy and morphometry such as airway dimensions, location of target cells in the bronchial epithelium, thickness of the mucus layer covering the airways, and rate of mucociliary clearance. To a degree, these parameters will vary across the population, being dependent on age, gender, smoking status, and other factors.

Many details and parameters must be assumed to model dose to the human respiratory tract (ICRP, 1994; NAS/NRC, 1999b), and different assumptions lead to different dose conversion coefficients. Assumptions must be made about aerosol characteristics, including: the equilibrium factor; the presence or absence of cigarette smoke or other aerosols; the amounts of potential alpha-energy concentration present in the unattached, nucleation, accumulation, and coarse fractions; and aerosol size, dispersion, hygroscopic growth factor, particle density, and shape factor (Marsh and Birchall, 2000; Marsh et al., 2002; 2005). These parameters have been measured in only a limited, possibly unrepresentative, sample of homes, and certainly vary from home to home.

Variability in parameter values persists regardless of how well an average value is known. There are age- and gender-dependent variabilities that have not been well characterized, and differences in nose and mouth breathing. Recent developments include accounting for cigarette smoke and other aerosols, hygroscopic particle growth in the respiratory tract, and absorption rates for radon decay products. The identity, location, and depth of target cells are important as well. These differences in assumptions as well as model structure result in differences in calculated dose conversion coefficients.

Dose conversion coefficients expressed as absorbed dose per unit potential alpha-energy exposure (E_p) must be converted to effective dose per E_p. The dose conversion coefficient may apply to the entire respiratory tract or to only the bronchial (BB) and bronchiolar (bb) regions. The ICRP Human Respiratory Tract Model (ICRP, 1994) apportions the 0.12 w_T for the respiratory tract as 0.1 % to the thoracic lymph nodes, and 33.3 % each to the BB, bb, and alveolar-interstitial region. For a dose conversion coefficient calculated for only the BB and bb regions, a tissue weighting factor w_{BB+bb} = (0.333 + 0.333) (0.12) = 0.08 is used, while for dose conversion coefficients calculated for the whole lung, w_{Lung} = 0.12 is used. Also, the alpha-particle w_R of 20 must be applied. NCRP (1984a) apportioned the whole-lung weighting factor of 0.12 between the bronchial tree (0.08) and the pulmonary region (0.04). There is an additional minor contribution of dose to the extrathoracic-1 compartment, but that has not been considered here.

UNSCEAR (2000) published a review of dose conversion coefficients expressed in absorbed dose per unit equilibrium equivalent radon concentration [nGy (Bq h m^{-3})$^{-1}$] listing 15 calculated values published between 1956 and 1998 using different models and assumptions. To compare with more recent publications, these have been converted to absorbed dose per E_p (mGy WLM^{-1}). There were no significant trends with year of publication, breathing rate, or depth of target cells. There was a suggestion of a linear increase with unattached fraction (correlation coefficient: $r^2 = 0.59$), but only if a single extreme result at unattached fraction of 35 % is included. Without that data point, $r^2 = 0.077$. The UNSCEAR (2000) results averaged 11 ± 10.4 mGy WLM^{-1} and were roughly lognormally-distributed with a GM of 8.47 mGy WLM^{-1} and a GSD of 1.98.

Since UNSCEAR (2000), six papers or documents were published or drafted with 15 additional dose conversion coefficient values. Harley[11] computes a value of 6 ± 3 mGy WLM^{-1} (1 SD) to the upper airways. Using a w_T of 0.08 and a w_R of 20, this becomes 9.6 ± 4.8 (1 SD) mSv WLM^{-1}. For homes, Marsh and Birchall (2000) calculate 15 mSv WLM^{-1}, while Marsh *et al.* (2002) give 11 mSv WLM^{-1} and Marsh *et al.* (2005) arrive at 12.9 mSv WLM^{-1}. NAS/NRC (1999b) addressed only comparative dosimetry between mines and houses and published values for all houses (10.5 mSv WLM^{-1}), houses with smokers (10.2 mSv WLM^{-1}), and houses without smokers (10.6 mSv WLM^{-1}). Winkler-Heil *et al.* (2007) compared three calculational methods and reported results of 7.8, 8.3, and 11.8 mSv WLM^{-1}.

The NAS/NRC dosimetry model, however, did not actually employ the aerosol particle size assumptions that were published in NAS/NRC (1999b), as detailed by James *et al.* (2004). Performing dosimetry calculations based on the assumptions published in NAS/NRC (1999b), James *et al.* (2004) obtained eight dose conversion coefficient values from 15.5 to 21.4 mSv WLM^{-1}, using full respiratory tract (four values) or BB + bb (four values) models, based on the presence or absence of cigarette smoke, and with or without hygroscopic growth. These values are almost twice as high as the other results reviewed by NCRP, because the assumptions about particle size distributions differ significantly from those used by all other investigators before and since.

Despite the flaws in the absolute values of dosimetric results that appeared in Table B-3 of NAS/NRC (1999b), the NAS/NRC uncertainty analysis is essentially correct, because it is based on underlying variability studies of equilibrium factors and many

[11]Harley, N.H. (2007). Personal communication (New York University Medical Center, New York).

other parameters that are included in NAS/NRC (1999b) and is expressed as a lognormal distribution with a GSD. On the basis of the NAS/NRC uncertainty analysis, and on statistical analysis of other dose conversion coefficients, NCRP concludes that a logarithmically-distributed uncertainty distribution with a GSD of 1.6 encompasses the range of models, assumptions and opinions on dose conversion coefficients of the past two decades.

The analyses of James *et al.* (2004), Marsh *et al.* (2005), and NAS/NRC (1999b) confirm the longstanding result that relatively little effective dose is produced by irradiation of the alveolar-interstitial region of the respiratory tract (NCRP, 1987b).

For indoor exposure in the United States, it is necessary to apply an average value of the dose conversion coefficient. Individuals are exposed to radon decay product aerosols that, depending on such factors as particular residence, aerosol characteristics, smoking habits, nose- and mouth-breathing habits, age, gender, and disease state, produce different doses for the same potential alpha-energy concentration, as well as different doses for the same radon-gas concentration.

Furthermore, there has been a difference in the dose conversion coefficient derived from epidemiological results expressed per E_p and that from dosimetric results derived using the ICRP detriment coefficient, w_Ts, and w_Rs (Brenner *et al.*, 1995; IAEA, 1996; ICRP, 1993; NAS/NRC, 1999b). Analysis of epidemiological results by ICRP (1993) suggested that either a w_T (lung) = 0.12, a w_R (alpha particles) = 20, or both, are too high to result in agreement between a dosimetric approach and an epidemiological approach. However, Tomasek *et al.* (2008) indicate that new analyses of the Czech Republic and French epidemiological studies of uranium miners yield dose conversion coefficients in closer agreement with the dosimetric results than was the case with earlier epidemiological results.

Based on the calculations of dose conversion coefficients by the independent scientists cited above, a lognormally distributed dose conversion coefficient with an *arithmetic* mean of 10 mSv WLM^{-1} and a GSD of 1.6 is assumed for the purpose of dose assessment and uncertainty estimation in this Report. Such a distribution has a SD of 5 mSv WLM^{-1} and a GM of 9 mSv WLM^{-1} using the methods of Strom (2007) and Strom and Stansbury (2000). This distribution centers on recently published values, includes the highest estimates from NAS/NRC (1999b) at the 95th percentile, and includes all others within a 90 % confidence interval of GM. This results in an estimate of effective dose per E_p that is more than two times higher than the 4 mSv WLM^{-1} value recommended for exposure in homes by ICRP (1993).

Based on the estimate of annual radon potential alpha-energy exposure of 0.207 WLM and a dose conversion coefficient of 10 mSv WLM^{-1}, the average adult in the United States receives an annual effective dose to the bronchial epithelium of 2.07 mSv (with a GSD of 1.6), where the uncertainty in the average is dominated by the uncertainty in the dose conversion coefficient. Variability in the annual effective dose is addressed in Section 3.5.11.

3.5.11 *Sources of Variability, Bias and Uncertainty*

The largest source of variability in individual doses from radon progeny, by far, is the variation in radon concentration among geographic areas and houses within the same area. Overall, according to NRRS, nearly 60 % of all homes have an annual average radon level <37 Bq m^{-3}, ~6 % have a level above 148 Bq m^{-3} and ~0.7 % have a level >370 Bq m^{-3}. In rare cases, indoor radon concentrations may exceed 37,000 Bq m^{-3}. Although, for most purposes, a lognormal function adequately describes the distribution of radon concentrations in U.S. homes, the derived lognormal distribution significantly understates the number of homes with highly-elevated concentrations.

As noted above, NRRS estimates of indoor radon concentrations may be biased slightly high because no account was taken of the differences in time spent on the different living levels of the home. Another source of bias is that the alpha-particle track detectors employed in NRRS were sensitive to airborne ^{220}Rn (thoron) as well as ^{222}Rn (radon). Given the limited information available on indoor thoron levels, the magnitude of this bias cannot be accurately assessed. UNSCEAR (2000) estimates that the average indoor ^{220}Rn concentration is 10 Bq m^{-3}, ~20 % of the average measured ^{222}Rn level in NRRS. The efficiency of the employed alpha-particle track detectors was found to be almost as high for ^{220}Rn (~80 %) as for ^{222}Rn (Tokonami *et al.*, 2001). Hence, the upward bias in NRRS measurements may have been roughly 20 %.

3.5.12 *Dose from Inhaled Radon Gas*

Unlike its progeny, radon is chemically inert, and does not deposit in the airways of the lung. Nevertheless, the lung will receive a dose from radon gas decaying within its airspace. In addition, a certain fraction of inhaled radon passes into the bloodstream, and partitions into all the tissues of the body. Given its hydrophobic nature, it will be at highest concentration in lipid rich regions such as fat cells and bone marrow. It has been estimated that, overall, the annual effective dose per unit radon-gas concentration is 1.4×10^{-3} mSv $(\text{Bq m}^{-3})^{-1}$, about half of which is to the lung (Kendall and Smith, 2002; Khursheed, 2000). Using the values cited above for average occupancy factors and radon-gas concentrations out- and indoors (Section 3.5.9), the average radon concentration is estimated to be:

$$\bar{C} = (46.3)(0.7) + (14.8)(0.2) + (15)(0.1) = 36.9 \text{ Bq m}^{-3}$$

The average annual effective dose from radon gas is then calculated to be 0.05 mSv. This brings the average annual total for radon and radon decay products (2.07 mSv, Section 3.5.10) to 2.12 mSv.

3.5.13 *Thoron*

Radon-220 (thoron), formed from alpha-particle decay of ^{232}Th, like ^{222}Rn, exists as a noble gas and decays into a series of short-lived progeny that deposit in and irradiate the lung with alpha particles. Measurements of thoron and its decay products in indoor air have been limited. There is often substantial variation of thoron gas within a room because of its short half-life (55.6 s). Thoron and radon progeny levels have been found to have some correlation (Chen *et al.*, 2008; Gunning and Scott, 1982; Rannou, 1987; Schery and Grumm, 1992; Tschiersch *et al.*, 2007; Tu *et al.*, 1992), but, thoron is unlikely to be an important source of exposure in homes with high ^{222}Rn (NAS/NRC, 1999b; Tu *et al.*, 1992). Tu *et al.*, (1992) indicate that ^{222}Rn comes primarily from soil gas and ^{220}Rn comes primarily from building materials.

In general, the potential alpha-energy concentration associated with thoron progeny is lower than for radon; moreover, the estimated dose conversion coefficient for thoron progeny is one-third that for radon progeny (NEA, 1983), which would lead to an estimate of 3.3 mSv WLM^{-1} [*i.e.*, (10 mSv WLM^{-1}) / 3]. Birchall[12] gives a value of 3.8 mSv WLM^{-1}. UNSCEAR (2000) estimated that the annual effective dose from inhaled thoron and its decay products is ~0.1 mSv, compared with the estimate of 2.12 mSv for ^{222}Rn gas and its progeny given in Sections 3.5.10 and 3.5.12. Although the contribution of ^{220}Rn and its decay products to the average effective dose is probably small compared with that from ^{222}Rn and its progeny, additional measurements would be warranted to better assess

---

[12]Birchall, A. (2008). Personal communication (Health Protection Agency, Chilton, United Kingdom).

the extent of exposure to thoron and its potential health risks (Steinhausler, 1996). The lingering difficulty is that the presence of ^{220}Rn increases the apparent value of ^{222}Rn measurements, but the usually unquantified ^{220}Rn decay products also truly produce alpha-particle dose to the respiratory tract. Therefore, it is necessary to disaggregate the two effects of: (1) ^{220}Rn gas causing upward bias in ^{222}Rn gas measurements; and (2) real irradiation of the human respiratory tract by ^{220}Rn decay products. Studies that jointly consider these two effects should be undertaken, with a goal of helping to interpret the vast body of historical measurements.

Different measurement technologies exhibit significantly different responses to ^{220}Rn when they purport to measure ^{222}Rn. Many alpha-track detectors cannot distinguish between the two, nor can liquid scintillation counting of activated charcoal. However, early measurements of charcoal detectors, both open-face and diffusion barrier, relied on gamma spectroscopy, which was specific for ^{222}Rn decay products. Unless an adequate diffusion barrier is included, alpha-particle track detectors for measuring radon gas will also register a contribution from thoron, leading to a spuriously high measured radon concentration. In particular, as noted above, the alpha-particle track detectors used in NRRS failed to completely screen out ^{220}Rn.

NAS/NRC (1999b) reported that $E_{\text{p,Rn-220}} / E_{\text{p,Rn-222}}$ averages ~0.5; UNSCEAR (2000) reported $E_{\text{p,Rn-220}} / E_{\text{p,Rn-222}}$ ranges from 0.3 to 0.5. For the dose conversion coefficient per E_{p} of 3.33 mSv WLM^{-1}, the average relative contribution from thoron decay products to dose is ~17 % in the United States, rather than the ~10 % quoted by UNSCEAR (2000). Measurements reported by Tu *et al.* (1992), $E_{\text{p,Rn-220}} / E_{\text{p,Rn-222}} = 0.47$ for all houses, or 0.0949 WLM y^{-1}, yielded an annual effective dose of 0.32 mSv. This dose cannot be added directly to the ^{222}Rn gas and decay product dose because of the unknown contribution of ^{220}Rn to the ^{222}Rn measurement results. In the absence of any data to inform this question, this Report assumes that about half of this annual effective dose, or 0.16 mSv, should be added for an average adult in the United States. Thus, the average annual effective dose for radon and thoron and their decay products is 2.28 mSv.

3.6 Radionuclides in the Body

This section focuses on measurements of tissue contents of ^{40}K, the ^{232}Th series, and the ^{238}U series. Potassium is a natural element, a small amount of which is radioactive ^{40}K, present in food. Thus, the source of almost all ^{40}K in the body tissues is food, primarily fruits and vegetables. The sources of radionuclides from the ^{232}Th and ^{238}U series are food and water. Brazil nuts are a significant single source of dose from these series (~1 %), but ~39 % of the dose may result from radionuclides from these series in domestic water supplies (Section 3.6.3 and Appendix B).

3.6.1 *Potassium-40*

Potassium concentration (C_K) values, expressed as mass of potassium (grams) divided by body mass (kilograms) (or parts per thousand by mass) were calculated based on *in vivo* ^{40}K measurements of 248 adult females and 2,037 adult males at the DOE Hanford Site (Strom *et al.*, 2009). The potassium concentration in males is generally higher than the concentration in females due to a higher percentage of lean body mass in males. The average potassium concentration values for both adult males and adult females decrease with increasing age (Figure 3.15) and with increasing values of body mass index (BMI) expressed as mass/height^2 (kg m^{-2}) (Figure 3.16), both with significant individual variation. Statistical properties of the data are given in Tables 3.9 and 3.10.

Dosimetry was performed from the fundamental physical properties of ^{40}K and its decay processes, as well as using the methods of Stabin and Siegel (2003). Standard phantoms from Cristy and Eckerman (1987) were used with the addition of the adult female phantom of Stabin and Siegel (2003).

Radioactive ^{40}K emits a 0.56 MeV beta particle (average energy) in 89.3 % of decay transitions, and a 1.46 MeV photon in 10.7 % of transitions (NNDC, 2008b). With a ^{40}K fractional abundance of 0.0117 atom percent or 0.01196 mass percent (NNDC, 2008c), natural potassium has a specific activity of 31.72 Bq g^{-1}. The possible energy per transition that can be absorbed ranges from 8×10^{-14} J if none of the 1.46 MeV photons are absorbed to 10.5×10^{-14} J if all of those photons are absorbed. In NCRP (1987b), an absorbed fraction of 0.8 appears to have been used.

Using dose conversion coefficients (mGy MBq^{-1} s^{-1}) for ^{40}K in seven different phantoms from the Radiation Dose Assessment Resource (RaDAR, 2008) and the Hanford age- and gender-dependent potassium data (Strom *et al.*, 2009), yields the results in Table 3.11. The dose conversion coefficients were for uniform source distributions irradiating the whole body. On average, adult males have 19 % more potassium per unit body mass, and receive 21 % more absorbed dose than adult females, due to the increased absorption of the 1.46 MeV photon in more massive men. None of the phantoms currently incorporate a variable BMI. The adult male phantom has a BMI of 26.4, compared with the Hanford male

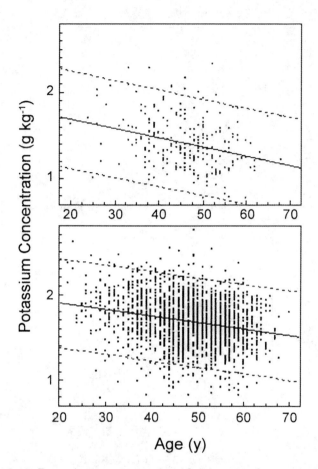

Fig. 3.15. Potassium concentration (C_K) (grams of potassium per kilogram of body mass) decreases with increasing age in adults (NCRP; 1987b; UNSCEAR, 1972). These data are for 248 women (top panel) and 2,037 men (bottom panel) (Strom *et al.*, 2009). Dashed lines show upper and lower 95 % confidence intervals for the population.

average of 30.9. The dose conversion coefficient approach is consistent with a first-principles approach assuming an absorbed fraction of 0.34 for the 1.46 MeV photon.

Figure 3.17 shows a modest increase in the effective dose with body mass, primarily due to increased absorption of the 1.46 MeV photon as mass increases. Trends in age dependence of average ^{40}K effective doses calculated using the phantoms specified in Table 3.11 for males and females are shown in Figure 3.18 for the data from NCRP (1987b) and (Strom *et al.*, 2009). Doses to adult males are ~8 % lower using the Hanford data than for NCRP data,

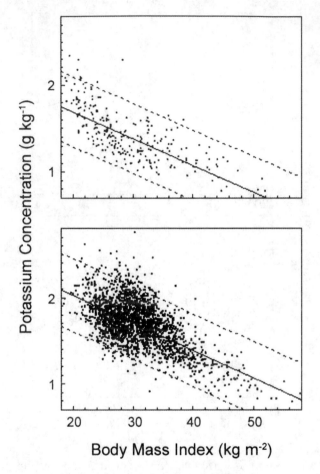

Fig. 3.16. Potassium concentration (C_K) decreases with increasing BMI in adults. These data are for 248 women (top panel) and 2,037 men (bottom panel) (Strom *et al.*, 2009). Dashed lines show upper and lower 95 % confidence intervals for the populations.

probably due at least in part to the decreased ^{40}K concentrations associated with the higher average BMI of Hanford males. Doses to adult males are higher than those to adult females by an average of 32 % in NCRP data compared with 21 % noted above for the Hanford data.

Very little data on potassium concentrations are available for people under the age of 20 y. More information is needed for this age group; lower body masses would result in lower doses for a given potassium concentration, due to the greater escape probability of the 1.46 MeV photon.

TABLE 3.9—*Summary statistics for potassium concentration (C_K) (grams of potassium per kilogram of body mass), age, and BMI distributions (adult males and females).*

Potassium Concentration

Gender	Number	Average (g kg^{-1})	SD (g kg^{-1})	Geometric Mean (g kg^{-1})	GSD
Males[a]	2,037	1.68	0.27	1.66	1.19
Females[b]	248	1.41	0.30	1.38	1.23

Age and BMI

Gender	Parameter	Average	SD	Minimum	Maximum
Males	Age (y)	48.8	8.58	22	70
Females	Age (y)	46.1	8.56	20	68
Males	BMI (kg m^{-2})	30.9	5.32	18.5	57.8
Females	BMI (kg m^{-2})	29.2	6.96	18.9	52.1

[a]Potassium-concentration data for males were more skewed in the positive direction than a normal distribution, but were not a lognormal distribution.
[b]Potassium-concentration data for females were lognormal.

TABLE 3.10—*Single and double linear regression results of potassium content as a function of gender, age and BMI.*

Gender	Intercept (g kg⁻¹)	Slope: Age (g kg⁻¹ y⁻¹)	Slope: BMI [g kg⁻¹ (kg m⁻²)⁻¹]	Correlation Coefficient (r^2)	GSD[a]
Males	2.664		−0.0318	0.384	
Females	2.306		−0.0307	0.524	
Males	2.047	−0.00747		0.055	
Females	1.897	−0.01058		0.094	
Males	2.946	−0.00620	−0.0311	0.421	1.133
Females	2.500	−0.00512	−0.0292	0.544	1.148

[a]The individual variation from the value predicted by these equations is lognormally-distributed about the *arithmetic* mean with this GSD. The *geometric* mean of the lognormal distribution is equal to the arithmetic mean multiplied by $e^{-(\ln GSD)^2/2}$ (Strom and Stansbury, 2000).

TABLE 3.11—*Results using dose conversion coefficients from the RaDAR Site with Hanford potassium data for adult males and females. The adult female data were used for children.*

Phantom[a]		Dose Conversion Coefficient (mGy MBq⁻¹ s⁻¹)	Phantom Mass (g)	Potassium Concentration (g kg⁻¹)	^{40}K Activity per Unit Body Mass (Bq kg⁻¹)	^{40}K Activity in the Body (Bq)	Annual ^{40}K Transitions (MBq s y⁻¹)	Annual Absorbed Dose (mGy y⁻¹)
C&E	Adult male	1.20×10^{-6}	73,700	1.682	53.36	3,933	1.24×10^{5}	0.149
S&S	Adult female	1.54×10^{-6}	56,800	1.409	44.70	2,539	8.01×10^{4}	0.123
C&E	15 y old	1.54×10^{-6}	56,800	1.409	44.70	2,539	8.01×10^{4}	0.123
C&E	10 y old	2.61×10^{-6}	33,200	1.409	44.70	1,484	4.68×10^{4}	0.122
C&E	5 y old	4.35×10^{-6}	19,800	1.409	44.70	885	2.79×10^{4}	0.122
C&E	1 y old	8.76×10^{-6}	9,720	1.409	44.70	435	1.37×10^{4}	0.120
C&E	Newborn	2.33×10^{-5}	3,600	1.409	44.70	161	5.08×10^{3}	0.118

[a] C&E = Cristy and Eckerman (1987)
S&S = Stabin and Siegel (2003)

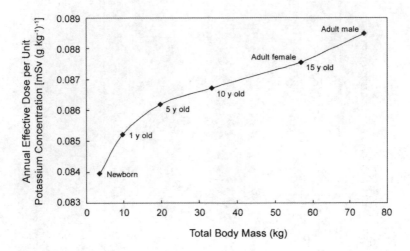

Fig. 3.17. Annual effective dose per unit potassium concentration (E / C_K) as a function of body mass for the phantoms in Table 3.11. Increasing mass is correlated with increasing age. Adult female and 15 y old have the same value of E / C_K.

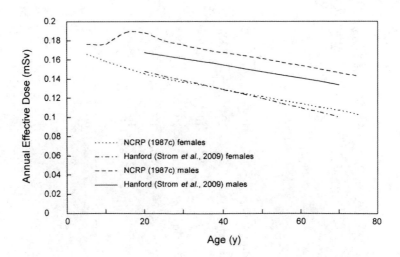

Fig. 3.18. Trends in age dependence of average ^{40}K effective doses calculated using phantoms in Table 3.11 for males and females.

In summary, the ubiquitous background radionuclide ^{40}K produces radiation doses that have significant trends with gender, age, body mass, and BMI, with significant individual variability. The annual effective dose for average adult males as a function of age (years) and BMI (kg m^{-2}) is:

$$E_{\text{Average adult male}} = 0.0885(2.946 - 0.0062\ age - 0.0311\ BMI), \quad (3.10)$$

and for average adult females is:

$$E_{\text{Average adult female}} = 0.0876(2.5 - 0.00512\ age - 0.0292\ BMI). \quad (3.11)$$

Individual variability about these arithmetic mean values is described by a lognormal distribution with a GSD of 1.133 for males and 1.148 for females. The *geometric* means of these lognormal distributions are equal to the arithmetic means multiplied by $e^{-(\ln GSD)^2/2}$ (Strom and Stansbury, 2000).

Ignoring the effects of age, height and body mass, average annual values are 0.149 and 0.123 mSv for men and women, respectively. Averaged over both men and women, the annual effective dose is 0.136 mSv. Annual effective doses range from 0.069 to 0.243 mSv for adult males, and 0.067 to 0.203 mSv for adult females, a roughly threefold variation for each gender.

3.6.2 *Thorium-232 and Uranium-238 Series*

Annual effective doses from the uranium and thorium series in the body (excluding inhalation of radon and thoron decay products) to members of the U.S. population were calculated based on data published by UNSCEAR (2000). UNSCEAR (2000) presented annual effective doses to reference individuals by two methods. The first was to estimate intakes by inhalation and ingestion, and then infer doses. The second was to perform dosimetry based on the radionuclide content of tissues and organs.

For this Report, doses from the uranium and thorium series to persons in the United States were scaled from reference values in UNSCEAR (2000) and data for the United States. The results are shown in Tables 3.12 and 3.13. Table 3.12 shows the relative contributions of members of these series to tissues for which data are available, with most of the annual effective dose due to ^{210}Pb/^{210}Po.

In Table 3.13, the "tissue content" method uses ICRP (2007a) w_Ts, while the "intake" method employed by UNSCEAR (2000) uses ICRP (1991) w_Ts. The differences in w_Ts result in <10 % difference in effective dose, but cannot be evaluated directly with the data given.

TABLE 3.12—*Average annual equivalent doses (H_T) to U.S. adults from natural radionuclides of the uranium and thorium series contained in the body, with contributions to annual effective dose (E^*) based on ICRP (2007a) tissue-weighting factors.*[a]

Tissue	H_T (μSv)							w_T	$w_T H_T$ (μSv)
	238/234U	230Th	226Ra	210Pb/210Po	232Th	228/224Ra	Sum		
Bone surfaces	8.48	3.23	107	250	0.59	53.2	423	0.01	4.2
Lung[b]	17.2	6.40	4.85	88.5	7.07	62.9	187	0.12	22.4
Kidney	7.73	4.08	4.85	242	1.40	9.44	269	0.0092	2.5
Liver	2.76	4.32	4.85	504	1.20	9.60	527	0.04	21.1
Other[c]	1.45	0.84	4.87	59.1	0.75	1.98	69	0.70	48.3
Bone marrow	2.68	66.5	13.9	101	41.1	8.68	234	0.12	28.0
E^*									126.6
									0.127 mSv

[a]Values are derived from reference values in Annex B, Table 20 of UNSCEAR (2000) and U.S. data in Annex B, Table 15, 16 and 19 of UNSCEAR (2000).

[b]Excluding ^{222}Rn, ^{220}Rn, and their short-lived decay products.

[c]Other tissues are all the remaining tissues in the ICRP (2007a) list: colon, stomach, breast, gonads, bladder, esophagus, thyroid, brain, salivary glands, skin, adrenals, extrathoracic region, gall bladder, heart, lymphatic nodes, muscle, oral mucosa, pancreas, prostate (male), small intestine, spleen, thymus, uterus/cervix (female).

TABLE 3.13—Annual effective doses from the uranium and thorium series (excluding inhalation of radon and thoron decay products) to members of the U.S. population based on UNSCEAR (2000) data.

Age Group	Calculation Method							
	E (mSv) Ingestion Method[a]				E^* (mSv) Tissue Content Method[b]			
	AM[c]	Low	High	GSD[c]	AM[c]	Low	High	GSD[c]
Infants	0.132	0.119	0.143	1.058	—	—	—	—
Children	0.114	0.098	0.127	1.081	—	—	—	—
Adults	0.058	0.050	0.064	1.075	0.127	0.115	0.138	1.057

[a]The tissue content method uses ICRP (2007a) w_Ts.
[b]The ingestion method uses ICRP (1991) w_Ts. The difference in weighting factors results in <10 % difference in effective dose.
[c] AM = arithmetic mean
   GSD = geometric standard deviation

Ingestion doses are clearly age-dependent, with infants receiving the highest doses, and children receiving slightly lower doses, but still twice the adult values. For adults, the tissue content method yields doses comparable to the doses for children obtained by the ingestion method. However, the adult doses using the tissue content method are over twice the doses using the adult ingestion method. One is forced to conclude that there is significant uncertainty in these results, perhaps a coefficient of variation of 0.3 or more. More data are needed in order to assess doses more accurately, and to assess both variability and uncertainty when comparing the two methods.

The variability in doses is far less in the data cited by UNSCEAR (2000) than, for example, in a recent set of uranium and thorium measurements reported by LaRiviere *et al.* (2007), who compared 68 measurements of uranium and thorium in human vertebrae from two Canadian cities with other reported measurements. There was no clear trend with age, but a threefold variability was evident. Some of the variability in the Canadian data can be explained by differences in the uranium and thorium content of drinking water (LaRiviere *et al.*, 2007).

The average annual values are 0.132 and 0.114 mSv for infants and children, respectively (ingestion method). Averaged over both men and women, the annual effective dose is 0.127 mSv for the tissue content method. Using the two different methods of calculation the annual effective doses range from 0.050 to 0.138 mSv for adults, a roughly threefold variation.

3.6.3 Radionuclides in Domestic Water Supplies

A separate assessment for the collective effective dose from radium, uranium and radon concentrations in drinking water for both public and private supplies and private wells is presented in Appendix B. The result was 33,700 person-Sv for 2006. However, an unquantified contribution from radionuclides in drinking water is already included in the overall estimate derived from the previous assessment for radionuclides in the body [87,000 person-Sv (Table 8.1)] which accounts for all intakes from food and water. The separate assessment in Appendix B provides an estimate for the proportion of S included in the ubiquitous background radiation component from radionuclides in the body that is due to ingestion of drinking water (~39 %).

3.6.4 Cosmogenic Radionuclides

The production of ^{14}C by cosmic-ray interactions in the upper atmosphere is latitude- and time-dependent, but the resulting radioactive carbon dioxide mixes throughout the atmosphere and is uniformly distributed at ground level where it is a source of human exposure. This source gives an annual H_E of ~0.01 mSv to the whole body, mostly from ^{14}C in tissues (NCRP, 1987b).

3.7 Summary and Conclusions

The population-weighted average annual effective doses to U.S. adult males resulting from the various sources described in this section are summarized in Table 3.14. Average annual effective doses to women and children are comparable, but, as discussed above, the data are too sparse to produce equally detailed summaries for women and children.

Rows in Table 3.14 are labeled as external irradiation from space and terrestrial radiation; internal irradiation from ingested radionuclides, separated as ^{40}K, the ^{232}Th and ^{238}U series, and other (^{14}C and ^{87}Rb); and internal irradiation from inhaled radionuclides, listed as ^{222}Rn and its short-lived decay products and ^{220}Rn and its short-lived decay products.

The average annual effective dose is useful to gain perspective for most individuals, but some will receive significantly less or far more than this dose. To illustrate this, the uncertainty and variability are displayed both quantitatively and qualitatively. Quantitative measures include arithmetic means, SDs, GMs, and GSDs. The 95 % confidence limits, that is, the 2.5 and 97.5 percentiles, are also given.

Qualitative characterizations of variability are described as "unknown," "very small," "small," "moderate" and "large." Very small means a GSD of no more than 1.02, small up to 1.1, moderate up to 1.5, large greater than 1.5. Variability assessments are given for age, gender, BMI, geographical location, amount of time spent out- and indoors at home or elsewhere, and building nature and construction. The latter is complex, because it affects shielding from radiation originating from space and from external terrestrial radiation, as well as radon entry and irradiation from natural radioactive material in building materials.

Uncertainty is assessed separately from variability, using the same categories, with the additional category of "very large," denoting a GSD of over two. Moderate and greater uncertainties generally arise from modeling uncertainties and lack of data.

For an individual drawn at random from the U.S. population, given no other information, the variability combines with the uncertainty to become the overall uncertainty in the dose for the individual. It is this overall uncertainty that is characterized in

TABLE 3.14—*Annual effective doses (millisievert) (E_{Exp})[a] to U.S. adult males (averaged over all adult ages) from various background sources.[b,c,d]*

Source	AM	SD	GM	GSD	Percentiles		Factors Affecting Variability							Comments
					2.5	97.5	Age	Gender	BMI	Geography	Time-Use	Building	Uncertainty	
External irradiation														
Space (99 of the most populated U.S. urban areas)	0.33	0.08	0.32	1.28	0.20	0.52	S	S	S	M	M	M	S	Urban areas show less variability than the entire country. Building shielding and time-use are variable.
Terrestrial (by state)	0.21	0.06	0.20	1.32	0.12	0.35	S	S	S	L	M	M	M	Dose conversion coefficients not resolved. Building shielding and time-use are variable. Variability shown here is only by state; GSDs for individual regions within states are *much* larger (1.61 – 2.09).
Internal irradiation (primarily ingestion)														
^{40}K	0.15	0.02	0.15	1.13	0.11	0.21	S	S	S	VS	N	N	S	Effect of high BMI on dosimetry unclear.
^{232}Th and ^{238}U series	0.13	0.007	0.13	1.06	0.11	0.14	U	S	U	M	N	N	M	Sparse data for U.S. populations. Variability probably much larger. Different dosimetric approaches give different answers.
Other: ^{14}C, ^{87}Rb	0.01	0.001	0.01	1.10	0.008	0.01	VS	VS	VS	VS	VS	VS	S	NCRP (1987b).

Internal irradiation (primarily inhalation)

^{222}Rn (radon) and its short-lived decay products	2.12	3.99	1.00	3.41	0.09	11.1	M	S	U	L	M	L	L	GSD (uncertainty) = 1.6; GSD (variability) = 3.11. Does not account for variability in equilibrium factor, aerosol and dosimetry differences in smoky environments.
^{220}Rn (thoron) and its short-lived decay products	0.16	0.30	0.08	3.41	0.007	0.8	M	S	U	L	M	L	VL	Paucity of data; confounding with ^{222}Rn measurements.
Composite[e]	3.11	3.61	2.33	1.95	0.94	12.1	M	S	S	L	M	L	L	

[a] Conversion of these values for E_{Exp} to S and E_{US} for the U.S. population of 300 million are provided in Table 8.1.

[b] Values in italics have some degree of subjective estimate.

[c] Doses to women from ^{40}K are lower; doses to women from external irradiation are slightly higher.

[d] AM = arithmetic mean
SD = standard deviation
GM = geometric mean
GSD = geometric standard deviation

Codes in variability and uncertainty columns:
U = unknown
VL = very large
L = large
M = moderate
S = small
VS = very small
N = none

[e] All composite values are from a Monte-Carlo simulation summing the seven contributions. All distributions were assumed to be lognormal except space, which was assumed to be normal. The 2.5 and 97.5 percentiles were computed assuming lognormality

the composite exposure. Figure 3.19 shows the distribution of doses from the various sources of ubiquitous background radiation using the arithmetic means presented in Table 3.14.

Because contributions from each of the seven sources in Table 3.14 are assumed to be statistically independent and there is no analytical method of adding lognormally-distributed variables, the best way to sum the distributions is with a Monte-Carlo simulation. The results are given in the last line of the table, and plotted in Figure 3.20, based on a U.S. population of 300 million. The annual effective dose to adult males in the United States is 3.11 mSv (arithmetic mean) with a SD of 3.61 mSv. As shown in Figure 3.20, it is not a normal distribution, nor is it strictly lognormal (there is a deficit of very low values). Approximately 2.5 million Americans receive annual doses from ubiquitous background radiation in excess of 20 mSv. The lowest annual doses are just over 0.5 mSv.

In most parts of the United States, the dominant annual tissue dose equivalent is that to the bronchial epithelium from the decay products of radon. The differences in the average annual effective dose reported here and H_E in NCRP (1987b) are not large.

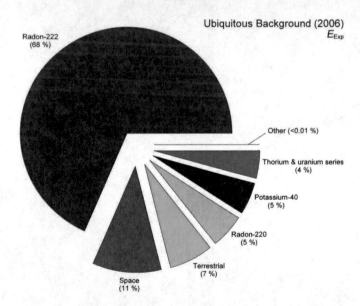

Fig. 3.19. Percent contribution of various sources of exposure to the annual E_{Exp} for ubiquitous background radiation (3.1 mSv) for 2006. The same percentages apply for S and E_{US}. The percent values have been rounded to the nearest 1 %, except those <1 % [see Table 3.14 for the values of E_{Exp} (millisievert)].

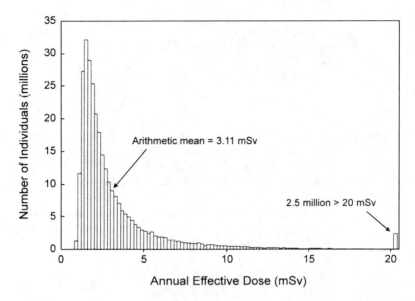

Fig. 3.20. Frequency distribution of annual effective dose (millisievert) for ubiquitous background radiation for members of the U.S. population, 2006.

Despite progress in systematic surveys of indoor radon, and many developments in dosimetry, the greatest uncertainty and variability both originate from radon, thoron, and their short-lived decay products. There are uncertainties associated with the estimated dose from internally-deposited uranium and thorium due to a scarcity of human tissue data, particularly for women, children and infants. Because of the complexity of intake routes, and differing uptakes of the various radionuclides in the natural series decay chains, different approaches have yet to be reconciled. There are uncertainties for external irradiation associated with shielding by buildings, irradiation by building materials, and portions of time spent out- and indoors.

4. Medical Exposure of Patients

Thumbnail Sketch (for 2006) (rounded values):

- collective effective dose (S): 900,000 person-Sv
- effective dose per individual in the U.S. population (E_{US}): 3 mSv
  - percent of total S or E_{US} for the U.S. population (48 %)
- subcategories included (percent of total S and E_{US} for medical exposure of patients)
  - computed tomography (49 %)
  - nuclear medicine (26 %)
  - interventional fluoroscopy (14 %)
  - conventional radiography and fluoroscopy (11 %)
  - external-beam radiotherapy (evaluated in Table 4.17 but not included in the total above)[13]
- average effective dose for the exposed group (E_{Exp}): not determined because the number of patients exposed (N_{Exp}) is not known, only the number of procedures
- group characteristics: for many situations, skewed to higher age groups and often to patients with serious health conditions and limited remaining lifespans

4.1 Introduction

Exposure to patients from medical procedures is of considerable interest because medical diagnostic and interventional procedures contribute significantly to the collective effective dose of the U.S.

---

[13]For radiotherapy, the estimates (limited to external-beam therapy) are: S = 350,000 person-Sv, E_{US} = 1.2 mSv, and E_{Exp} = 0.4 Sv. E_{Exp} is derived from absorbed doses to organs and tissues outside the treatment volumes and exceeds the E_{Exp} levels for all other sources, and the exposed population is small and being treated for a life-threatening illness. Also, absorbed doses to some tissues or portions of tissues outside but nearby the treatment volume could approach or exceed 1 Sv. For these reasons, it may be inappropriate to include this source of exposure in an assessment of effective dose to the U.S. population.

population. Patients exposed to medical sources have a distribution that is much different from that of the population as a whole. It is skewed in age to older individuals and in health status to sicker individuals. There also may be a skewed gender distribution. To the extent that information is available the distributions of medical procedures by age and gender are presented. In Section 4, available data have been amassed and evaluated for various medical radiation sources, primarily:

- x-ray sources used in CT, conventional radiography and fluoroscopy, interventional fluoroscopy, and radiation therapy; and
- gamma-ray sources used in nuclear medicine and radiation therapy.

Radiation exposure to the U.S. population from medical procedures was estimated using two data elements: number of medical procedures and effective dose per procedure. For each group, estimates of effective dose were combined with estimated numbers of procedures to estimate collective effective dose. The collective effective doses were estimated independently for each modality. The total exposure from all medical procedures was obtained as the sum of exposure across modalities. The sources of information for both number of procedures and effective doses varied by procedure, and are discussed below.

4.1.1 Exposure Categories

The data in this section are grouped by type of medical modality, as follows:

- computed tomography (Section 4.2);
- conventional radiography and fluoroscopy (including dental and chiropractic radiography, and bone densitometry) (Section 4.3);
- interventional fluoroscopy (Section 4.4);
- nuclear medicine (Section 4.5); and
- external-beam radiotherapy (Section 4.6).

Procedures within each modality were placed into relevant groups by body part or organ system, as discussed in the respective sections.

4.1.2 *Sources of Data on the Estimates of the Number of Procedures*

The number of procedures in each category was based on a main data source (Section 4.1.2.1) that contained estimates of the number of procedures performed in all facilities in the United States. A number of additional sources supplemented and validated the information obtained from the main source. Section 4.1.2 describes the data sources and the methods used to reconcile numbers across sources and to map them into the desired procedure categories.

4.1.2.1 *Main Data Source.* The number of procedures was derived mainly from commercial market benchmark reports produced by IMV. Nine of these reports were obtained that cover the following procedure categories: cardiac catheterization (IMV, 2004), CT (IMV, 2005a; 2006a), mammography (IMV, 2006b), nuclear medicine (IMV, 2006c), positron emission tomography (PET) (IMV, 2006d), radiographic fluoroscopy (IMV, 2006e), interventional angiography (IMV, 2006f), and radiation oncology (IMV, 2005b).

For each of the procedure categories, IMV used a survey to collect information on procedure volume by body part and organ system and a number of practice characteristics (such as productivity, staffing, equipment type). With the exception of the radiographic fluoroscopy and interventional angiography reports (which only covered hospitals with 150 beds or more), the data cover all hospital and nonhospital facilities performing the respective procedures. The surveys had high response rates (~60 % for most modalities). For modalities other than radiographic fluoroscopy and interventional angiography, the numbers of procedures are projected to represent all sites performing such imaging in the United States and, therefore, utilization by the entire U.S. population. The most recent year of data available varied by report, and ranged from 2003 to 2006. As a result, patients of all ages are represented in these procedure counts. Each of the reports contains an estimate of the proportion of procedures performed on pediatric patients. The unit of data collection is a facility, and the data are nationally representative.

4.1.2.2 *Supplementary Data.* The following data sources were used to validate information on the distribution of procedures across body parts and organ systems within modalities, for example, percent of CT procedures of the abdomen or head and neck.

4.1.2.2.1 *Medicare Physician Supplier Procedure Summary Files.* These files (CMS, 2006) are summarized administrative claims data for Medicare fee-for-service enrollees and are publicly available for analysis from the Centers for Medicare and Medicaid Services.

Summarized procedure counts for each modality were obtained from the American College of Radiology, sorted by the Healthcare Common Procedure Coding System Common Procedural Terminology (CPT) (AMA, 2004) code of the Health Care Financing Administration (now Centers for Medicare and Medicaid Services). Procedure counts were grouped by modality and body part or organ system as appropriate for analysis.

These data include all Medicare claims from 1997 through 2005 and account for procedures performed on nearly 40 million Medicare fee-for-service enrollees over the entire country. However, because the data mainly cover persons of age 65 y and older and the disabled Medicare enrollees, these numbers represent approximately one-third of all utilization and one-seventh of the U.S. population (NCHS, 2006; USCB, 2006a).

The estimates for conventional radiographic and fluoroscopic procedures were mainly based on the Medicare data.

4.1.2.2.2 *U.S. Department of Veterans Affairs.* Data from summarized administrative claims for all VA enrollees were provided by the VA under the Freedom of Information Act. Procedure counts were available for fiscal years 1991 to 2006, and were grouped by CPT code, patient age, and gender. Procedures were grouped by modality and body part or organ system as appropriate for analysis. Summarized claims data from the VA from 2003 to 2006 were used for some comparisons. The VA health plan had between four and seven million enrollees between 1999 and 2004 (CBO, 2005); the actual enrollment in each year was not available.

While the data are nationwide, women and children are underrepresented (<0.01 % of the VA claims are from those under age 15 y, and ~8 % are women; one-fourth of the U.S. population is under 18 y and over half are women) (USCB, 2006b).

4.1.2.2.3 *Large National Employer Plan.* Administrative claims data from a large national employer plan (LNEP) were used to spot-check distributions of procedures for some modalities. Claims data were available for 2003 and were summarized by modality and body part or organ system by the American College of Radiology. These data included claims for four million covered individuals, are nationally distributed, and include enrollees of all ages and both genders. The data are, however, not nationally representative because all the enrollees had health insurance (thus, not reflecting the uninsured in the U.S. population), and the population in this data set was skewed towards older ages compared with the U.S. population.

4.1.2.2.4 *Commercial Sources.* A commercial source provided information regarding the number of dental bitewing film packets sold in the United States.[14] These values were used to estimate the dose to the population from intraoral radiography.

4.1.2.3 *Reconciling Data from Supplementary Sources with Data from IMV.* Procedure counts from IMV provided the primary information for numbers of procedures. Where the distribution of procedures across body part or organ system in the IMV data failed to match the distribution in the other data sources, the distributions in the other data sources were used to estimate the possible range of values for population exposure, as supplemental estimates to the IMV data.

In some cases, such as radiography, the IMV reports did not categorize procedures in a format that would allow determination of collective effective dose. In those cases, the calculations were based on the Medicare data. The total utilization for radiographic procedures was estimated as 3.6 times the Medicare utilization, derived through a multistep process as follows. The procedure counts included Medicare fee-for-service enrollees except the 15 % in managed care (Table 144 of NCHS, 2006). Since managed care enrollees are expected to have a lower level of utilization than fee-for-service enrollees, an estimate of radiography utilization for all Medicare enrollees was made by applying a multiplier of 1.1 (rather than 1.15) to the Medicare fee-for-service utilization. Medicare utilization is ~30 % of all utilization (Table 124 of NCHS, 2006). Thus, the total of Medicare fee-for service utilization was estimated from 3.3 multiplied by 1.1. As a test, a comparison of IMV estimates of utilization to Medicare utilization where available confirmed that 3.6 was an appropriate multiplier.

4.1.2.4 *Limitations in Data Availability.* There is very little information available on the volumes of chiropractic and dental imaging. Chiropractic imaging procedures are not covered under Medicare, and form a very small part of the imaging procedures in the other data sources noted in Section 4.1.2. Data used to estimate the number of dental visits that included x rays for imaging were derived from survey data from the Medical Expenditure Panel Surveys

---

[14]Gray, J.E. (2007). Personal communication (DIQUAD, LLC, Steger, Illinois).

(AHQR, 2007), data from the Nationwide Evaluation of X-Ray Trends (NEXT) surveys on number of patients at dental facilities (FDA, 2003), the National Oral Health Surveillance System estimates of dental visits (CDC, 2006), and personal communication with industry staff.[15] The sources did not agree; therefore the number of dental intraoral films sold in the United States was used to determine the number of intraoral (bitewing and full-mouth survey) images (Section 4.3.1).

4.1.2.5 *Projecting Estimates to 2006.* Data on procedure counts were not always available for 2006; in those cases, data for the most recent year available were used with projected annual growth in procedures to estimate utilization of radiology procedures in 2006.

4.1.3 *Sources of Data for Effective Dose per Procedure*

Effective doses for procedures were derived by a variety of methods, each of which is described in the respective discussion for the five subcategories of medical exposure. For:

- CT, data on dose length product and age and body region specific conversion coefficients were utilized;
- conventional radiography and fluoroscopy, a published survey of effective dose was applied;
- interventional fluoroscopy, data on *KAP* and protocol specific dose conversion coefficients were utilized;
- nuclear medicine, data on dose conversion coefficients expressed as effective dose per unit administered activity were utilized; and
- external-beam radiotherapy, published values for absorbed dose to organs and tissues located outside the treatment volumes were utilized.

The values of effective dose for various procedures are informed "averages" made with the realization that for any given procedure, actual values in practice may vary by an order of magnitude.

The effective doses presented for medical exposure of patients were derived from various literature sources that all use the ICRP (1991) w_Ts and formulation for effective dose. In its latest recommendations, ICRP (2007a) approved new w_Ts that change the formulation of effective dose. There has been a decrease in w_T applied

---

[15]Gray, J.E. (2007). Personal communication (DIQUAD, LLC, Steger, Illinois).

for hereditary effects (gonads; from 0.2 to 0.08) and an increase in w_Ts for other tissues (notably the female breast; from 0.05 to 0.12). In particular, effective doses for procedures in which the female breast is essentially the only organ irradiated (*i.e.*, mammography) or in which the female breast receives the dominant absorbed dose (*e.g.*, chest procedures that include irradiation from the anterior direction), would be higher using the ICRP (2007a) formulation. When the gonads are directly irradiated (*e.g.*, pelvic procedures), effective doses would be lower. ICRP (2007a) also includes tissues not previously listed separately (brain, salivary glands) or previously included in the remainder category (extrathoracic region, lymphatic nodes, and oral mucosa) that impact doses from dental examinations. For two cases (mammography, and dental bitewing and full-mouth surveys), an indication of the difference in the effective dose value due to the revised ICRP (2007a) w_Ts is noted.

4.2 Computed Tomography

Computed tomography (CT) is fundamentally a method for acquiring and reconstructing images of thin cross-sections of an object. It differs from conventional radiography in two significant ways: (1) CT eliminates the superimposition of structures that occurs in radiography because of the projection of three-dimensional body structures onto the two-dimensional recording system, and (2) the sensitivity of CT to subtle differences in x-ray attenuation is about a factor of 10 higher than normally achieved by radiographic imaging systems.

Since its introduction in 1972, CT has evolved into an essential diagnostic imaging tool for a continually increasing variety of clinical applications. Technological advances in CT and the ease of use of this technology have led to many clinical applications that have increased the use of CT at a rate of 8 to 15 % per year for the last 7 to 10 y.

Two major revolutionary advances in CT technology occurred in the past decade that have become the catalysts for the rapid growth of this imaging modality. The first of these was the introduction of helical CT, enabling more rapid acquisition of a volume data set. The second advance was the introduction of multidetector CT (MDCT). MDCT scanners have distinct advantages, such as: the ability to obtain a large number of thin slices during a single rotation of the x-ray tube around the patient (typically <0.5 s), resulting in high image quality (isotropic resolution images suitable for improved three-dimensional images); and the ability to image a large scan region each rotation of the x-ray tube, enabling scanning of the entire body in <30 s.

4.2.1 *Effective Dose from Computed Tomography*

4.2.1.1 *Calculation of the Effective Dose.* The effective dose is calculated from information about absorbed dose to individual organs and w_T assigned to each organ. Specific organ doses are determined through simulations of the absorption and scattering of x rays in various tissues by using a mathematical model of the human body.

In practical terms the effective dose in CT is derived from a quantity called the dose-length product (*DLP*). Although effective dose calculations require specific knowledge about individual scanner characteristics, a reasonable estimate of effective dose (*E*), independent of scanner type, can be achieved using the relationship:

$$E = k \, DLP \qquad (4.1)$$

where:

k = age and body region-specific conversion coefficient ($mSv \, mGy^{-1} \, cm^{-1}$) listed in Table 4.1 for adults

Shrimpton and Wall (2000) discuss age-specific pediatric conversion coefficients for newborns to age 15 y.

DLP (mGy cm) is the CT dose index based on volume ($CTDI_{vol}$) (milligray) multiplied by the scan length (L) (centimeters):

$$DLP = CTDI_{vol} \, L \qquad (4.2)$$

where *DLP* reflects the total energy absorbed from a specific scan acquisition; and $CTDI_{vol}$ is an index of dose based on a 100 mm range of integration, and this index corresponds to the average absorbed dose that would accrue in the phantom central section.

TABLE 4.1—*Head, neck, chest, abdomen, and pelvis values of k for adults (McCollough et al., 2008).*[a]

Region of Body	k ($mSv \, mGy^{-1} \, cm^{-1}$)
Head	0.0021
Neck	0.0059
Chest	0.014
Abdomen	0.015
Pelvis	0.015

[a]See also Bongartz *et al.* (2004), Jessen *et al.* (1999; 2000), and Shrimpton *et al.* (2006).

Descriptions of $CTDI_{vol}$ and other related CT dose indices ($CTDI$, $CTDI_w$) are given in Appendix C. The effective dose values per scan are calculated, while $CTDI_{vol}$ is measured using standard phantoms.

4.2.1.2 *Typical Effective Doses in Computed Tomography.* For the most common CT procedures, Table 4.2 lists the effective dose per scan for adults, where a scan refers to a single sequence of rotations, table movement, and data acquisition spanning one particular anatomic range of clinical interest. Table 4.2 values are based on values cited in published reports and also on computation of effective doses for CT studies with known technique factors (Bou Serhal *et al.*, 2001; Brix *et al.*, 2003; Broadhead *et al.*, 1997; Brugmans *et al.*, 2002; Burling *et al*, 2004; Chapple *et al.*, 1992; Cohnen *et al.*, 2001; 2003; Conway *et al.*, 1992; Crawley and Rogers, 1994; Geleijns *et al.*, 1997; Hart and Wall, 2004; Heggie and Wilkinson, 2000; Huda *et al.*, 2001; Hunold *et al.*, 2003; Hurwitz *et al.*, 2007; Javadi *et al.*, 2008; Jessen *et al.*, 1999; 2000; Kemerink *et al.*, 2003; Mahesh and Cody, 2007; Martin, 2007; McCollough, 2003; McCollough and Schueler, 2000; McCollough *et al.*, 2008; Mettler *et al.*, 2000; 2008a; Morin *et al.*, 2003; Nickoloff *et al.*, 2000; Nishizawa *et al.*, 1991; Shope *et al.*, 1981; Shrimpton *et al.*, 2006; Stern *et al.*, 2007; Szendro *et al.*, 1995; Teeuwisse *et al.*, 2001; Van Unnik *et al.*, 1997; Ware *et al.*, 1999). Table 4.2 gives the range of effective doses with the effective dose value per scan chosen for the collective effective dose estimation.

4.2.1.3 *Effects of Computed Tomography Technology on Effective Dose.* The demand for faster scans and images providing high spatial and temporal resolution has resulted in the development of CT scanners with high tube current, many (64 or more) thin detector rows, wide detector and x-ray beam dimensions (4 cm or more at the axis of rotation), and rapid tube and detector rotation (a half to a third of a second per rotation). According to national survey reports (IMV, 2005a; 2006a), the number of MDCT scanners in the United States increased from nearly 51 % of total scanners in 2004 to 71 % in 2006. In 2006, 52 % of MDCT scanners had the capability to yield 16 or more slices per gantry rotation. The radiation doses from the early MDCT scanners (four-slice MDCT) were higher than those from single-slice helical or nonhelical CT scanners due to poor geometric and detection efficiency. With improved detection and geometric efficiency, the radiation doses from 16- and greater-slice MDCT scanners are similar to or lower than those from

TABLE 4.2—*Ranges for effective dose per scan for CT categories and the effective doses used in the calculations for 2006 for collective effective dose (all values are for adults).*

CT Category	Range for Effective Dose (per scan) (mSv)	Effective Dose (per scan) Used in the Calculation (mSv)
Head	0.9 – 4	2[a]
Chest	4 – 18	7[a]
Abdomen and pelvis	3 – 25	10[b]
Extremity	0.1 – 1	0.1[c]
Virtual colonography	5 – 15	10[a]
Whole-body screening	5 – 15	10[d]
Calcium scoring	1 – 12	2[e]
Angiography: head	1 – 10	5[d]
Angiography: heart	5 – 32	20[f,g]
Other scans	1 – 10	5[d]

[a]Mettler *et al.* (2008a)

[b]McCollough *et al.* (2008) and Brix *et al.* (2003). McCollough *et al.* (2008) lists a range of 8 to 14 mSv. Brix *et al.* (2003) lists 9.7 mSv for multi-slice CT and 10.3 mSv for single-slice CT. A value of 10 mSv was selected as reflecting current clinical practice.

[c]The lower end of the range of effective doses. In the absence of a single citation listing actual values, the selected value was based on calculated effective doses from scan techniques used in routine extremity CT protocols.

[d]The mid-point of the range of effective doses was selected.

[e]McCollough *et al.* (2008) lists a range of 1 to 3 mSv. The mid-point of the McCollough *et al.* (2008) range was selected.

[f]Hurwitz *et al.* (2007) and Javadi *et al.* (2008); results from two large academic centers.

[g]A very recent study (post-2006) reports that a median value of 12 mSv (Hausleiter *et al.*, 2009) is more representative of current practice.

single-slice helical or nonhelical CT scanners. However, technological advances in CT have yielded many new clinical protocols resulting in additional numbers of CT scans, therefore increasing the collective effective dose.

4.2.2 *Estimating Computed Tomography Usage in the United States*

The number of CT scans performed in the United States has been estimated from a number of data sources that were discussed in Section 4.1.2.

4.2.2.1 *IMV Benchmark Reports.* The IMV CT benchmark report for 2006 is based on responses from 2,565 out of an identified universe of 7,649 hospital and nonhospital sites (IMV, 2006a). The IMV CT benchmark report for 2004 is based on responses from 4,478 out of an identified universe of 7,356 hospital and nonhospital sites (IMV, 2005a).

4.2.2.2 *Number of Computed Tomography Procedures.* From examining the information in the databases, the number of CT procedures performed in the United States during 2006 is estimated to be 62 million. This represents almost an 8 % growth from 2005 (57.6 million CT procedures). On average, the number of CT procedures increased ~10 to 11 % per year from 1993 to 2006 (Table 4.3 and Figure 4.1). The growth of CT shows similar trends within the various databases, as shown in Table 4.4. Medicare data show an annual increase in the number of CT procedures of 13 % from 2001 to 2004 (Table 4.5). Eight to 10 % of all CT procedures performed in the United States between 2004 and 2006 were pediatric procedures (IMV, 2005a; 2006a). However, the number of procedures for pediatric cases could not be determined separately because detailed information on the distribution of CT categories within the pediatric population was not available.

A number of newer CT applications, including PET-CT, single-photon emission CT (SPECT) CT, CT-fluoroscopy, and interventional applications, that are beginning to appear on surveys, are not accounted for separately in this Report due to lack of detailed data.

4.2.2.3 *Number of Computed Tomography Scans.* Medicare data were used to classify each CT procedure based on CPT codes. Some CT procedures consisted of two scans. To estimate the collective effective dose it is necessary to estimate the number of scans associated with these procedures. According to the IMV reports, 67 % of all CT procedures included contrast. Medicare data show that nearly 50 % of CT procedures had either one scan with contrast or two scans, one with and one without contrast. Nearly 13 % of Medicare procedures involved two scans (with and without contrast). CT procedures were classified into various categories and adjusted for the number of procedures with two scans. This yielded an estimate for the total number of CT scans that is ~8 % higher than the number of CT procedures in both 2003 and 2006, resulting in a total of 67 million CT scans for 2006. The effective doses per CT scan (Table 4.2) were then applied to calculate collective effective dose to the U.S. population (Section 4.2.3).

TABLE 4.3—Number of CT procedures in both hospital and nonhospital facilities (IMV, 2005a; 2006a).

Year	CT Procedures (in millions)			Increase from Previous Year (%)		
	Total	In Hospital	Not in Hospital	Total	In Hospital	Not in Hospital
1993	18.3	16.1	2.2			
1994	19.5	17.2	2.3	7	7	5
1995	21.0	18.4	2.6	8	7	13
1996	22.6	19.7	2.9	8	7	12
1997	25.1	21.6	3.5	11	10	21
1998[a]	26.3	22.8	3.5	5	6	0
1999	30.6	25.8	4.8	16	13	37
2000	34.9	29	5.9	14	12	23
2001	39.6	33.1	6.5	13	14	10
2002	45.4	37.9	7.5	15	15	15
2003	50.1	41.4	8.7	10	9	16
2004	53.9	44.3	9.6	8	7	10
2005	57.6	47.2	10.4	7	7	8
2006	62.0	51	11	8	8	6

[a]MDCT was introduced in 1998.

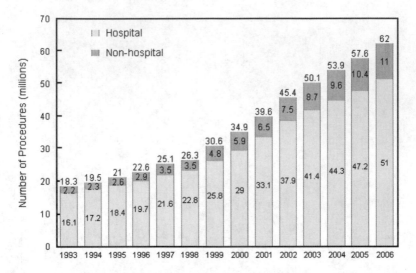

Fig. 4.1. Number of CT procedures per year in the United States (millions), 1993 to 2006. Average growth: >10 % y^{-1}.

4.2.3 *Collective Effective Dose Calculations*

The collective effective dose to the U.S. population was based on 2006 data starting with the CT procedures data from IMV (converted to number of CT scans). The various categories of CT procedures, the number of CT scans, and the selected effective doses per scan for each category are listed in Table 4.6. The number of CT scans and the collective effective doses for the categories are also shown graphically (in percent) in Figure 4.2. The annual collective effective dose to the U.S. population is ~440,000 person-Sv. With the U.S. population of 300 million for 2006, the annual E_{US} is ~1.5 mSv. For verification, similar calculations were performed on Medicare data extended to the U.S. population. Accordingly, the annual collective effective dose to the U.S. population based on the 2004 Medicare data was ~400,000 person-Sv and E_{US} was ~1.4 mSv.

4.2.4 *Sources of Uncertainty in the Dose*

The main sources of uncertainty in the estimates of S and E_{US} are the number of procedures, estimation of the number of scans from the number of procedures, and the effective dose per scan for each category.

TABLE 4.4—*Percentage of CT procedures in various categories among the four data sets (IMV, Medicare, VA and LNEP).*

Category	IMV			Medicare				VA		LNEP	
Year →	1998	2003	2006	1998	2003	2004	1997	2003	2006	2001	2003
Head and neck[a]	32	31	29	38	31	29	37	27	24	33	29
Chest	17	16	16	14	18	19	18	21	22	15	15
Abdomen/pelvis[b]	40	38	36	46	49	50	43	50	52	50	53
Extremity	6	5	5	1	1	1	1	1	1	1	1
Miscellaneous[c]	6	10	7	1	1	1	1	1	1	1	1
CT angiography	—	—	7								
Total[d] (in millions)	26.3	50.1	62.0	8.9	15.9	18.4	0.27	0.58	0.80	0.61	0.98

(Procedures (%))

[a]Head: Includes brain, and head and neck.
[b]Abdomen/pelvis: Includes both abdomen-pelvis and spine.
[c]Miscellaneous: Includes interventional, whole-body screening, calcium scoring, other cardiac, virtual colonography, and miscellaneous.
[d]Total: Total number of procedures in millions among eligible population.

TABLE 4.5—*Number of CT procedures performed among the Medicare population (data extracted based on the CT procedures listed among various CPT codes).*

Year →	2001	2002	2003	2004	2001	2002	2003	2004
Beneficiaries Eligible for These Services →	31,453,591	32,486,122	33,240,563	34,005,096				
Category	Nonduplicate Procedure Counts				Medicare Procedures per 1,000 Beneficiaries			
Head and neck	4,526,852	4,979,270	5,374,299	5,857,566	144	153	162	172
Chest	2,051,099	2,491,644	2,914,239	3,331,130	65	77	88	98
Abdomen/pelvis	5,590,300	6,503,828	7,350,546	8,340,532	178	200	221	245
Extremity	84,990	109,776	142,059	177,939	3	3	4	5
Other	115,440	120,188	111,076	107,874	4	4	3	3
Total procedures	12,368,681	14,204,706	15,892,219	17,815,041				
Annual growth		14.8 %	11.9 %	12.1 %				

TABLE 4.6—*Effective doses and collective effective doses for CT.*

Categories	Number of Scans (millions)	Scans (%)	Effective Dose per Scan (mSv)	Collective Effective Dose (person-Sv)	Collective Effective Dose (%)
Head [a]	19.0	28.4	2	38,044	8.7
Chest	10.6	15.9	7	74,326	17.0
Abdomen/pelvis	21.2	31.7	10	212,538	48.6
Extremity	3.5	5.2	0.1	515	0.1
CT angiography: heart	2.3	3.4	20	46,000	10.5
CT angiography: head	2.0	3.0	5	10,000	2.3
Spine	4.1	6.2	10	41,369	9.5
Interventional	2.3	3.4	0.1	230	0.05
Whole-body screening	0.2	0.3	10	2,000	0.5
Calcium scoring	0.5	0.8	2	1,000	0.2
Cardiac [b]	0.3	0.5	20	6,000	1.4
Virtual colonography	0.2	0.3	10	2,000	0.5
Miscellaneous	0.7	1.1	5	3,500	0.8
Total [c]	67.0			437,523	

2006 U.S. population E_{US} from CT

300 million
1.46 mSv

[a]Head: Includes brain and head and neck.
[b]Cardiac: Procedures other than CT angiography of the heart.
[c]Total: The 62 million procedures for 2006 as listed in IMV (2006a) adjusted by category for procedures with two scans.

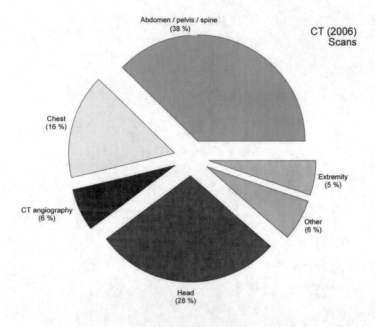

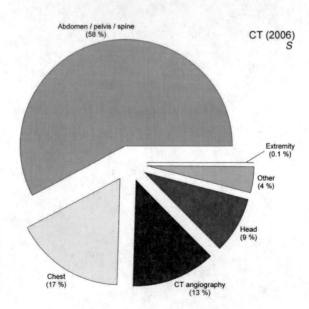

Fig. 4.2. Percent contribution of various CT categories to total number of scans (67 million) (top) and S (440,000 person-Sv) (bottom) for 2006. The percent values have been rounded to the nearest 1 % [see Table 4.6 for the number of scans and the values for S (person-sievert)].

As noted above, IMV reports are based on the survey information gathered from various hospital and nonhospital sources and extrapolated to the identified universe of hospital and nonhospital sites in the United States for the main categories of CT procedures. The number of procedures included in the computation, however, was further subdivided by the CPT codes listed in the Medicare data. In addition, the total number of CT scans was estimated by adjusting the number of procedures in each category by a small percentage to account for those procedures with two scans.

For this Report the methodology of determining the effective dose was based on measurements made using standardized *CTDI* phantoms and *DLP*-to-effective dose conversion coefficients derived from Monte-Carlo simulations. These simulations use a mathematical model of a standard adult. Hence, the effective dose per scan values reported here are for a standard adult and may not adequately reflect the effective dose values for children or very large adults. The simulations do take into account gender-specific organs however, and provide an estimate of effective dose that is averaged over both genders. These estimates of effective dose are typical of current MDCT scanner technology, and may not reflect past or future variations in CT scanner technology or user preferences in scanning protocols at any individual scanning facility.

4.2.5 *Trends in the Next Ten Years*

While the greatest growth in the number of CT procedures occurred in the late 1990s and early 2000s, the use of CT technology in the United States is likely to continue to increase over the next 10 y. Many new clinical applications are being developed; CT technology can be used with ease, perform a patient scan in a very short time (few seconds), and provide high quality images for diagnosis. The majority of CT scanners in the United States are MDCT systems and the percentage of scanners that are MDCT systems will continue to increase.

4.3 Conventional Radiography and Fluoroscopy

Conventional radiography and fluoroscopy comprise the largest number of x-ray examinations of patients in the United States. However, the collective effective dose from these examinations is now only a relatively small portion of the medical dose in the United States. For the purposes of this Report, conventional radiography is defined as the use of x-ray imaging systems such as those using screen-film image receptors, computed radiography, digital radiography, direct exposure x-ray film (as used in intraoral radiography), or any other type of system producing two-dimensional x-ray projection images. Conventional fluoroscopy is real-time projection imaging used for diagnostic purposes for examinations, such as upper GI studies or barium enemas. Section 4.4 addresses interventional applications of fluoroscopy.

4.3.1 Estimates of the Number of Procedures

The numbers of conventional radiographic and fluoroscopic examinations used to estimate the collective effective dose to the U.S. population were derived primarily from two sources, the Medicare data (CMS, 2006) and a commercial source (for number of dental bitewing exposures).[16] The information in IMV (2006e) for conventional radiographic and fluoroscopic examinations did not include imaging in nonhospital settings or in hospitals with fewer than 150 beds, and did not have adequate specificity on imaging by body part for use in this Report. Though the Medicare data include, for the most part, only procedure counts for the elderly, this was the only comprehensive data source available for these procedures. Utilization for the country was estimated, as described in Section 4.1.2.3 previously, as 3.6 times the Medicare utilization for each procedure category.

NEXT studies (CRCPD, 2008) provide estimates of average procedures per week performed in each facility. These were used as a second source to validate estimates of procedures per year and the number of U.S. facilities.

Estimates of the number of mammography procedures were obtained from the FDA website for the Mammography Quality Standards Act (FDA, 2007a) that documents the number of mammograms reported by accredited facilities. The total number of mammography procedures in 2006 was 34.5 million, which is the number used for calculating S for mammography. IMV (2006b) estimates mammography volume as 37.7 million in 2005. Medicare accounts for just under one-third of mammography volume, and Medicare enrollees accounted for 11.1 million mammograms in 2005 (CMS, 2006).

Difficulties were encountered in determining the number of dental x-ray examinations or exposures per year. Several sources of data provided estimates of this number, varying from 60 to 200 million (CDC, 2006; Moyal et al., 2007; Suleiman et al., 1999). A commercial source provided an estimate of the number of dental

---

[16]Gray, J.E. (2007). Personal communication (DIQUAD, LLC, Steger, Illinois).

bitewing exposures in 2005 as ~500 million.[17] This includes both direct film x-ray exposure and digital bitewing exposures. This latter estimate was chosen for the number of intraoral (bitewing and full-mouth survey) images in the United States.

The number and type of projections used for diagnostic x-ray examinations plays a significant role in the radiation dose to the patient. For example, if one assumes that a lumbar spine examination consists primarily of one antero-posterior (AP) and one lateral projection, the dose will be significantly lower than if the examination consists of one AP, one lateral, two oblique, and one spot projection. In the latter case the higher dose to the patient is due to both the greater number of projections and to the fact that the oblique projections and the spot projection require higher radiation exposures than the AP projection.

The number of projections used for these examinations is not stated in the Medicare database. The number and types of projections used for calculation of the effective dose were selected based on experience in the clinical environment and are shown in Table D.1 in Appendix D. Often there are several different CPT codes for the same examination, with each CPT code representing a different number of projections. The numbers of particular examinations are given in Table 4.7.

4.3.2 *Estimates of Effective Dose per Procedure*

Mettler *et al*. (2008a), based on a survey of the international and U.S. literature, was the primary source of information for effective doses for conventional radiographic and fluoroscopic examinations. Supportive information for dose calculations is available from several sources of data including the applicable surveys of NEXT (CRCPD, 2008), the Michigan Department of Community Health website (MDCH, 2007), New Jersey Department of Environmental Protection (NJDEP),[18] Mayo Clinic,[19] and the Conference of Radiation Control Program Directors, Inc. white paper on bone mineral measurements (Hawkinson *et al*., 2006). The data appear consistent among the sources, with a few exceptions. Some details for the NEXT and state agency surveys are given in Sections 4.3.2.1 and 4.3.2.2.

---

[17]Gray, J.E. (2007). Personal communication (DIQUAD, LLC, Steger, Illinois).

[18]Lipoti, J.A. (2007). Personal communication (New Jersey Department of Environmental Protection, Trenton, New Jersey).

[19]Schueler, B.A. (2007). Personal communication (Mayo Clinic, Rochester, Minnesota).

Table 4.7—*Effective doses (or effective dose equivalents) per examination, number of examinations, and collective doses for conventional radiographic and fluoroscopic examinations, 1980 and 2006.*

Examination	For 1980 (NCRP, 1989a)			For 2006 (this Report)			
	Effective Dose Equivalent (mSv)	Number (thousands)	Collective Effective Dose Equivalent (person-Sv)	Effective Dose (mSv)	Number [thousands (%)]	Collective Effective Dose (person-Sv)	Collective Effective Dose (% of total)
Chest	0.08	64,000	5,120	0.1	128,944 (44.0)	12,894	12.8
Breast[a]	0.22			0.18[a]	34,500 (11.8)	6,210	6.2
Skull	0.20	8,200	1,800	0.1	329 (0.1)	33	0.03
Cervical spine		5,100	1,020	0.2	5,800 (2.0)	1,160	1.2
Biliary				1.7	573 (0.2)	974	0.1
Thoracic spine				1.0	2,590 (0.9)	2,590	2.6
Lumbar spine	1.27	12,900	16,400	1.5	11,197 (3.8)	16,796	16.7
Upper GI[b]	2.44	7,600	18,500	6.0	4,044 (1.4)	24,264	24.1
Abdomen (kidney, ureter and bladder)	0.56	7,900	4,420	0.7	14,964 (5.1)	10,475	10.4
Barium enema[b]	4.06	4,900	19,900	8.0	656 (0.2)	5,248	5.2
IVP[b]				3.0	1,180 (0.4)	3,540	3.5
Pelvis	0.44			0.6	8,185 (2.8)	4,911	4.9
Hip	0.83			0.7	11,778 (4.0)	8,245	8.2
Pelvis and hip	0.64[c]	4,700[d]	3,010[e]				
Extremities	0.01	45,000	450				

Hands and feet	0	26,677 (9.1)	0	0.0
Knees	0.005	19,364 (6.6)	97	0.1
Shoulders	0.008	9,213 (3.1)	74	0.07
Other head and neck films	0.22	1,975 (0.7)	435	0.4
Dental: bitewing and full-mouth survey[f]	0.005 per image[g]	500 million images[g]	2,500[h]	2.5
Dental panoramic	0.01	1,841 (0.6)	18	0.02
Dental cephalometric	0.012	806 (0.3)	10	0.01
DEXA, axial only	0.001	8,734 (3.0)	9.0	0.01
Total (for 1980)			70,620	
Total (for 2006)		293,350[i]	100,483[j]	

[a] Based on FDA data for all mammography units in the United States (FDA, 2006) and a w_T for breast of 0.12, the effective dose (E^*) would be 0.42 mSv. Using the ICRP (2007a) w_T of 0.05 (ICRP, 1991).

[b] These procedures include a fluoroscopic component.

[c] Weighted value (equally) for pelvis and hip.

[d] Sum of pelvis and hip.

[e] Weighted value (by number of examinations) for pelvis and hip.

[f] Based on data for number of images from a commercial source (see Footnote 17, Section 4.3.1), and data for dose from Gibbs (2000). Using the ICRP (2007a) $w_{T}E$, an effective dose (E^*) was estimated at 0.021 mSv (Ludlow et al., 2008) for commonly used round collimation and D-speed film.

[g] Number of images, not examinations.

[h] Based on number of images.

[i] Excludes the number of examinations associated with the 500 million images for dental bitewing and full-mouth procedures.

[j] Includes 2,500 person-Sv from the 500 million dental bitewing and full-mouth images.

Effective doses for each procedure are given in Table 4.7 and are calculated as a weighted average of the effective doses for similar CPT codes, weighted by the number of examinations for each CPT code in the database.

Mammography in the United States is unique in that it is the only medical x-ray imaging procedure regulated by FDA. As a result dose and image quality data are available for all mammography facilities in the United States (*i.e.*, the mean glandular doses are based on measurements of all mammography units). The effective dose from mammography is 0.18 mSv [two views of each breast, a mean glandular dose for the total breast tissue of 1.8 mGy per view (FDA, 2006), and a w_T of 0.05 (ICRP, 1991)]. Using the ICRP (2007a) w_T for breast of 0.12, E^* would be 0.42 mSv. NCRP Report No. 149 (NCRP, 2004a) provides detailed technical and clinical information on the practice of mammography.

Effective doses from extremity examinations (hands, arms, feet, legs) are quite low, because the most radiation-sensitive organs are not directly exposed. The only radiation dose to these organs is from scattered radiation that is typically <1 % of the entrance skin exposure. The w_Ts recommended by ICRP (1991) for the skin and bone surfaces are 0.01 for each. Huda and Gkanatsios (1998) concluded that the upper limits for effective dose for adult examinations ranged from 0.17 to 2.7 μSv, with pediatric doses (for a 1 y old) being a factor of three lower. Consequently, the effective dose to a patient from these examinations is on the order of 1 to 10 μSv.

For dental exposures, the dose per image data were derived from Gibbs (2000) and are comparable to Ludlow *et al.* (2008) using the ICRP (1991) formulation for E. ICRP (2007a) has included additional tissues to be considered when calculating E^* (brain and salivary glands separately; and extrathoracic region, lymphatic nodes, and oral mucosa in the remainder category). Ludlow *et al.* (2008) have incorporated this information and, based on measured doses in the relevant tissues and organs, estimate that the value of E^* would range from 1 to 22 μSv per image for a bitewing or full-mouth series, assuming 18 images in a full-mouth series. In particular, Ludlow *et al.* (2008) estimate E^* at 21 μSv for commonly used round collimation and D-speed film. The Ludlow *et al.* (2008) E^* value for a panoramic examination ranges from 14 to 24 μSv and the value for a cephalometric examination is ~5 μSv.

The effective dose for dual-energy x-ray absorptiometry (DEXA) (used for bone mineral measurement) is very low (Table 4.7), and the procedure is carried out primarily on postmenopausal females, although similar examinations are carried out on the entire spectrum of adult and pediatric patients. Hawkinson *et al.* (2006)

provides an in-depth discussion of all types of bone mineral measurement techniques and a summary of doses from each technique. Only DEXA studies that expose the trunk are included here, since other methods contribute little to effective dose.

4.3.2.1 *Nationwide Evaluation of X-Ray Trends and the Mammography Quality Standards Act.* The NEXT program is a partnership between the Conference of Radiation Control Program Directors, Inc. and the FDA Center for Devices and Radiological Health to characterize the radiation doses patients receive during diagnostic x-ray examinations (FDA, 2003). The program documents the state of the practice of diagnostic radiology. The NEXT survey program selects a particular radiological examination for study and captures entrance exposure data[20] from a nationally representative sample of U.S. clinical facilities. The number of facilities selected varies by study, averaging ~300 facilities nationwide. The exception is mammography, where, after passage of the Mammography Quality Standards Act (MQSA, 2005), data became available on all mammography facilities, resulting in data on 8,867 facilities in 2006 (FDA, 2008). State radiation control personnel from ~45 states conduct the surveys using reference phantoms, which were designed to represent the radiation attenuation presented by an average-size patient. Surveys are repeated periodically to track trends as technology and clinical practices change. The survey results are captured and published in their entirety and as user-friendly pamphlets to share with practitioners and members of the public. The results summarize the data from actual practice and not from clinical trials. These studies are independent from user or manufacturer bias.

NEXT protocols provide methodologies for capturing technical data associated with the practice of the surveyed diagnostic x-ray procedure, including patient skin-entrance air kerma, image quality, clinical technique factors, quality of film processing, and general quality control or quality assurance practices. NEXT protocols must be used in conjunction with the associated NEXT phantom (FDA, 2003) in order to compare recently acquired data with existing NEXT survey results.

4.3.2.2 *Data from State Agencies.* Data from many more facilities than considered in the NEXT studies may be available from individual states. For instance in the 2001 NEXT survey (FDA, 2003),

---

[20]Except in the case of mammography, where absorbed dose to the glandular tissue in the breast is determined.

adult chest data were provided from only 220 x-ray machines. Survey data available from New Jersey include 1,863 chest machines, 2,998 units used for foot studies and 6,736 units for lumbosacral spines (Lipoti, 2008). Michigan also provides data from a large number of surveys on their website (MDCH, 2007). However, data from a single state could demonstrate a regional bias. Therefore these data were used mainly for validation and comparison. If data were not available from the NEXT study, such as for podiatric examinations, available information from states was used.

4.3.3 *Calculation of the Collective Effective Dose from Conventional Radiography and Fluoroscopy*

The collective effective dose for conventional radiography and fluoroscopy is the product of the number of examinations (including multiple projections) and the effective dose for the examination, summed over all radiographic (including dental) and fluoroscopic examinations.

The collective effective dose to the U.S. population from conventional radiography and fluoroscopy (Table 4.7) for 2006 is 100,480 person-Sv compared with 70,620 in 1980 (NCRP, 1989a), a factor of 1.4 increase. The increase in collective effective dose is due primarily to increases for four examinations (chest, abdomen, pelvis and hip) and the inclusion of breast examinations, which did not have an entry for 1980. There was a 25 % increase in the effective dose per chest examination with the number of examinations doubling. There was also a 25 % increase in the effective dose per abdomen examination with the number of examinations also about doubling. The largest increase in the collective effective dose was for pelvis and hip examinations. There was an increase of 36 % in the effective dose per pelvis examination and a 16 % decrease per examination of the hips. The increase in the collective effective dose for the combined pelvis and hip examinations is primarily due to a large increase in the total number of examinations. NCRP (1989a) listed the number of pelvis and hip examinations as 4,700,000. Present data indicate a total of 19,963,000 pelvis and hip examinations, an increase of a factor of 4.25. This increase is probably due to better data sources (*i.e.*, the use of the Medicare data). This may also be the case for the apparent increase in the number of chest and abdomen examinations. An additional reason may simply be the aging population requiring more of these procedures. The annual number of procedures and collective effective doses for specific examinations is provided in Table 4.7 and summarized in Figure 4.3.

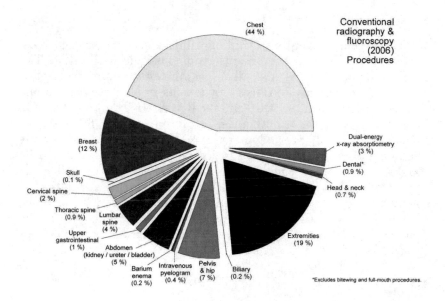

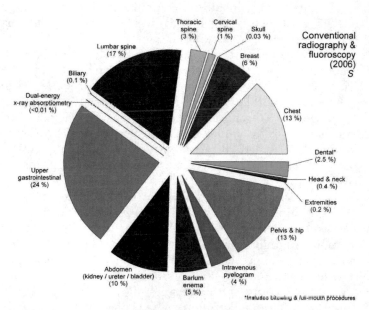

Fig. 4.3. Percent contribution of various subcategories of conventional radiographic and fluoroscopic procedures to number of procedures (293 million) (top) and S (100,000 person-Sv) (bottom) for 2006. The percent values have been rounded to the nearest 1 %, except for those <1 % [see Table 4.7 for the number of procedures and the values for S (person-sievert)].

4.3.4 *Sources of Uncertainty*

Doses from conventional radiographic and fluoroscopic procedures are based on measurements using a standard phantom. The dose to any individual may differ significantly from that determined using a phantom. Larger variations in dose occur from one facility to another and within one facility. As an example, the 2002 NEXT Survey shows a maximum to minimum ratio for entrance skin exposure of 49 for abdomen examinations with a ratio of the entrance skin exposure at the third versus the first quartile of 1.33 (Moyal *et al.*, 2006). Such a broad spread is typical of all x-ray examinations and introduces uncertainty into the calculation of collective effective doses. Table 4.8 presents some ranges for effective dose for various adult conventional radiographic and fluoroscopic examinations (Mettler *et al.*, 2008a), where the upper values are from ~2 to ~28 times the lower value.

4.3.5 *Trends Over the Next Ten Years*

Digital radiography, including computed radiography, is growing. In 2006, it was being used for only a relatively small proportion of the examinations in medical imaging.

Data from Michigan indicate that from 2002 to 2006, 16 % of the radiographic facilities used digital imaging for chest radiography (MDCH, 2007). Of the facilities performing lumbar spine examinations, 9.6 % used digital imaging. In dental radiography the proportion of facilities with digital imaging is ~14 % (MDCH, 2008). These percentages refer to the number of facilities and not the number of examinations performed. Typically, it is the larger, higher-volume facilities that are making the transition to digital radiography most rapidly. Consequently, one would expect that the proportion of digital examinations would be higher than the proportion of facilities using digital equipment. In the future, however, it would be expected that increasing numbers of facilities will use these digital systems.

The impact of digital imaging on the collective effective dose to the population is expected to be relatively minor. Although the Michigan data for 2002 to 2006 indicate that there has been an increase in the entrance skin exposure of 67 % for a PA chest projection and 28 % for an AP lumbar spine projection for digital imaging when compared with screen-film imaging (MDCH, 2007), it is not clear that these increases in entrance skin exposure to patients are necessary. With experience, the proper adjustment of technical factors may result in equivalent or even lower entrance skin exposures per examination for digital imaging compared with screen-film imaging.

TABLE 4.8—*Ranges for effective dose for various adult conventional radiographic and fluoroscopic examinations (Mettler et al., 2008a).*

Examination	Average Effective Dose (mSv)	Range for Effective Dose (mSv)
Skull	0.1	0.03 – 0.22
Cervical spine	0.2	0.07 – 0.3
Thoracic spine	1	0.6 – 1.4
Lumbar spine	1.5	0.5 – 1.8
PA and LAT chest	0.1	0.05 – 0.24
PA chest	0.02	0.007 – 0.050
Abdomen	0.7	0.04 – 1.1
Pelvis	0.6	0.2 – 1.2
Hip	0.7	0.18 – 2.71
Intravenous pyelogram	3	0.7 – 3.7
Upper GI series[a]	5	1.5 – 12
Barium enema[a]	8	2 – 18

[a]Includes fluoroscopy.

The introduction of digital imaging using charged-coupled devices has the potential to decrease entrance exposure per image in dental radiography because these systems are inherently faster than either D- or F-speed film. This increased speed is gained largely from the scintillators applied to the surface of the charged-coupled device. Further, systems that use photostimulable phosphor plates are comparable in speed to F-speed film and thus their use results in less exposure that when using D-speed film systems. For example, according to data for 2002 to 2006 collected in Michigan, at 70 to 79 kVp the median entrance skin exposure for digital imaging systems (type unspecified) was 34 % of that associated with use of D-speed film (MDCH, 2008).

4.4 Interventional Fluoroscopy

In this Report, interventional fluoroscopy refers to any procedure in which the use or application of a medical device is fluoroscopically guided in the body, and includes procedures that are performed for diagnostic and therapeutic purposes. During these procedures, typical fluoroscopic absorbed-dose rates in the skin can range from 20 to >50 mGy min^{-1} (FDA, 1994). The effective dose may reach 1 to 10 mSv. Long interventional procedures may result in effective doses of 10 to 50 mSv and may also produce localized radiation-induced skin injuries (Koenig *et al.*, 2001a; 2001b; Shope, 1996; Vlietstra *et al.*, 2004).

Federal regulations (FDA, 2007b) require that the maximal air-kerma rate at the specified measurement point not exceed 44 mGy min^{-1} (5 R min^{-1} exposure rate) for systems without automatic exposure rate control; not exceed 88 mGy min^{-1} (10 R min^{-1} exposure rate) for systems with automatic exposure rate control; and not exceed 176 mGy min^{-1} (20 R min^{-1} exposure rate) for equipment having an optional high-level control, when the high-level control is activated. The requirements apply differently for equipment manufactured before May 19, 1995 and that manufactured on or after May 19, 1995. FDA regulations apply to manufacturers and not to users of equipment, and the requirements on air-kerma rates do not apply during recording of fluoroscopic images. Consequently, in practice the dose rate may be significantly higher and vary among facilities by an order of magnitude (Balter *et al.*, 2004).

Air-kerma rate surveys of high-level control fluoroscopy at six institutions reported 200 to 900 mGy min^{-1} (Cagnon, 1991). Serial-imaging (cinefluorography) air-kerma rate is typically a factor of 10 greater than the fluoroscopic air-kerma rate for a given projection. There is a wide variation in air-kerma rate with projections in cardiovascular and digital subtraction angiography, where oblique projection angles increase tissue thickness, resulting in a very-high cinefluorography air-kerma rate. For example, Cusma *et al.* (1999) reported that using an anthropomorphic phantom the air-kerma rate for fluoroscopy and cineangiography in the left anterior oblique cranial projection was about four times that of the AP projection.

Image-intensifier based fluoroscopic equipment is rapidly being replaced with flat-panel detector technology and many interventional-fluoroscopic laboratories are becoming completely digital imaging departments.

4.4.1 *Dose Indices and Effective Dose in Fluoroscopy*

ICRP Publication 85 (ICRP, 2000) defined dosimetric quantities for interventional fluoroscopy. These include beam air kerma, incident beam air kerma, kerma-area product (*KAP*), entrance surface air kerma, entrance skin dose, local skin dose, and maximum local skin dose.

In this Report, the effective dose for interventional procedures using fluoroscopy has been determined through the product of two quantities. The first quantity is *KAP* (similar to the formerly used roentgen-area product and dose-area product), which is the incident air kerma (in gray or milligray) multiplied by the cross-sectional area of the x-ray beam (in cm²). The second quantity consists of dose conversion coefficients published in the literature to estimate the effective dose from *KAP*. However, published dose conversion coefficients vary due to differences in protocols (number and projection angle of the fluoroscopic and cinefluorographic views) at various facilities and with differences in technical and geometric factors (*e.g.*, tube voltage, total filtration, focus-to-skin distance, and field size). *KAP* is a surrogate measurement for the amount of radiation that the patient absorbs. The effective dose is computed as follows:

$$E = DCC_E \, KAP, \tag{4.3}$$

where:

E = effective dose (millisievert)
DCC_E = dose conversion coefficient from *KAP* to E (mSv Gy⁻¹ cm⁻²)
KAP = kerma-area product (Gy cm²)

Section 4.4.2.2 discusses the estimation of DCC_E and *KAP* for adults.

4.4.2 *Estimation of the Number of Procedures and Effective Dose*

4.4.2.1 *Sources of Information for the Type and Number of Procedures.* Three IMV benchmark reports served as the basis for the annual U.S. frequency of procedures. These were the reports for cardiac catheterization (IMV, 2004), radiographic fluoroscopy (IMV, 2006e), and interventional angiography (IMV, 2006f). IMV (2006f) for interventional angiography has two broad classifications (*i.e.*, diagnostic and therapeutic) and a total of 14 procedures. IMV (2004) for cardiac catheterization lists six categories of procedures (*i.e.*, coronary diagnostic, coronary therapeutic, combined diagnostic and therapeutic, electrophysiology, pacemaker, and other). From IMV (2006e) for radiographic fluoroscopy, only selected procedures (*i.e.*, urinary studies, myelography, endoscopic retrograde cholangiopancreatography, arthrograms and other orthopedic and joint procedures, obstetrics and gynecology, peripheral vascular, biopsy, vertebroplasty, and "other") were included in the interventional-fluoroscopic category. Other radiographic fluoroscopy procedures, such as barium swallow and upper GI contrast examinations are considered in Section 4.3 on conventional radiography and fluoroscopy. Table 4.9 summarizes the 2006 annual number of interventional-fluoroscopic procedures performed in the United States. The procedures in the three IMV reports were placed in four groups as listed in Table 4.9: nonvascular procedures, noncardiac diagnostic arteriography, noncardiac interventional vascular procedures, and cardiac procedures. The groups were selected to be consistent with the terminology used in clinical practice.

The various IMV reports employed different volume indices, such as the number of procedures or the number of cases for different time periods. For example, the 2004 to 2005 survey reported the number of x-ray procedures in interventional angiography (IMV, 2006f). The IMV cardiac catheterization survey (IMV, 2004) reported the number of procedures until 1999, but as of that year, the reports gave the number of cases (defined as a patient's visit to the catheterization laboratory on any given day), regardless of the number of procedures performed during the visit. Thus, in this Report, the number of cases reported was increased by 25 % to obtain the number of procedures during the period from 1999 through 2003, based on IMV (2004). Further, the average annual increase of 4 % was applied to the 2003 survey to project the 2004 cardiac catheterization data. In order to project cardiac catheterization data for 2006, the 2004 estimates were increased by 8 % based on the average rate of increase from 1999 through 2003. In radiographic fluoroscopy, the survey used the number of patient visits as a volume index. The 2004 to 2005 survey (IMV, 2006e) reported 19.33 million procedures in radiographic fluoroscopy for an estimated 12.43 million patient visits. Consequently, the number of patient visits was converted to the number of procedures using a multiplier of 1.56. To estimate 2006 radiographic fluoroscopy procedures, a multiplier of 1.5 was applied to the 2004 estimates. This correction was extrapolated from the trend data from 2002 through 2004. The number of interventional angiography procedures for 2006 was estimated from the same report based on a review of the trend data from the period 1999 through 2004. A multiplier of 1.10 was applied to the 2004 data.

4.4.2.2 *Sources of Information for Effective Dose.* As shown in Equation 4.3, an estimate of the effective dose for each type of procedure requires input data for KAP and DCC_E. Data for KAP and DCC_E are available in the literature for interventional-fluoroscopic procedures (Hart and Wall, 2002; Schultz and Zoetelief, 2005). Miller *et al.* (2003) published dose survey results for interventional-fluoroscopic procedures at seven academic medical centers in the United States. The paper lists KAP values for 21 specific procedures. The National Radiological Protection Board (Hart and Wall, 2002) tabulated a typical effective dose for each one

TABLE 4.9—*Effective dose, collective effective dose and E_{US} for fluoroscopically-guided diagnostic and interventional procedures (2006).*[a]

Groups/Subgroups	Number of Procedures	Number of Procedures (% of grand total)	Effective Dose[b] (mSv)	Collective Effective Dose (person-Sv)	Collective Effective Dose (% of grand total)
Nonvascular procedures					
Urinary studies	2,691,000	16.1	2	5,382	4.2
Myelography	2,035,800	12.2	4	8,143	6.3
Endoscopic retrograde cholangiopancreatography	1,427,400	8.5	4	5,710	4.4
Arthrograms, orthopedic and joints	1,404,000	8.4	0.2	281	0.2
Obstetrics and gynecology	748,800	4.5	1	749	0.6
Biopsy	163,800	1.0	1	164	0.1
Vertebroplasty	93,600	0.6	16	1,498	1.2
Other	70,200	0.4	4[c]	281	0.2
Total	8,634,600	51.6		22,208	17.3
Noncardiac diagnostic arteriography					
Peripheral vascular (including runoffs)	837,700	5.0	5	4,189	3.3

TABLE 4.9—(continued).

Groups/Subgroups	Number of Procedures	Number of Procedures (% of grand total)	Effective Dose[b] (mSv)	Collective Effective Dose (person-Sv)	Collective Effective Dose (% of grand total)
Neurologic (including carotid)	264,000	1.6	5	1,320	1.0
Renal	264,000	1.6	5	1,320	1.0
Carotid and aortic arch	231,000	1.4	15	3,465	2.7
Other peripheral	198,000	1.2	5	990	0.8
Neurologic (excluding carotid)	110,000	0.7	1	110	0.1
Pulmonary	71,500	0.4	6	429	0.3
Other	49,500	0.3	6[c]	297	0.2
Total	2,025,700	12.1		12,120	9.4
Noncardiac interventional vascular procedures					
Vascular access	363,000	2.2	7	2,541	2.0
Angioplasties	330,000	2.0	5	1,650	1.3
Stents	242,000	1.4	40	9,680	7.5
Inferior vena cava filters	192,500	1.2	14	2,695	2.1

Embolization	159,500	1.0	55	8,773	6.8
Thrombolytic therapy	143,000	0.9	3.5	501	0.4
Total	1,430,000	8.5		25,840	20.1
Cardiac procedures					
Diagnostic arteriography	2,137,050	12.8	7	14,959	11.7
Percutaneous intervention	498,150	3.0	23	11,457	8.9
Combined diagnostic and intervention	1,323,000	7.9	30[d]	39,690	30.9
Electrophysiology studies	264,600	1.6	3.2	847	0.7
Pacemaker	361,800	2.2	1	362	0.3
Other	60,750	0.4	15[c]	911	0.7
Total	4,645,350	27.8		68,226	53.1
Grand total	16,735,650			128,394	

2006 U.S. population 300 million

$$E_{US} = 0.43$$

[a] A more detailed version of Table 4.9 (Table D.2) is found in Appendix D.
[b] See Section 4.4.4 for a discussion of uncertainty in the range of values for effective dose.
[c] Effective dose for Other subgroup was estimated by taking the unweighted average of all effective doses in the respective group.
[d] Sum of effective doses for diagnostic arteriography and percutaneous intervention.

of 150 x-ray procedures in the United Kingdom. The reports also list estimated mean values for KAP and DCC_E. Regulla and Eder (2005) reported patient exposure in medical imaging in Europe. In addition, many published research articles were consulted to estimate the mean effective dose, KAP, and DCC_E. If an estimate of the effective dose was not possible for a specific procedure due to lack of published KAP and DCC_E values, an estimate was made from published data by comparison with similar procedures. Also used in the calculation were data from Betsou et al. (1998), Bogaert et al. (2008), Bor et al. (2004), Chu et al. (1998), Delichas et al. (2003), Efstathopoulos et al. (2006), Lindsay et al. (1992), Marshall et al. (2000), McFadden et al. (2002), McParland (1998), Miller et al. (2003), Neofotistou et al. (1998), Pukkila and Karila (1990), Rosenthal et al. (1998), Thwaites et al. (1996), Williams (1997), and Zweers et al. (1998). The DCC_E values (available only from the European literature) were in general agreement among the different European publications, although some variations existed. For this reason, the DCC_E values from the European publications were applied to the KAP data for the United States (mainly from Miller et al., 2003).

In cases where a category simply reflects a general description of various procedures in the same category, the unweighted average of effective doses for the procedures was assigned for this category; for example, a category of "therapeutic cardiac catheterization" may include several different procedures rather than one single procedure. Table 4.9 summarizes the effective doses for interventional-fluoroscopic procedures compiled for this Report.

Pediatric procedures were not included in the calculations for interventional fluoroscopy. This is in part due to the lack of available data on the mean effective dose for all pediatric procedures in the IMV cardiac catheterization, interventional angiography, and radiographic fluoroscopy reports. Also, the percentage of pediatric patients for cardiac catheterization laboratories was <1 % of the cases (IMV, 2004). For interventional angiography, it was assumed that 100 % were adult cases. For radiographic fluoroscopy categories, the IMV report estimated 15 % pediatric cases and 85 % adult cases. However, E_{US} was estimated assuming 100 % adult procedures. This was due, in part, to the lack of:

- detailed data giving the breakdown between adult and pediatric procedures in each category; and
- age distribution data for specific procedures, because specific disease distributions and procedures may vary between adults and pediatric patients.

Table 4.10 summarizes the sources of information and the assumptions with respect to the patient population.

4.4.3 Estimation of the Mean Effective Dose to an Individual and Collective Effective Dose

Table 4.9 tabulates data for interventional-fluoroscopic procedures for 2006. The first column identifies the clinical groups (nonvascular procedures, noncardiac diagnostic arteriography, noncardiac interventional vascular procedures, cardiac procedures) and subgroups of procedures, the second column shows the number of procedures for the subgroups, the third column shows the percentage of the total procedures for each subgroup, the fourth column lists the average effective dose in millisievert for each subgroup, the fifth column shows the collective effective dose in person-sievert, and the last column shows the percentage of the total collective effective dose for each subgroup. As shown, the total collective effective dose (S) for 2006 in interventional fluoroscopy was 128,000 person-Sv and E_{US} was 0.43 mSv. Figure 4.4 shows the distributions for the number of procedures and for collective effective dose for the four groups for 2006. It is of interest to note that the cardiac procedures comprise only 28 % of the total number of procedures, yet the collective effective dose is 53 % of the total for all interventional procedures.

TABLE 4.10—*Sources of information and assumptions for patients exposed for interventional-fluoroscopic calculations.*

IMV Category	IMV Benchmark (reference)	Adults (%)	Pediatric (% of total)	U.S. Population (millions)
Cardiac catheterization[a]	2003 (IMV, 2004)	100	<1	291
Interventional angiography	2004 – 2005 (IMV, 2006f)	100	NA	294
Radiographic fluoroscopy (partial)	2004 – 2005 (IMV, 2006e)	100 assumed	15 actual	294

[a]Cardiac catheterization data extrapolated to 2004 from 2003 data.

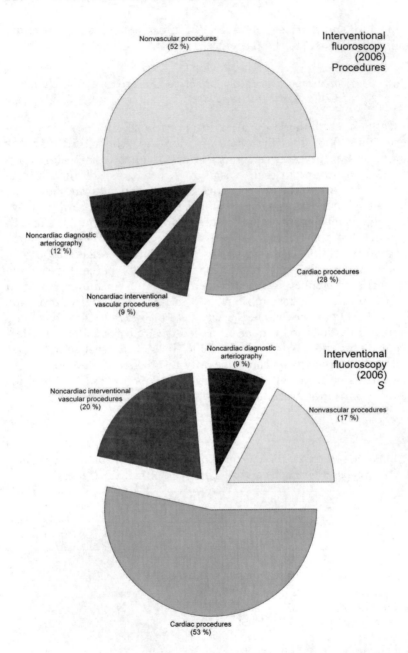

Fig. 4.4. Percent contribution of various groups of interventional-fluoroscopic procedures to number of procedures (16,700,000) (top) and S (128,000 person-Sv) (bottom) for 2006. The percent values have been rounded to the nearest 1 % [see Table 4.9 for the number of procedures and the values for S (person-sievert)].

4.4.4 *Sources of Uncertainty in the Dose*

The uncertainty in the estimate of the annual value of E_{US} in interventional fluoroscopy is a combination of the uncertainties from various components in the calculation. Two main sources of uncertainty are the number of procedures and the effective dose for each type of procedure.

Uncertainty in the number of procedures was introduced because two different volume indices were reported, as noted in Section 4.4.2.1. Consequently upward adjustments of reported cases were used to estimate the number of procedures for cardiac catheterizations and radiographic fluoroscopy. It should be noted that the conversion from patient visits to procedures assumed a constant increase across all the various procedures. Furthermore, all data are extrapolated to 2006.

Uncertainty in determining the effective dose results because of the dose variation within a given procedure. In interventional procedures the variation in the effective dose can be as much as a factor of 300 (Regulla and Eder, 2005). The effective dose variation within a given procedure is shown in Table D.2 for a large number of procedures. Variations in dose may be in part due to differences in clinical techniques used at various hospitals, equipment, and complexity of a given procedure. The issue becomes even more complex when data from outside the United States are consulted. Thus, one must keep in mind the difficulty and limitation in estimating the average effective dose from interventional-fluoroscopic procedures.

Estimates of DCC_E have been reported to have a wide variation for the same interventional procedures at different facilities. This is due to variations in clinical factors such as the number and orientation of the fluoroscopic and cinefluorographic views, and in technical factors associated with equipment such as tube voltage, filtration, focus-to-skin distance, and field size. For example, Table D.2 in Appendix D lists a range of values from 0.1 to 0.23 mSv Gy^{-1} cm^{-2} for cardiac radiofrequency ablation. Thus, one must keep in mind the variation of DCC_E in adopting a value for a specific interventional-fluoroscopic procedure.

4.4.5 *Case Volume Trend in the IMV*
Benchmark Reports

The trends discussed below are for the data as presented in the three IMV reports and using the IMV terminology for assigning a site as a radiographic fluoroscopy room, an interventional angiography laboratory, or a cardiac catheterization laboratory.[21] Other procedures are performed at a given site that overlap those at other types of sites and therefore the terminology does not fully reflect all the procedures performed at the site. The trends are presented in order to illustrate the general growth in interventional fluoroscopy in recent years. The assignments here are not to the more specific clinically-recognized procedure groups presented in Table 4.9.

4.4.5.1 *Trend in Procedures and Patient Visits to Radiographic Fluoroscopy Rooms.* In the 2004 to 2005 survey, 19.3 million procedures in radiographic fluoroscopy were estimated to have involved 12.4 million patient visits (IMV 2006e), an increase in procedures of 54 %, from the 12.5 million procedures in 2002. The total number of patient visits increased 25 % during the same period. Based on the rate of increase from 2002 to 2004, the patient visits for 2004 were increased 50 % to obtain the number of visits in 2006. The trend for radiographic fluoroscopy is shown in Figure 4.5 for 2001 through 2006.

4.4.5.2 *Trend in Procedures in Interventional Angiography.* From 2000 to 2004, the total procedures performed in angiography laboratories grew ~5 % annually, from 3.39 million to 4.02 million procedures (IMV, 2006f). For estimation of the numbers of procedures in 2005 and 2006, a 5 % increase per year was applied to the 2004 survey data and the 2005 estimate, in sequence. Figure 4.6 shows the trend in interventional angiography from 2000 through 2006.

4.4.5.3 *Trend in Cases in Cardiac Catheterization Laboratories.* From 1998 to 2002, total cases in the catheterization laboratory increased 17 %, from 3.28 to 3.85 million, but were essentially flat from 2001 to 2002. The number of cases from 1998 through 2002 was converted to the number of procedures by applying a multiplier

---

[21]The IMV assignment criteria were:
- *Radiographic fluoroscopy*: At least 50 % nonvascular radiographic fluoroscopy procedures performed on fixed radiographic fluoroscopy equipment.
- *Interventional angiography*: Cardiac catheterizations or coronary angiography procedures <50 % of total angiography volume, and at least one fixed x-ray imaging unit with a C-arm.
- *Cardiac catheterization*: Either a dedicated cardiac catheterization laboratory or an angiography suite whose cardiac catheterization volume is >50 % of its total volume.

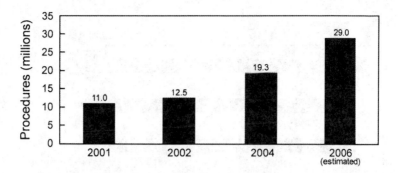

Fig. 4.5. Trend in total number of procedures for radiographic fluoroscopy (2001 to 2006) (IMV, 2006e).

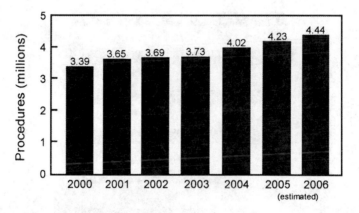

Fig. 4.6. Trend in total number of procedures for interventional angiography (2000 to 2006) (IMV, 2006f).

of 1.25. The average increase in the number of procedures was 4 % per year from 1993 through 2002. Therefore, to estimate the number of procedures for 2006, a multiplier of 1.04 y^{-1} was applied to the 2004 IMV data and the 2005 estimate, in sequence. Figure 4.7 shows the trend in cardiac catheterization procedures from 1993 through 2006.

Since the introduction of the helical MDCT scanner in 1998, CT imaging is used increasingly for many diagnostic and therapeutic procedures where fluoroscopic equipment was used in the past. For example, CT has found applications in some traditional interventional procedures, such as coronary CT angiography, and CT fluoroscopy during treatment for pain relief to list a few. This trend is

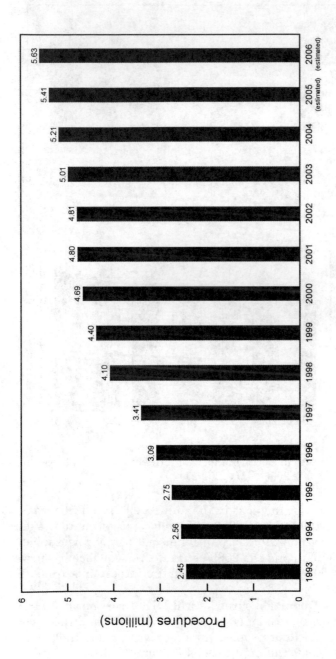

Fig. 4.7. Trend in total number of procedures for cardiac catheterization (1993 to 2006) (IMV, 2004).

expected to continue into the future and, in some cases, CT may replace traditional fluoroscopy-based angiography.

4.5 Nuclear Medicine

Nuclear medicine is the medical specialty in which unsealed radionuclides are used for diagnosis and treatment. Nuclear-medicine images have less spatial or anatomic resolution than do radiographic or magnetic resonance examinations but nuclear-medicine techniques are better able to display physiologic and metabolic mechanisms. Nuclear-medicine techniques are widely used to assess regional blood flow, regional pulmonary ventilation, organ function, cellular metabolism, and other *in vivo* biologic processes.

Nuclear medicine has grown steadily since the end of World War II. There has been continuing evolution of instrumentation, development of new radiopharmaceuticals, and competition with other imaging techniques. This section assesses the type and frequency of nuclear-medicine procedures and estimates E_{US} and the collective effective doses associated with the practice of nuclear medicine.

Radionuclides are usually chemically manipulated to form radiopharmaceuticals that are administered orally, by inhalation or, most commonly by injection. Radiopharmaceuticals localize in various target tissues and organs in the body. The mechanisms of localization are shown with examples in Table 4.11. Table 4.12 lists the radionuclides commonly used in nuclear medicine.

4.5.1 *Nuclear-Medicine Procedures*

The majority of nuclear-medicine procedures are diagnostic examinations. Therapeutic nuclear-medicine procedures represent a small percentage of all radionuclide use and by the nature of the high therapeutic doses cannot be evaluated with the quantity effective dose. As a result, the frequency of therapeutic procedures has been estimated but therapeutic procedures have not been included in either E_{US} or the collective effective dose estimates. NCRP Report No. 124 (NCRP, 1996) assumed that in 1991 treatment of hyperthyroidism and thyroid cancer was 2 % of the number of diagnostic procedures. The Medicare 2004 data (CMS, 2006) indicate that <0.1 % of all procedures were for unsealed radionuclide therapy. However, the age distribution of the Medicare population likely excludes most hyperthyroid and thyroid cancer patients.

There are very little data on the use of nuclear-medicine procedures in medical research protocols. The data on number of procedures used in this Report (Section 4.1.2) are predominantly

TABLE 4.11—*Mechanisms of localization in nuclear medicine and examples.*

Mechanisms of Localization	Examples
Active transport	Iodocholesterol in adrenal scanning Iodine or pertechnetate (accumulation by choroid plexus, Meckel's diverticulum, salivary gland, stomach, and thyroid) ^{99m}Tc iminodiacetic acid analogs in liver/biliary tract Orthoiodohippurate in renal tubules Thallous ions in myocardium
Antibody-antigen reactions	Tumor imaging, monoclonal antibodies
Capillary blockade	Macroaggregated albumin in lung
Compartmental containment	Labeled red blood cells (RBC) for gated blood pool studies
Compartmental leakage	Labeled RBC for detection of GI bleeding
Diffusion	Filtration of diethylenetriamine pentaacetic acid (DTPA) by kidney
Metabolism	Fluorodeoxyglucose imaging of brain, tumor, myocardium
Phagocytosis and lymph nodes	Colloid scanning for liver and spleen, bone marrow
Physicochemical adsorption	Phosphate bone-scanning agents
Receptor binding	Neuroreceptor imaging
Sequestration	Leukocytes for abscess scanning Labeled platelets (damaged endothelium) Heat-damaged RBC for splenic scanning

from financial reimbursement sources and procedures performed solely for research would not be paid by insurance companies. Those procedures in research protocols that can be termed as "clinically indicated" and billed to insurance companies or Medicare are already included in the data used for this Report.

4.5.1.1 *Diagnostic Examinations.* The type of instrumentation employed is often used to describe types of diagnostic nuclear-medicine examinations. Planar imaging uses a gamma camera which

TABLE 4.12—*Characteristics of radionuclides commonly used in nuclear-medicine procedures.*

Radionuclide	Physical Half-Life	Emissions
Photon-emitting radionuclides for imaging		*Approximate Gamma-Ray Energies (keV)*
^{99m}Tc	6 h	140
^{123}I	13.2 h	159
^{131}I	8.0 d	364
^{133}Xe	5.3 d	81
^{67}Ga	78.3 h	90, 190, 290, 390
^{111}In	67 h	173, 247
^{113m}In	1.7 h	392
^{201}Tl	73.1 h	69, 81 (x rays from mercury daughter)
^{81m}Kr	13 s	191
Positron-emitting radionuclides for imaging		*Maximum positron energy (MeV)*[a]
^{11}C	20 min	0.96
^{13}N	10 min	1.19
^{15}O	2 min	1.73
^{18}F	110 min	0.635
^{68}Ga	68 min	1.90
^{82}Rb	1.3 min	3.15
Unsealed radionuclides used for therapy		*Beta particles*[b] *and gamma rays*
^{32}P	14.3 d	1.71 MeV maximum and 0.7 MeV mean beta
^{89}Sr	50.5 d	1.46 MeV maximum and 0.58 MeV mean beta, 910 keV gamma (0.01 %)
^{90}Y	64 h	2.2 MeV maximum and 0.93 MeV mean beta
^{131}I	8.0 d	0.19 MeV mean beta, 364 keV gamma (82 %)
^{153}Sm	46 h	0.81 MeV maximum and 0.23 MeV mean beta, 103 keV gamma (28 %)
^{186}Re	90 h	0.34 mean beta, 186 keV gamma (9 %)
^{198}Au	2.7 d	0.96 MeV maximum and 0.31 MeV mean beta, 412 keV gamma (96 %)

[a]Two gamma rays, each with 511 keV energy, are associated with the annihilation of a positron.

[b]The approximate range (centimeter) of a beta particle in tissue is the energy (million electron volt) divided by two.

stays on one side of the patient and records gamma rays emanating from the patient to produce a two-dimensional projection image, usually in anterior, posterior or lateral projections. In SPECT imaging, the gamma camera is rotated about the patient collecting projection images from many angles that are subsequently displayed after computer manipulation in "slices" through the patient or less commonly in a three-dimensional format. Both planar and SPECT imaging usually use radionuclides that emit gamma rays in the range of 80 to 200 keV. Recently there has been rapid growth of another technique, PET, in which a ring-shaped PET camera detects pairs of oppositely-directed 511 keV annihilation photons from positron-emitting radiopharmaceuticals. PET scanning now is almost always performed in conjunction with a CT scan so that the PET images, displaying information about physiological function, can be "fused" with CT images that depict anatomy.

Diagnostic nuclear-medicine examinations can be divided into general classes based on organ systems, or less commonly, by diagnostic purpose. The most common uses and indications are described in Appendix E.

4.5.1.2 *Therapeutic Procedures.* Compared with diagnostic nuclear-medicine applications, therapeutic nuclear-medicine applications are much fewer in number, but often use higher administered activities (*e.g.*, when treating malignancies), and commonly use radionuclides with longer biological and physical half-lives. Therapeutic radiopharmaceuticals in current clinical use are usually beta-particle emitters but many also have gamma-ray emissions.

The use of unsealed radiopharmaceutical therapies has almost doubled over the last decade. In developed countries, UNSCEAR (2000) estimated that worldwide the annual number of procedures increased from 210,000 in the period 1985 to 1990 to 380,000 in the period 1991 to 1996.

The common types of therapy with unsealed radionuclides are oral or intravenous administration of liquids or capsules (systemic therapy) or instillation of colloidal suspensions into closed body cavities (intracavitary therapy). Examples of systemic therapy include treatment for hyperthyroidism, thyroid cancer, and bone metastases. Examples of intracavitary therapy include treatment of malignancies of the pleural and peritoneal cavities and intra-articular administration for synovectomy. The estimated number of common types of therapeutic procedures with unsealed radionuclides is shown in Table 4.13. Similar information for the United States is not available. The various techniques of radiopharmaceutical therapy with unsealed radionuclides are briefly described in Appendix E.

TABLE 4.13—*Nuclear-medicine therapy: Estimated worldwide annual procedures 1991 to 1996 (adapted from UNSCEAR, 2000).*

Condition	Radiopharmaceutical and Route	Procedures per Million Population	
		(developed countries)	(worldwide)
Thyroid malignancy	^{131}I sodium iodide (oral or i.v.[a])	35	15
Hyperthyroidism	^{131}I sodium iodide (oral or i.v.)	110	42
Polycythemia vera	^{32}P phosphate (oral or i.v.)	3	1
Bone metastases	^{89}Sr chloride (i.v.)	5	2
	^{153}Sm ethylene diaminomethylene phosphoric acid (i.v.)		
Synovitis	^{90}Y colloid	7	2
	^{169}Er colloid (intra-articular)		
Malignant disease (other than thyroid cancer and polycythemia vera)	^{131}I m-iodo-benzylguanidine (i.v.)	—[b]	—[b]
	^{90}Y colloid (intracavitary)		

[a]i.v. = intravenous administration.
[b]Unknown.

4.5.2 *Estimate of the Annual Number of Procedures*

The primary data set used for the detailed estimation of specific procedures in nuclear medicine was provided by Medicare (Table D.3 in Appendix D). Based on the 2005 IMV report (IMV, 2006c), the 2004 Medicare data source appears to have about one-third to one-fourth of the national data for procedures (Table D.4 in Appendix D). The Medicare data are based on billing codes. In some instances there is more than one CPT code for a given procedure. Thus counting discrete CPT-based billing data as visits or procedures without excluding the "add on" codes would result in an over-estimate. This is a particularly important issue for estimation of nuclear-medicine procedures and doses. The most common nuclear-medicine examination (cardiac perfusion) has three CPT codes (78465 as the primary code and 78478 and 78480 as add on codes) for a single procedure. For this Report, the "add on" codes have been identified and have not been counted in total number of procedures or in calculating effective dose.

The Medicare data set is complemented with more general data from IMV, from VA (Table D.4 in Appendix D), and from a LNEP. The IMV data set is judged to be the best available estimate for the total number of studies. For purposes of dose estimation the specific Medicare procedure counts were multiplied by the value of 3.41, which is slightly lower than the 3.6 multiplier specified in Section 4.1.2.3, but reflects the ratio in total visits reported by IMV compared with the Medicare data.

As can be seen from Table D.4, the annual number of nuclear-medicine visits in 2005 was just over 17.2 million, and these represent 19.7 million procedures (IMV, 2006c) (some patient visits may include more than one procedure). The agreement regarding distribution of studies by general category is very good between the Medicare and IMV data sets.

4.5.3 *Characteristics and Age Distribution of the Patient Population Exposed*

The number of patients cannot be approximated with much certainty from the available data. One might analyze the procedures and determine which procedures are performed in conjunction. For example, most lung scans include both a ventilation and perfusion component. On billing records and financial data these may or may not be separate CPT codes and charges. More importantly, similar bundled codes are found in cardiac nuclear medicine which comprise over half of all nuclear-medicine procedures. Some of the data sets reviewed report "visits" to nuclear-medicine departments. It is often not clear exactly what is meant by this term but it appears to be examinations as defined by financial records or billing codes. Finally, it is not known how many patients have repeat or additional procedures within the same year.

IMV (2006c) indicates that of the 17.2 million visits in 2005, 11.5 million were done in hospital settings and 5.7 million at non-hospital sites. Overall 23 % of examinations were done on inpatients and 77 % were done on outpatients.

The distribution of nuclear-medicine examinations by age and gender for 1980 (Bunge and Herman, 1985; NCRP, 1989a) given in Table 4.14 shows that 77 % of nuclear-medicine procedures were performed on persons age 45 y or older. There have been a few articles showing that taking the actual age distribution into account results in a lower age-weighted collective dose (e.g., NCRP, 1989a).

The age distribution of all diagnostic nuclear-medicine procedures for 2003 derived from a large insurance plan (adjusted to be representative of the age distribution of the U.S. population)[22] is shown in Figure 4.8 and that for cardiac nuclear-medicine procedures is shown in Figure 4.9.

The age distribution shown in Figure 4.8 is very similar to the age distribution found for all nuclear-medicine procedures in 1980. At that time 37.8 % of procedures were done on persons 45 to 64 y and 39.0 % on persons over the age of 64 y. These can be compared with 41.2 and 38.8 % respectively found for the same age groups in 2003.

TABLE 4.14—*Age and gender of those in the U.S. population having nuclear-medicine examinations in 1980 (adapted from NCRP, 1989a).*

Age (y)	Male (%)	Female (%)	Both (%)
<15	0.9	0.8	1.7
15 – 29	3.4	4.6	8.0
30 – 44	5.4	8.1	13.5
45 – 64	17.5	20.4	37.9
>64	17.7	21.4	39.1

[22]The population of the large insurance plan did not have the same age distribution as the U.S. population. The distribution of the number of procedures by age for that population was adjusted to estimate what the number of procedures by age would have been if the age distribution did match that of the U.S. population.

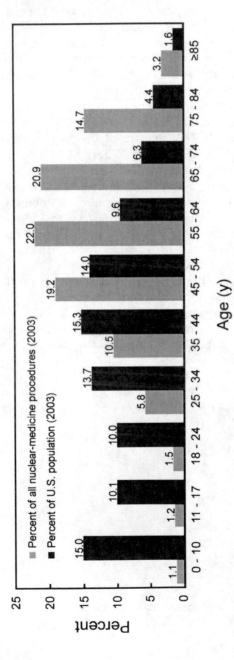

Fig. 4.8. Age distribution for patients having nuclear-medicine procedures (all types) compared with the age distribution of the U.S. population, both for 2003. The number of procedures has been adjusted to be representative of the U.S. population (see footnote 22).

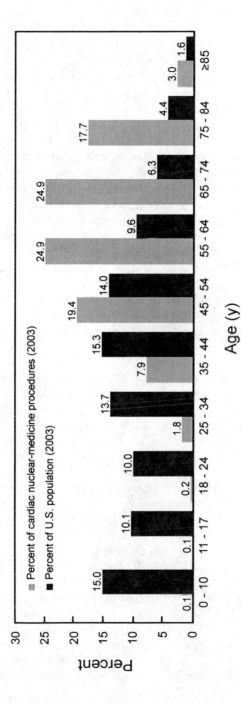

Fig. 4.9. Age distribution for patients having cardiac nuclear-medicine procedures compared with the age distribution of the U.S. population, both for 2003. The number of procedures has been adjusted to be representative of the U.S. population (see footnote 22).

4.5.4 *Effective Dose, Collective Effective Dose and Effective Dose to an Individual in the U.S. Population*

4.5.4.1 *Discussion of the Effective Doses for the Procedures.* Organ doses in patients and effective doses are not measurable quantities. They are estimated by a variety of methods and are available from a number of sources. The dose conversion coefficient is expressed as effective dose per unit of administered activity. Previously, the Monte-Carlo dosimetric model of the Medical Internal Radiation Dose Committee of the Society of Nuclear Medicine (SNM) was utilized (Snyder *et al.*, 1975). However, now there are more sophisticated Monte-Carlo dosimetric models. The most commonly used dose conversion coefficients are from ICRP (1998), which also take into account the metabolic models and biokinetic data for the radiopharmaceuticals. In addition, dose conversion coefficients are available from FDA required inserts for approved radiopharmaceuticals (commonly based on information from SNM) and a more limited amount of information is available in textbooks and on the SNM website (SNM, 2008). The radionuclides, administered activities, dose conversion coefficients, and effective doses per procedure in nuclear medicine, listed by CPT code, are presented in Table D.5 in Appendix D. For certain CPT codes and procedures there are different radiopharmaceuticals that can be used and when this occurs both are shown.

The percentage ratio when more than one radiopharmaceutical can be used for a procedure is shown in Table D.5 in Appendix D, and the effective dose per procedure is weighted accordingly. With the exception of cardiac nuclear medicine these assumptions would have little effect on total population exposure. As an example, the methodology used in Table D.5, for CPT code 78460 (Column 2) performed for evaluation of myocardial perfusion (Column 3), is as follows. This procedure can be done using either ^{99m}Tc sestamibi or ^{201}Tl chloride and it was assumed that in 2005 the proportion of each radiopharmaceutical used was 75 % / 25 % (Column 4). The administered activity was estimated to be 1,480 MBq for ^{99m}Tc sestamibi and 150 MBq for ^{201}Tl chloride (Column 5). The dose conversion coefficient for ^{99m}Tc sestamibi is 0.0085 mSv MBq^{-1} and for ^{201}Tl chloride is 0.22 mSv MBq^{-1} (Column 6). The effective dose for this procedure performed with ^{99m}Tc sestamibi is then 1,480 MBq × 0.0085 mSv MBq^{-1} = 12.6 mSv. For this procedure using ^{201}Tl chloride the effective dose is 150 MBq × 0.22 mSv MBq^{-1} = 33 mSv. With the stated assumption for use, the weighted average effective dose for the procedure can be obtained as (12.6 mSv × 0.75) + (33 mSv × 0.25) = 17.7 mSv (Column 7). The procedure can also be performed with ^{99m}Tc tetrofosmin.

The choice of using an administered activity at the high end of the "suggested" ranges is consistent with most clinical practices. If lower average amounts are actually administered, the dose estimates could be 10 to 20 % too high, but this is unlikely. For example, the most common activity ordered for a bone scan is 1.11 GBq, with the suggested range in the literature being 0.74 to 1.11 GBq (SNM, 2008).

4.5.4.2 *Estimate of Collective Effective Dose and Effective Dose to an Individual in the U.S. Population.* The collective effective dose for individual procedures has been estimated by using dose conversion coefficients, using the high end of the "suggested" range for administered activity and multiplying by the estimated numbers of that specific procedure. The collective effective doses for all procedures were then added and divided by the population of the United States (in this case 300 million). The results are shown in Table 4.15, Figure 4.10, and Table 4.16.

4.5.5 *Uncertainties Affecting Dose Estimation*

There are a number of sources of uncertainty in the dose estimates. Assumptions have been made and are implicit in the ICRP and other models regarding the transfer of the radionuclide between different metabolic or physiologic compartments in the human body as well as excretion rates. These factors are perturbed by pathophysiological processes present in different disease states. There is uncertainty in the modeling of radiation transport as well as in the amount of impurities (*i.e.*, other radionuclides) in the radiopharmaceutical. These uncertainties could result in uncertainties of 50 % or more in the effective dose. Uncertainties also arise in determining the amount of administered activity, although these are unlikely to affect effective doses by >10 %.

In the source data and review of surveys, there is some uncertainty in the distribution or percentage of procedures for a category of studies (such as GI). Only the Medicare data provided CPT codes that allowed the precise evaluation of nuclear-medicine subcategories (*e.g.*, whether cardiac procedures were myocardial perfusion studies, ejection fraction, or shunt studies). These Medicare distribution percentages for subcategories were assumed to apply to the national datasets (such as IMV) to obtain S and E_{US} estimates.

Other sources of uncertainty arise because:

- doses to individuals will vary a small amount based on patient size for the same amount of administered activity;

TABLE 4.15—*Summary of 2005 doses to the U.S. population from various diagnostic nuclear-medicine procedures.*[a]

Category	Collective Effective Dose (person-Sv)	Percent of Total
Cardiac	187,915	85.2
Bone	20,517	9.3
Tumor	3,925	1.8
GI	3,534	1.6
Lung	2,012	0.9
Infection	1,329	0.6
Renal	643	0.3
Thyroid	397	0.2
Brain	259	0.1
Total	220,533 (220,500)	100

[a]The weighted average effective dose for each nuclear-medicine procedure in a given category is provided in Table D.5 in Appendix D and the method of weighting is discussed in Section 4.5.4.1.

- disease states and personal habits (*e.g.*, frequent urination, higher iodine content in the diet) will affect the retention as well as distribution of the radiopharmaceutical; and
- more than one radiopharmaceutical can be used for the same procedure (*e.g.*, use of ^{99m}Tc pertechnetate or ^{123}I for thyroid scanning).

In extreme circumstances the actual dose to a very ill individual could be several-fold different from that projected for normal persons. In these circumstances, this Report used a best estimate of current clinical practice.

There is a small amount of uncertainty in leaving out procedures with very small numbers such as those listed as "other" or "miscellaneous" categories in the source data. This would likely lead to an underestimation of only a few percent.

Another source of uncertainty arises because dose conversion coefficients are age dependent. Dose conversion coefficients incorporate age-specific H_Ts to the exposed organs and tissues, but use w_T values for a population of all ages and both genders.

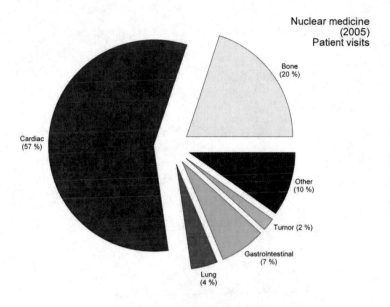

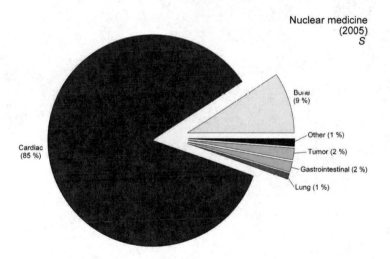

Fig. 4.10. Percent contribution of various subcategories of nuclear-medicine procedures to number of patient visits (17,220,000) (top) and to S (220,500 person-Sv) (bottom) for 2005. The "other" subcategory includes thyroid, renal, brain and infection. Estimates for 2006 for number of procedures and S were projected from these data (Table 4.16). The percent values have been rounded to the nearest 1 % [see Table D.4 for the number of patient visits and see Table 4.15 for the values for S (person-sievert)].

TABLE 4.16—*Number of nuclear-medicine examinations performed or estimated in the United States from 1972 through 2006.*

Year	Procedures (millions)	U.S. Population (millions)	Exams or Visits per 1,000 Population	E_{US} (mSv)	Collective Effective Dose (person-Sv)
1972[a]	3.3	209.9	15.7		
1973[a]	3.5	211.9	15.6		
1974[a]		213.9			
1975[a]	4.8	216.0	22.2		
1976[a]		218.0			
1977[a]		220.2			
1978[a]	6.4	222.5	28.8		
1979[a]		225.0			
1980[a]	(5.8 – 6.4)	226.5			
1981[a]	7.0	229.5	30.5		
1982[a]	7.6 (7.4 – 7.7)	231.6	32.6	0.14	32,100
1983[a]		233.0			
1984	6.3[b]	235.8	26.7		
1985	6.2[b]	237.9	26.2		
1986	6.7[b]	240.1	27.9		
1987	6.8[b]	242.3	28.1		
1988	7.1[b]	244.5	29.0		

Year					
1989	7.1[b]	246.8	28.9		
1990		249.7			
1991		252.1			
1992		255.0			
1993		257.7			
1994		260.3			
1995	10.2[c]	262.8	38.8		
1996	10.5[c]	265.2	39.6		
1997	10.9[c]	267.7	40.7		
1998	11.8[c]	270.2	43.7		
1999	12.6[c]	272.7	46.2		
2000	13.5[c]	282.1	47.9		
2001	14.5[c]	284.8	50.9		
2002	14.9[c]	287.9	51.8		
2003	15.7[c]	290.8	54.0		
2004	16.5[c]	294.7	56.0		
2005	17.2[c]	296.0	58.1	0.74	220,500
2006	18.1[d]	300.0	60.3	0.77	~231,000[d]

[a]Mettler et al. (1985).
[b]NCRP (1991).
[c]Data for 2005 (IMV, 2006c) reflects patient visits and not procedures.
[d]Data extrapolated assuming ~5 % annual growth from 2005.

4.5.6 *Discussion of Trends*

Table 4.16 shows that between 1982 and 2006, the estimate of E_{US} from *in vivo* diagnostic nuclear medicine increased by 450 % and the collective effective dose increased by 620 %. During the period 1972 through 2006, diagnostic nuclear-medicine procedures increased by a factor of 5.5 while the U.S. population increased by ~50 %. During the last decade there was 5 % annual growth in the number of nuclear-medicine procedures while the U.S. population grew <1 % annually.

Table D.6 in Appendix D and Figure 4.11 (histogram of Table D.6) also show a marked shift in the type of procedures, with the studies of the brain and thyroid decreasing from a combined percentage of over 56 % of all procedures in 1973 to <4 % in 2005. The most dramatic increase occurred in cardiac procedures increasing from 1 % in 1973 to 57 % in 2005. Cardiac studies are relatively high-dose procedures and account for over 85 % of the effective dose to the patient population. Currently, over 75 % of all studies fall into two categories, cardiac and bone and these two types of examinations account for almost 95 % of the collective effective dose.

There are a number of recent trends that are new enough that their impact has not been evident in survey data from 2005. One of these is the marked shift from ventilation-perfusion nuclear-medicine scans to the use of MDCT scans for evaluation of pulmonary embolism. As a result, nuclear-medicine lung scans have become rare. This has almost certainly reduced the dose in nuclear medicine but only by ~1 %. The dose to the patients for evaluation of pulmonary embolism, however, has almost certainly increased as CT scans of the chest have an effective dose of ~5 mSv (compared with ~2.5 mSv for a lung scan) and because the CT examination is easier to perform, many more examinations are being ordered.

Another trend which is occurring in cardiac-myocardial perfusion studies is the gradual replacement of ^{201}Tl chloride with ^{99m}Tc sestamibi or ^{99m}Tc tetrofosmin. Depending upon the activity injected, the effective dose per examination could be lower with technetium radiopharmaceuticals. The potential impact of CT coronary artery screening and calcium scoring on cardiac nuclear medicine is uncertain.

PET scans have been available clinically for several years, but the recent availability of more cyclotrons, an increase in the production and ease of availability of ^{18}F fluorodeoxyglucose (FDG), combined with the sales of PET/CT scanners and favorable reimbursement policies, will increase the number of PET/CT scans in

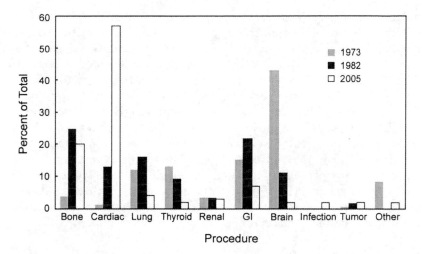

Fig. 4.11. Change in numbers of procedures (in thousands) and percentage since 1972 for *in vivo* diagnostic nuclear-medicine examinations.

the future. This will increase the radiation dose to the patients because the combined scans deliver an effective dose in the range of 40 mSv. IMV (2006d) indicated an annual growth rate in PET scans ranging from 25 to 50 %.

The increasing size and, more importantly, the increasing mean age of the U.S. population will likely increase the demand for tumor scans (for localization, staging, and monitoring response to therapy), bone scans (looking for metastatic disease), and cardiac scans. The potential use of newer techniques in molecular imaging, gene- and antibody-targeted cancer therapies remains largely uncertain.

4.6 Radiotherapy (External Beam)

4.6.1 *Applicability of Radiotherapy Exposures to this Report*

Radiotherapy, the use of radiation for the treatment of disease, differs from other medical exposures of patients for several reasons. A sample analysis for external-beam radiotherapy has been performed to illustrate the issues associated with estimating effective dose from radiotherapy modalities.

4.6.1.1 *Injury to Normal Tissues.* Consideration of injury to normal structures and the symptoms that may accompany the injuries forms part of the decision to undergo treatment. However, for many patients, the treatments are life saving; for others the treatments may sustain a higher quality of life.

4.6.1.2 *Extremely-High Treatment Doses.* While the number of patients undergoing radiotherapy is just under 1 % of the number having diagnostic procedures, the therapeutic absorbed dose to the target volume (*i.e.*, the treatment dose) is on the order of 5,000 to 50,000 times as large as the tissue doses resulting from diagnostic procedures. Subsequently, effective doses for radiotherapy calculated in the usual manner would be extremely high. Also, the concept of effective dose applies only to stochastic effects (such as cancer) and does not apply at the levels of radiotherapy treatment doses that result in deterministic effects. A possible approach to a more relevant estimate of the effective dose resulting from radiotherapy would be to exclude the very-high tissue doses within the treatment volume and only consider the tissue doses in structures outside the treatment volume. This approach is explored in Section 4.6.3.

4.6.2 *Problems in Assessing Effective Doses for the Radiotherapy Population*

4.6.2.1 *Tissue Doses Vary Greatly.* While data on the number of radiotherapy procedures performed may be available by anatomical treatment site, the treatment dose that each radiotherapy patient receives is customized to the patient's disease and condition. As an example, treatments to the brain range from a palliative absorbed dose of 8 Gy to a curative absorbed dose of 70 Gy. Simply sorting the number of patient visits by anatomical site fails to give the dosimetric information necessary to calculate a collective effective dose.

4.6.2.2 *Location and Extent of Fields Vary.* The actual location of the radiation field for a given anatomical site varies among patients, increasing the uncertainty in tissue doses from radiotherapy procedures. Again using the brain as an example, the target may be in the temporal lobe or in the brain stem. In addition, the radiation field might cover the whole brain or focus tightly on a small feature. Both the location and the size of the field would have a major impact on the dose to nearby structures.

4.6.2.3 *Neutrons.* Radiotherapy beams >10 MV produce secondary neutrons, primarily in the treatment unit that impinge on the patient. The magnitude of secondary neutron absorbed dose varies more than does the secondary (leakage and scatter) photon absorbed dose as a function of beam energy and field size. While the absorbed dose to tissues from such neutrons at higher accelerating potentials is about a tenth of that from photons, w_R for neutrons can result in an H_T (to the tissues) close to that for photons.

4.6.3 *Possible Estimation Techniques for Collective Effective Dose*

Task Group 158 of the American Association of Physicists in Medicine is conducting an analysis of the absorbed dose to nontarget organs in radiotherapy. However, the analysis is not yet complete and therefore was not available for this Report. With all the uncertainty involved with estimating a collective effective dose for the population of radiotherapy patients, and the lack of correspondence to the other procedures covered in this Report, only a very rough estimate of collective effective dose can be made. For each treatment site, the number of courses of treatment for 2004 reported in IMV (2005b) was increased by 3 % to obtain an estimate for 2006. The number of courses of treatment was used as the estimate for the number of patients.

Table 4.17 presents the results for a typical treatment dose, beam energy, and field size for the procedures performed at each treatment site.[23] The mean absorbed dose to the listed organs and tissues was calculated from published peripheral dose information outside of the treatment volumes (Fraass and van de Geijn, 1983; Stovall et al., 1995), based on a typical distance from the treatment site to the organ, and organ size. For those anatomical sites usually treated with beam energies >10 MV, no adjustment was made for the neutron contribution (*i.e.*, $w_R = 1$). Finally, each H_T (the values listed in Table 4.17) was multiplied by the appropriate w_T (ICRP, 1991) and the products were summed to give effective dose.

The analysis did not include treatment of bone metastases or soft-tissue sarcomas. In these cases, the anatomical site may be anywhere in the body, therefore distances to target sites become indeterminate.

The uncertainty in this estimate is greater than the estimate. While typical distances and depths were used, no data exist to provide realistic guidelines. Factors of two to three in the values for any of the quantities used could easily be argued. Given all these qualifications, the rough estimate of collective effective dose in 2006 for external-beam radiotherapy is ~350,000 person-Sv.

4.6.4 *Current Trends in Radiotherapy Exposure*

4.6.4.1 *Intensity Modulated Radiotherapy.* One of the biggest changes in radiotherapy practice over the last few years has been

---

[23]Uselmann, A. and Thomadsen, B.R. (2009). Personal communication (University of Wisconsin-Madison, Madison, Wisconsin).

TABLE 4.17—*Number of patients, equivalent doses (H_T), effective doses, and annual collective effective dose for external-beam radiotherapy in the United States in 2006.*[a]

Treatment Site	Percent of Total Patients[c]	Number of Patients	Organ or Tissue[b] H_T (Sv)											Effective Dose (Sv)	Collective Effective Dose (person-Sv)
			Gonads	Colon	Lung	Active Bone Marrow	Stomach	Esophagus	Breast	Bladder	Liver	Thyroid	Remainder		
$w_T \rightarrow$			0.20	0.12	0.12	0.12	0.12	0.05	0.05	0.05	0.05	0.05	0.05		
Breast	21.7	212,558	0.06	0.08	0.58	0.35	0.59	0.48	—[d]	0.04	0.77	0.58	0.76	0.337	71,632
Prostate	20.2	197,865	2.37	1.43	0.07	1.30	0.15	0.10	0.00	1.72	0.23	0.05	0.32	0.949	187,774
Lung	13.7	134,196	0.05	0.07	—[d]	0.28	0.31	0.56	0.34	0.05	0.33	0.25	0.44	0.187	25,095
Head and neck	7.1	69,547	0.04	0.04	0.46	0.87	0.09	0.52	0.45	0.04	0.09	1.18	0.46	0.319	22,185
Colorectal	5.9	57,792	0.52	—[d]	0.08	0.33	0.15	0.04	0.09	0.62	0.19	0.05	0.74	0.258	14,910
Gynecological	5.4	52,895	—[d]	0.63	0.07	0.40	0.16	0.04	0.08	0.81	0.16	0.06	0.60	0.240	12,695
Brain metastases	5.0	48,977	0.00	0.01	0.05	0.05	0.01	0.04	0.04	0.01	0.01	0.14	0.04	0.031	1,518

Brain primaries	4.0	39,181	0.01	0.02	0.11	0.11	0.03	0.08	0.08	0.02	0.03	0.30	0.04	0.059	2,312
GI	3.6	35,263	0.29	—[d]	0.15	1.58	0.30	0.06	0.18	0.45	0.32	0.03	1.00	0.233	8,216
Lymphoma, leukemia	2.4	23,509	0.03	0.05	0.00	1.14	0.37	0.26	0.28	0.05	0.28	0.45	1.44	0.333	7,828
		871,783 (total in this table)												Total	354,165
														E_{US}	1.18 mSv
														per patient	0.41 Sv

[a] Uselmann, A. and Thomadsen, B.R. (2009). Personal communication (University of Wisconsin-Madison, Madison, Wisconsin).

[b] Tissues in the effective dose calculation that are not included here are: skin, bone surface.

[c] The total number of radiotherapy patients is taken as 979,530, which includes patients with bone metastases and soft-tissue sarcomas that are not included in this table.

[d] A value for the target organ is not included, but for a pair of organs with only one being treated (e.g., lungs, breasts), there would be a relevant value to the other member of the pair.

the increase in the use of intensity modulated radiotherapy (IMRT). These treatments use small collimating leaves to selectively irradiate small sections of the treatment volume to create dose distributions that closely conform to the small sections and avoid very close normal structures. Because the whole volume requires treatment using many subvolumes, the total time the accelerator runs increases six times, on average. Thus, while this treatment approach spares the neighboring structures from high tissue doses, the absorbed dose in the whole patient from the leakage radiation increases. In general, while the integral absorbed dose for IMRT remains approximately the same as for conventional radiotherapy, IMRT exposes large volumes of the patient to moderate absorbed doses, compared with smaller volumes receiving high absorbed doses with conventional therapy.

4.6.4.2 *Imaging for Field Localization.* In the past, the tissue dose a patient received from radiographs required to localize the treatment volume was small compared with the treatment dose, and was limited to tissues close to the treatment site, exposing few other organs. As the precision of the radiotherapy treatments improves, imaging becomes more frequent and may use in-room or cone-beam CTs for daily positioning. While not approaching the absorbed dose in the treatment volume, CT increases the doses to neighboring structures.

4.6.5 *Trends over the Next Ten Years*

The two competing trends in radiotherapy discussed in Section 4.6.4 make prediction for the near future difficult. On one hand, image guidance and dynamic collimation has been, and will continue, to decrease the margin around targets and reduce the volume of the patient that receives high tissue doses. Often the tighter margins will lower the effective dose by reducing the tissue doses to neighboring organs. On the other hand, IMRT treatments tend to use more fields, and sometimes fields that continuously rotate around a patient over great lengths. IMRT treatments can deliver tissue doses to much of the patient that would not have received a significant tissue dose with conventional radiotherapy approaches. While the tissue doses outside of the target remain low compared with the prescribed treatment dose, they often are large compared with tissue doses received during imaging procedures.

Image guidance will continue to increase in use over the next 10 y. While some of the guiding imaging uses ultrasound, much uses x rays. The imaging component of effective dose, which has not been included in Table 4.17, will continue to increase.

4.6.6 *Summary*

In NCRP Report No. 93 (NCRP, 1987a), the following statement was made, "From the absorbed doses per organ outside of the field per unit of exposure given by the UNSCEAR (1982) and from estimates of the frequency of these treatments in the U.S., it seems likely that the individual annual H_E is below 0.01 mSv (1 mrem) for the U.S. population." Since that time more data are available concerning absorbed dose to organs and tissues outside the treatment volume, derived from measurement data and calculations.

In 2006, the effective dose estimate per radiotherapy patient (E_{Exp}) was high (0.4 Sv). The estimated annual collective effective dose was 350,000 person-Sv and E_{US} was 1.2 mSv, but the uncertainties are large. These values are comparable to those for diagnostic and interventional procedures. However, the population exposed is small (<0.3 % of the total U.S. population) and is a special group for whom high doses are necessary for treatment of their life-threatening disease. Also, absorbed doses to tissues or portions of tissues outside but nearby the treatment volumes could approach or exceed 1 Sv. Therefore, the inclusion of this source of exposure in the estimate of effective dose to the U.S. population may not be applicable. The estimates for external-beam radiotherapy are not included with the results for the other subcategories of medical exposure of patients.

4.7 Summary and Conclusions

Table 4.18 presents a summary of annual collective effective dose and E_{US} for 2006 from diagnostic and interventional medical procedures that use ionizing radiation. The values in Table 4.18 have been updated since the preliminary 2006 results in Mettler *et al.* (2008b). Figure 4.12 compares the percentage of collective dose (and E_{US}) due to medical exposure as reported in NCRP Report No. 100 (NCRP, 1989a) and in this Report. Table 4.19 presents the comparison in tabular form. Note there is not an analysis for E_{Exp} because the information used is for number of procedures performed rather than number of individuals exposed. A separate analysis for external-beam radiotherapy is given in Section 4.6 and presented in Table 4.17, but is not included in Table 4.18 or other summaries for S and E_{US} in this Report. A comparable analysis for nuclear-medicine therapy (Section 4.5.1) or for brachytherapy was not attempted.

NCRP (1989a) applies to doses in 1980 for radiography and in 1982 for nuclear medicine. The 2006 data in Table 4.19 clearly show the marked increase in collective dose and E_{US} in the ~25 y

Table 4.18—*Estimated number of procedures, S, and E_{US} for various categories of diagnostic and interventional procedures utilizing ionizing radiation for 2006.*[a]

Category	Number of Procedures (millions)	Number of Procedures (percent)	S (person-Sv)	E_{US} (mSv)	S and E_{US} (percent)
Computed tomography	67[b]	17	440,000	1.5	49
Conventional radiography and fluoroscopy	293[c]	74	100,000[d]	0.3	11
Interventional fluoroscopy	17	4	128,000	0.4	14
Nuclear medicine	18	5	231,000	0.8	26
Total	395	100	899,000	3.0	100

[a]Values have been updated since the preliminary 2006 results in Mettler *et al.* (2008b).
[b]In the case of CT, this is the number of CT scans (Section 4.2).
[c]Excludes dental bitewing and full-mouth procedures (see Footnote i of Table 4.7).
[d]Includes a small contribution (2,500 person-Sv) from dental bitewing and full-mouth procedures (see Footnote j of Table 4.7).

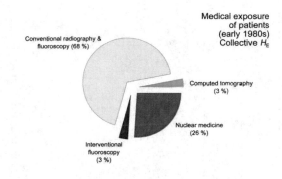

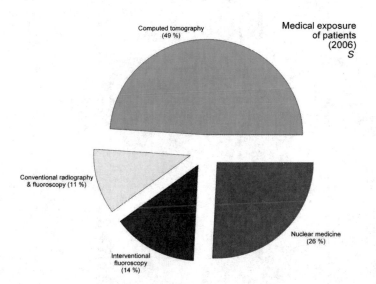

Fig. 4.12. Comparison of collective dose values for CT, conventional radiography and fluoroscopy, interventional fluoroscopy, and nuclear medicine (as percent of total collective dose) as reported for the early 1980s (123,700 person-Sv) (top) (NCRP, 1989a) and for 2006 (this Report) (899,000 person-Sv) (bottom). For E_{US}, the same percentages apply. Collective dose quantities are S for 2006 and collective H_E for NCRP (1989a) [see Table 4.19 for values of the collective dose quantities (person-sievert) and E_{US} (millisievert) for each period].

TABLE 4.19—*Comparison of annual values for E_{US} and collective dose as reported in NCRP Report No.100 (NCRP, 1989a) and in this Report for 2006.*

Procedure	1980/1982[a] (NCRP, 1989a)		2006 (this Report)		Ratio (2006) / (1980/1982)	
	E_{US} (mSv)	Collective H_E (person-Sv)[b]	E_{US} (mSv)	S (person-Sv)	E_{US}	Collective Dose
U.S. Population (millions)	(1980) 226.5 (1982) 231.6		300		1.32 1.30	
Computed tomography	0.016	3,660	1.47	440,000	92	120
Conventional radiography and fluoroscopy	0.36	83,700	0.33	100,000	0.9	1.2
Interventional fluoroscopy[c]	0.018	4,200	0.43	128,000	24	31
Nuclear medicine	0.14	32,100	0.77	231,000	5.5	7.2
Total	0.53	123,700	3.00	899,000	5.7	7.3

[a]Conventional radiography and fluoroscopy, CT, and interventional-fluoroscopic data apply to 1980; nuclear-medicine data apply to 1982.
[b]Values differ slightly from those reported in NCRP (1987a) and Tables 8.2 and 8.3.
[c]Noted as "Other" in NCRP (1989a).

between the two reports. Some of the increase in collective dose is due simply to the 30 % increase in population between 1980 to 1982 and 2006. Removing the effect of population growth leaves the increase in E_{US} that is due mostly to the higher utilization of various medical imaging modalities, particularly CT, nuclear medicine, and interventional fluoroscopy. Earlier CT systems had just become available before 1980, therefore the increase for CT accompanies its development as an essential modality in the modern practice of medicine. Likewise, interventional-fluoroscopic procedures did not become a significant modality until after 1980. The nuclear medicine increase of a factor of 5.5 in E_{US} is driven by nuclear cardiology, a procedure also in its infancy in 1982. Without nuclear cardiology, the number of nuclear-medicine procedures increased only by ~1,000 over 24 y, even though the U.S. population increased by 30 %. Use of conventional radiography and fluoroscopy decreased slightly over this time, reflecting the shift from this modality to CT and magnetic resonance imaging. Some particular radiographic examinations did increase, such as mammography, which was also just becoming accepted medical practice in 1980, and chest imaging, which as a screening tool for admissions may simply reflect an increase in the number of patients in the health care system. Thus, most of the increase in E_{US} for medical applications represents utilization of new tools since the assessment in NCRP (1989a).

5. Consumer Products and Activities

Thumbnail Sketch (for 2006) (rounded values):

- collective effective dose (S): 39,000 person-Sv
- effective dose per individual in the U.S. population (E_{US}): 0.1 mSv
  - percent of total S or E_{US} for the U.S. population (2 %)
- subcategories included (percent of total S and E_{US} for consumer products and activities)
  - cigarette smoking (35 %)
  - building materials (27 %)
  - commercial air travel (26 %)
  - mining and agriculture (6 %)
  - other sources (3 %) (Section 5.1)
  - combustion of fossil fuels (2 %)
  - highway and road construction materials (0.6 %)
  - glass and ceramics (<0.03 %)
  - television and video; sewage sludge and ash; self-illuminating signs (all negligible)
- average effective dose for the entire exposed category (E_{Exp}): not determined
  - variation in E_{Exp} among the included categories: 1 to 300 µSv (0.001 to 0.3 mSv)
- group characteristics: relatively large numbers of individuals, exposed to low doses

5.1 Introduction

An extensive discussion of radiation exposure from consumer products is contained in NCRP Report No. 95 (NCRP, 1987d). Much of that information is still relevant. In this Report exposures from some of the more significant sources have been updated and information is included about some additional sources. Potential sources that are not discussed further in this Report (refer to Table 5.1 of NCRP, 1987d) include:

- dental prostheses
- opthalmic glass
- luminous watches and clocks
- gas and aerosol (smoke) detectors
- electron tubes
- thorium products (including gas mantles and welding rods)

The estimated annual collective dose from these sources in NCRP Report No. 95 (NCRP, 1987d) was ~700 person-Sv. Adjusting for the 2006 population (300 million compared with 230 million), the estimated 2006 annual collective dose from these sources (referred to as "other sources" in this Report) is ~1,000 person-Sv.

This section covers exposure from television receivers and video terminals, sewage sludge and ash, radioluminous products, commercial air travel, tobacco products, glass and ceramics, building materials, and other miscellaneous sources (highway and road construction materials, mining and agriculture products, combustion of fossil fuels). Some of these sources of radiation are either few in number, or the resulting radiation doses are very low, and make a negligible if any contribution to collective dose, but may contribute a determinable dose to certain individuals.

There are no measured doses or dose rates for individuals or groups of individuals that can be used to estimate average or collective effective dose to the U.S. population from these sources. Consequently, one must rely primarily on measurements of activity or radionuclide concentrations associated with these sources, and uncertain assumptions that provide order-of-magnitude calculations of the low doses to the exposed population.

5.2 Television Receivers and Video Terminals

Television and display monitors currently utilize display technologies that no longer employ cathode-ray tube components (the source of x-ray emissions). Most of the radiation reported earlier from these sources (NCRP, 1987d) was from receivers manufactured before the federal performance standard (FDA, 2007c) (originally published in 1968) was issued. X-ray emissions from receivers manufactured under the standard are essentially zero. Technologies such as liquid crystal, plasma, and other such display monitors have no potential for generating x rays.

5.3 Sewage Sludge and Ash

Radionuclides may concentrate in sewage sludge and ash. NORM also may be concentrated from domestic and commercial water usage that depends on groundwater sources containing such radioactive material. Source, byproduct, and accelerator-produced radioactive material may also be concentrated from the regulated discharge of radionuclides into publicly-owned treatment works (POTW) from state, Agreement State, or NRC licensees. The Interagency Steering Committee on Radiation Standards (ISCORS) Sewage Sludge Subcommittee performed a national sewage sludge and ash survey for radionuclides (ISCORS, 2003), developed and performed modeling to assess the radiation doses from sewage sludge and ash (ISCORS, 2005a), and provided recommendations to POTW operators for determining whether the presence of radioactive material in sewage sludge or ash could pose a threat to the health and safety of POTW workers or members of the public (ISCORS, 2005b). With regard to radiation exposure, POTW workers are viewed for the purpose of this Report as being members of the public.

The levels of radioactive material reported in sewage sludge and ash (ISCORS, 2003) indicate that at most POTWs, radiation exposure to workers or to members of the public, including from land application of sludge for growing food crops, is very low and consequently is not likely to be a concern (ISCORS, 2005b).

Dose modeling was used to convert the radionuclide concentrations in the sewage sludge and ash to the total peak dose (TEDE) for several selected scenarios. A description of each scenario is provided in Table 5.1. These generic scenarios were developed to represent situations in which members of the public or POTW workers might be exposed to sewage sludge or ash through typical sludge management practices. The scenarios were intended to represent realistic situations that are likely to lead to conservative, but not worst-case, radiation exposure assessments (ISCORS, 2005a).

The sewage sludge and ash national survey results were used as the source for the dose calculations. For each scenario, the total dose corresponding to every sample was calculated using an upper-bound (95th percentile) conversion coefficient from concentration to dose. This means that there is only a 5 % chance that the conversion coefficient (dose-to-source ratio) would be higher than the one used in these calculations. For each scenario, the distribution of dose values obtained from the survey results was used to estimate the median and upper-bound doses. The median and upper-bound values of TEDE (both with and without the indoor radon contribution) are presented in Table 5.2.

These results are not representative of the typical exposure of members of the public from sewage sludge, since the original survey was biased toward POTWs that were suspected to have source

TABLE 5.1—*ISCORS selected sludge management scenarios (ISCORS, 2005a).*

Scenario Name	Description
Onsite resident	Inhabits a home built on land previously used for farming and amended with sludge-based fertilizer.
Recreational user	Occasionally spends time on land that was severely disturbed by mining or excavation, followed by a reclamation effort that included a single large application of sewage sludge and other soil additives.
Nearby-town resident	Lives in a town, the proximal edge of which is located ~0.8 km downwind and downstream from an agricultural field where sludge has been applied for one or more years.
Landfill/surface impoundment neighbor	Two subscenarios were designed for the study of the near-surface burial of sludge and ash: (1) a 1 hectare, 2 m deep municipal solid-waste landfill; and (2) a surface impoundment of the same dimensions. The house is sited 150 m from the boundary.
Incinerator neighbor	A member of the public residing near a typical sewage sludge incineration facility. The incinerator burns dewatered sludge on an ongoing basis.
Sludge application worker	Typically drives or works on a truck, tractor or other vehicle that dispenses liquid, dewatered, or dried sludge at a constant rate on fields.
POTW workers	Three tasks that are representative and that may give rise to slightly higher exposures to the sludge are: (1) sludge sampling and sample transport to the laboratory for analysis; (2) sludge transport on an open conveyor belt; and (3) biosolids loading operations (e.g., filling trucks with sludge using a front-end loader).

TABLE 5.2—*Calculated annual TEDE (millisievert) to an individual based on radionuclide concentration from survey samples.*[a]

Scenario/Sub-Scenario	Median Sample[b] (mSv)		Upper Bound (mSv)		Dominant Radionuclides (pathways)
	TEDE (with indoor radon)	TEDE (no indoor radon)	TEDE (with indoor radon)	TEDE (no indoor radon)	
Onsite resident[c]					
1 y of application	5×10^{-3}	2×10^{-3}	0.03	0.01	
5	0.03	0.01	0.1	0.05	^{226}Ra (indoor radon)
20	0.09	0.03	0.6	0.2	
Recreational user[d]	4×10^{-4}	—	2×10^{-3}	—	^{226}Ra (external)
Nearby-town resident[c,d]					
1 y of application	6×10^{-6}	—	3×10^{-5}	—	
5	3×10^{-5}	—	1×10^{-4}	—	^{226}Ra (outdoor radon)
20	9×10^{-5}	—	5×10^{-4}	—	
Landfill neighbor					
MSW[e] sludge	5×10^{-5}	2×10^{-5}	3×10^{-4}	1×10^{-4}	
MSW ash	1×10^{-4}	3×10^{-5}	4×10^{-4}	1×10^{-4}	^{226}Ra (indoor radon)
Impoundment	2×10^{-3}	6×10^{-4}	0.01	4×10^{-3}	

Incinerator neighbor[d]	0.01		0.08	—	Multiple (multiple)
Application worker[c,d]					
1 y of application	3×10^{-4}		2×10^{-3}	—	^{226}Ra (external)
5	2×10^{-3}		8×10^{-3}	—	
20	6×10^{-3}		0.03	—	
POTW[e] workers					
Sampling (per sample)	1×10^{-9}		5×10^{-9}	—	^{226}Ra (external)
Transport	5×10^{-7}	1×10^{-7}	2×10^{-6}	6×10^{-7}	^{228}Th (indoor radon)
Loading[f] (radon only)	0.04 – 0.2 (0.01 – 0.1)	0.03	0.2 – 0.7 (0.04 – 0.6)	0.1	^{226}Ra, ^{228}Th (indoor radon)

[a]Results with and without indoor radon contribution (using 95th percentile dose-to-source ratios) (ISCORS, 2005a; Wolbarst et al., 2006).

[b]95 % dose-to-source ratios are used in all total peak dose calculations. TEDE values rounded to one significant figure.

[c]Doses for 50 and 100 y of application may be found in ISCORS (2005a).

[d]Radon contribution not separately calculated.

[e] MSW = municipal solid waste

 POTW = publicly-owned treatment works.

[f]Range represents results for nine combinations of air-exchange rates and ceiling heights; ranges presented in parentheses are for the radon pathway only.

water that contained radionuclides. Additionally, the dose-to-source ratios that were used for the dose estimates were the 95th percentile. A review of Table 5.2 shows that the radiation associated with NORM was the dominant contributor to dose, primarily from indoor radon for the onsite resident, and exposure from ^{226}Ra for the POTW worker.

As a verification of the ISCORS modeling, NJDEP undertook studies of radionuclides in sewage sludge (NJDEP, 2006a; 2006b). The NJDEP study found that levels of ^{226}Ra and ^{228}Ra in sewage sludge at several POTWs where the groundwater is known to contain elevated levels of radium (Szabo and dePaul, 1998) were above the 95th percentile of the national sewage sludge survey. Since several of these POTWs apply their sludge to land, soil samples were taken to determine if there was any buildup of radium in the fields where the sludge had been applied for the past 10 y. The levels of naturally-occurring radionuclides in soil where sludge was sprayed onto the field were the same as those in an agricultural field where no sludge was applied. Both fields received irrigation and fertilizer applications.

Air sampling for radon was also performed indoors at several POTWs using E-Perm® detectors. All radon concentrations were <148 Bq m^{-3}. Gamma-radiation surveys performed at several POTWs using a Model 19 MicroR Meter® (Ludlum Measurements, Inc., Sweetwater, Texas) demonstrated that there were no areas of the POTWs where the dose rate was above the ambient background.

The NJDEP study showed that occupational and public exposures to radionuclides in sewage sludge from these selected POTW sites was not a major concern, even though these sites were expected to have higher than average levels of radionuclides. These POTW sites were selected because they were known to have had radium-bearing sewage sludge applied for at least 10 y. These data may not be representative of other regions of the country, but the New Jersey results demonstrate that the estimated dose to members of the public and POTW workers from typical sludge management practices is negligible. Using the results of the upper bound from Table 5.2 (ISCORS modeling), dose estimates (Table 5.3) were made for the four scenarios that had results above NCRP annual negligible individual dose (values >0.01 mSv) (NCRP, 1993a).

5.4 Radioluminous Products (Tritium)

Distribution of self-illuminating tritium exit signs and pathway lighting has increased significantly. They are used as a safety feature in aircraft and large buildings in the event of a power outage.

TABLE 5.3—*Upper-bound annual dose estimates for sewage sludge.*

Scenario	Number of People Exposed[a]	TEDE per Person Exposed (E_{Exp}) (mSv)	Collective TEDE (person-Sv)
Onsite resident (20 y of application)	375	0.6	0.2
Incinerator neighbor	6,250	0.08	0.5
Application worker (20 y of application)	1,531	0.03	0.05
POTW workers (loading)	2,580	0.2 – 0.7[b]	0.3 – 0.9

[a]DOL (2005), EPA (1999; 2003b), ISCORS (2003; 2005a), USCB (2005), and USDA (2001a; 2001b; 2003; 2006).
[b]Based on range of air exchange rates and ceiling heights.

They have a useful life of 15 to 20 y and do not require maintenance. The exit signs present no radiation hazard to members of the public under normal use since the weak beta particles emitted by tritium are easily absorbed by the material containing the tritium. Exit signs may nominally contain 925 GBq of tritium and are obtained and used under an NRC or Agreement State general license.

The Product Stewardship Institute used the NRC database of registered tritium exit signs to estimate that an average of 108,400 signs per year were registered between 1983 and 2002 (PSI, 2003). The average number of registrations has decreased since the peak production years of 1988 through 1992. NRC estimates that 73,980 signs were registered on a nationwide basis in 2004.[24]

The number of exit signs that are currently >15 y old is ~755,000. By 2010, that number will have increased to 1,500,000 signs. The manufacturers will take back and properly dispose of the exit signs, although the current owner of the sign may be unaware of the age of the sign or proper method of disposition. Two of the manufacturers quoted by the Product Stewardship Institute (PSI, 2003) stated that they typically recycle ·25 % of the number they produce annually. If this is a typical return rate, it appears that 75 % of the obsolete signs are either still in use or have been discarded as trash and now reside in local landfills.

[24]Kirkwood, A. (2007). Personal communication (U.S. Nuclear Regulatory Commission, Rockville, Maryland).

The Nuclear Materials Events Database (NRC, 2007b) for the time period 2001 to 2005 shows that in 2005, there were six reports of tritium exit signs involving landfills and three reports per year for the three previous years.

The Commonwealth of Pennsylvania has done extensive sampling of leachate from 54 landfills having leachate collection systems (PDEP, 2005). In 2004, 50 % of the Pennsylvania landfills were found to contain tritium at a concentration >0.74 MBq m^{-3} in the leachate (the applicable or relevant requirement for this liquid effluent) (PDEP, 2005). A follow-up study in 2005 found a mean concentration of 0.77 MBq m^{-3} for the 93 % of the landfills where tritium was present, with one leachate sample over 7.4 MBq m^{-3} (PDEP, 2006). The reports conclude that the probable source of the tritium is improperly disposed exit signs and postulates that once the signs are broken, the gaseous tritium is oxidized into tritiated water that is captured as leachate. The leachate is not for public consumption. It must be treated onsite or go to a publicly operated treatment system, and adequately diluted in the receiving body of water. The dose to a member of the public from this source is therefore projected to be minimal. With regard to radiation exposure, the landfill workers are viewed for the purpose of this Report as being members of the public.

Other luminous products such as watches and clocks that contain tritium or radium are sources of exposure for members of the public. Individual exposures related to products containing radium may be of the order of 1 mSv annually, but the number of individuals exposed is small. Consequently, the annual collective effective dose from radioluminous products is not likely to exceed 0.1 person-Sv.

5.5 Commercial Air Travel

Radiation from cosmic and solar sources during airline travel can be a significant source of exposure for the frequent flyer. A discussion of the dose rates encountered during airline travel is given in Section 7.3. Table 7.5 in Section 7.3 provides a list of domestic and international city pairs with respective altitude, airtime, and calculated E values for a one-way flight, and is applicable to both public airline travel (discussed here) and occupational exposure to airline crew members (Section 7.3). The lower dose rates in general represent low altitude, low latitude flights while the higher dose rates in general represent high altitude, high latitude flights. Frequent business flyers that travel standard routes can review Table 7.5 and calculate their annual doses by multiplying the number of trips per year times the E per flight.

Total annual doses depend on the flight route patterns, flying altitude, and the total number of flying hours per year. The Bureau of Transportation Statistics (BTS, 2008) reported that in 2006 there were 660.7 million passengers on domestic and 84.8 million passengers on international airline travel on U.S. carriers. Thus, 89 % of all passenger flights are domestic, with 11 % international. The data in Table 7.5 indicate that the average dose rate for domestic flights is 3.30 μSv per air hour (with a SD of 1.81 μSv per air hour) and the average air time is 2.84 h. The average dose rate for international flights is 5.21 μSv per air hour (with a SD of 0.94 μSv per air hour) and the average air time is 9.35 h. An estimate of annual S for all passengers is obtained as follows:

- $(660.7 \times 10^6$ passengers$)$ $(3.30 \times 10^{-3}$ mSv h$^{-1})$ $(2.84$ h$)$ $(1$ Sv per 1,000 mSv$) = 6{,}192$ person-Sv (for domestic flights); and
- $(84.8 \times 10^6$ passengers$)$ $(5.21 \times 10^{-3}$ mSv h$^{-1})$ $(9.35$ h$)$ $(1$ Sv per 1,000 mSv$) = 4{,}131$ person-Sv (for international flights).

The annual value of S for commercial air travel is estimated to be ~10,300 (10,323) person-Sv for 2006, the sum of the domestic and international values.

5.6 Tobacco Products

5.6.1 *Smoking Population*

Maurice *et al.* (2005) analyzed self-reported data from the 2004 National Health Interview Survey and found that ~21 % of adults (45 million) were current smokers. About 36 million smoked every day, while 8.3 million smoked some days. The prevalence of heavy smokers (>25 cigarettes per day) has dropped over the past 11 y from 19 to 12 % (5.4 million). In 1993 the mean number of cigarettes smoked per day in the United States was 20. In 2004 this number had decreased to about 17 (18 for men and 15 for women). It is assumed that the smoking population did not change significantly between 2004 and 2006.

5.6.2 *Radionuclides in Tobacco Leaves*

In the natural decay chain from ^{226}Ra, ^{210}Pb decays to ^{210}Po (Figure 3.2). Lead-210 and ^{210}Po have been measured in both tobacco leaves and cigarette smoke. These airborne decay products of ^{222}Rn can attach to sticky trichomes or "hairs" on both sides of the tobacco leaf while the plant is growing and while drying after harvesting. These radionuclides can also be taken up through the root system

(Tso *et al.*, 1964; 1966) from phosphate fertilizers containing uranium and soils rich in humic substances. There have been many reported measurements of the content of radium and its progeny in tobacco and cigarettes. Table 5.4 gives the concentrations of ^{226}Ra, ^{228}Ra, ^{210}Pb and ^{210}Po in tobacco and Table 5.5 gives the ranges and averages of ^{210}Po activity per cigarette. The average mass of tobacco per cigarette is 0.7 to 0.8 g. It is clear that there is significant variation in the radionuclide content in tobacco, but all the reported measurements are in substantial agreement.

5.6.3 *Radionuclides in Tobacco Smoke*

Black and Bretthauer (1968) found no enrichment of ^{210}Po in the butts of cigarettes. About 6 % was found in the inhaled mainstream smoke, 44 % in side-stream smoke, 16 % in ashes, and 34 % in the remaining cigarette butt. This distribution may vary depending on the puff size. Larger puffs could result in double the amount of ^{210}Po inhaled. They estimated 2.8 mBq per cigarette would be inhaled in mainstream smoke. Filters were found to remove 30 to 60 % of ^{210}Po from mainstream smoke. Desideri *et al.* (2007) found 8 to 29 % of the ^{210}Po was absorbed in filters. Khater (2004) found ~75 % of the ^{210}Po content of a cigarette was transferred to the smoke. Only ~5 % is removed by filters. Of the amount in smoke, he assumed that 50 % of the ^{210}Po and ^{210}Pb is inhaled during smoking. Skwarzec *et al.* (2001) found the ^{210}Po content of cigarette smoke ranged from 2 to 21 mBq (mean 10 mBq) per cigarette. Filters only removed ~2.5 % of the ^{210}Po on average.

Clearly there is significant variation in the various reported measurements and assumptions about the amount of ^{210}Po in cigarette smoke and the effectiveness of filters in removing it. Two of the more recent reports, Khater (2004) and Skwarzec *et al.* (2001), are in reasonably good agreement on the fraction of ^{210}Po in cigarette smoke (70 to 75 %), based on an average of 14 mBq per cigarette from Table 5.5, and the effectiveness of filters (2.5 to 5 %).

5.6.4 *Inhalation*

The coal temperature of a burning cigarette averages ~700 °C (Black and Bretthauer, 1968). When a cigarette burns, both ^{210}Po and ^{210}Pb will volatilize and then form insoluble particles. Cohen *et al.* (1980) showed that ^{210}Po accounts for most of the alpha-particle activity in cigarette smoke and is not readily soluble in physiological saline. Martell (1974) found ^{210}Pb to be highly enriched in the insoluble fraction of inhaled mainstream smoke. Inhalation of ^{210}Pb may also be a long-term source of ^{210}Po exposures (Savidou *et al.*, 2006). Khater (2004) determined that a one-

TABLE 5.4—*Radionuclides in tobacco.*

Reference	Source of Tobacco	Concentration (Bq kg^{-1})			
		^{226}Ra	^{228}Ra	^{210}Pb	^{210}Po
Godoy et al. (1992)	Brazil	2 – 17		11 – 27	4 – 46
Black and Bretthauer (1968)	United States				18
	10 other countries				7 – 22
Skwarzec et al. (2001)	Worldwide				3 – 37
Abd El-Aziz et al. (2005)	Egypt	7		16	13
Hill (1965)	7 countries				8 – 25
Peres and Hiromoto (2002)	Brazil			11 – 30	11 – 30
Papastefanou (2007)	Greece	2 – 8	1 – 7	6 – 18	
Savidou et al. (2006)	Greece			7 – 18	4 – 17

TABLE 5.5—*Polonium-210 in cigarettes.*

Reference	Source of Tobacco	^{210}Po Content in a Single Cigarette (mBq)	
		Range	Average
Khater (2004)	Egypt	10 – 22	17
	Other countries[a]	4 – 23	
Khater and Al-Sewaidan (2006)	Saudi Arabia	6 – 22	14
	21 other countries	8 – 23	14
Skwarzec *et al.* (2001)	Poland	4 – 24	13
Desideri *et al.* (2007)		7 – 14	12

[a]Popular brands from other countries sold in Egypt.

pack-a-day smoker would inhale 120 mBq d^{-1} each of ^{210}Po and ^{210}Pb. Desideri *et al.* (2007) estimated that at 20 cigarettes per day a smoker would inhale 80 ± 30 mBq d^{-1} each of ^{210}Po and ^{210}Pb. Skwarzec *et al.* (2001) found that Polish smokers inhaled from 20 to 215 mBq of ^{210}Po and ^{210}Pb each for 20 cigarettes a day. Roessler and Guilmette (2007) estimated that 1.8 mBq ^{210}Po is inhaled with each cigarette, which is in the lower portion of the range reported by Skwarzec *et al.* (2001). From these data 100 mBq d^{-1} for each radionuclide, ^{210}Po and ^{210}Pb, is a reasonable estimate for intake for a one-pack-a-day smoker.

When inhaled these radionuclides will result in exposure to tissues of the bronchial epithelium, similar to inhalation of short-lived decay products of ^{222}Rn, or they could be slowly dissolved in the lung and carried to other parts of the body.

5.6.5 *Deposition*

A portion of the radionuclides inhaled with tobacco smoke will be retained in lung tissue. Khater (2004) estimated that ~50 % of the ^{210}Po inhaled is retained in the smoker's lungs. Roessler and Guilmette (2007) estimated that ~20 % of the ^{210}Po deposits in the lung. Similar or greater fractions of inhaled ^{210}Pb are likely to be retained in the smoker's lungs, especially if the ^{210}Pb is less soluble than the ^{210}Po. These radionuclides may concentrate at bifurcations of the segmental bronchi (Martonen *et al.*, 1987).

Cohen *et al.* (1980) found a statistically-significant excess of ^{210}Po in the alveoli of smokers compared with nonsmokers. Elevated levels of ^{210}Pb were found in alveolar tissues from former smokers who had not smoked for >5 y. Thus, the radiation dose from ^{210}Pb and ^{210}Po could continue for many years after cessation of smoking.

5.6.6 Organ Doses

For the inhalation pathway the primary determinant of the absorbed-dose pattern will be the in vivo solubility of the inhaled ^{210}Po and ^{210}Pb. Roessler and Guilmette (2007) calculated the absorbed doses that would result from an inhalation intake of 1 MBq ^{210}Po. At 30 d after intake, the absorbed doses for an inhaled Type-F compound (ICRP, 1995) (fast rate of solubility or release from lung tissue) would be 3.8 mGy for the lung, 137 mGy for the kidney, 71 mGy for the liver, 28 mGy for the active bone marrow, and 118 mGy for the spleen. In comparison, for a Type-S compound (ICRP, 1995) (slow rate of solubility or release from lung tissue), the 30 d absorbed doses would be, for the same tissues, 873, 1.5, 0.8, 0.3, and 1.3 mGy, respectively. The in vivo solubility greatly affects the partitioning of absorbed dose between the lung and systemic target organs. The systemic target organs for ^{210}Po are relatively well known, as there have been a significant number of published animal studies on inhaled, ingested and injected ^{210}Po and absorption through skin (Fink; 1950; Moroz and Parfenov, 1972; Stannard, 1988).

5.6.7 Effective Dose

To determine the total E, one has to consider the direct deposition of energy from radionuclides retained in bronchial epithelium along with the dose to various organs from both ^{210}Pb and ^{210}Po that may be slowly absorbed and carried to other parts of the body (Section 5.4.5). A number of investigators have used dose conversion coefficients from ICRP Publication 72 (ICRP, 1996) to estimate E for smokers. The values calculated for E have been normalized to one cigarette per day and are given in Table 5.6.

Papastefanou (2007) estimated the annual values of E for 30 cigarettes a day from ^{226}Ra, ^{228}Ra, and ^{210}Pb, and stated that E from ^{210}Po should be the same order of magnitude as from ^{210}Pb. He also provided the sum for E for the three natural radionuclides. Peres and Hiromoto (2002) assumed that 10 % of the ^{210}Pb and 20 % of the ^{210}Po in a cigarette are inhaled for their estimated annual value for E for a one-pack-a-day smoker. Skwarzec et al. (2001) estimated annual values for E for ^{210}Po and for ^{210}Pb for smokers in Poland.

Desideri et al. (2007) assumed 50 % retention in the lung and estimated the annual value for E for 17 cigarette brands at 20 cigarettes a day. Khater and Al-Sewaidan (2006) also estimated annual values of E from smoking 20 cigarettes a day.

TABLE 5.6—*Annual effective dose (microsievert) for one cigarette per day.*

Reference	E (µSv)					
	^{226}Ra	^{228}Ra	^{210}Pb	^{210}Po	Range	Average
Papastefanou (2007)	1.3 – 6.7	0.6 – 3.3	1.7 – 4.3	1.7 – 4.3	5.0 – 13.3	8.3
Peres and Hiromoto (2002)					6.0 – 20	8.0
Skwarzec et al. (2001)			3.5	1.7		
Desideri et al. (2007)					7.5 – 25	16.3[a]
Khater and Al-Sewaidan (2006)					20 – 35	27.5[a]
Derived from Roessler and Guilmette (2007)					—	30
Overall average						18

[a]Assumed as midpoint of range.

Using the estimate of absorbed dose to the lung from Roessler and Guilmette (2007) of 873 mGy in the first 30 d following an inhalation of 1 MBq of ^{210}Po and a Type-S compound, the annual value of E is estimated at ~30 µSv for one cigarette per day using a value of 14 mBq inhaled per cigarette.

Based on these reports, the annual E for a one-pack-a-day smoker (20 cigarettes) would range from 0.1 to 0.7 mSv with an average of 0.36 mSv. An estimate of S for the U.S. adult population is given in Table 5.7 based on a smoking population of 45 million adults (Section 5.6.1) and an average annual E of 18 µSv for one cigarette per day (Table 5.6).

5.6.8 Additional Impacts of Cigarette Smoking

Studies by Johnson *et al.* (1990; 1991) and Abu-Jarad and Fazal-ur-Rehman (2003) show that indoor cigarette smoking is a major source of aerosol particles carrying radon progeny. Martell (1974) also concluded that polonium and lead atoms adhere to smoke particles and remain suspended in room air to be breathed by smoker and nonsmoker alike. These results indicate that everyone in the home of a smoker is not only subject to direct, side-stream, or second-hand smoke, but they are also exposed to radon decay products attached to cigarette smoke. However, no information is available to estimate a dose from this exposure.

5.7 Glass and Ceramics

5.7.1 Uranium as a Coloring Agent in Glassware

Makers of glassware have used many materials to produce different colors. After his discovery of uranium dioxide in 1789, Martin Kapworth began experimenting with this new element as a

TABLE 5.7—*Annual collective effective dose (S) from cigarettes.*

	Cigarettes (d^{-1})	E per Smoker (mSv)	Smokers (millions)	S (person-Sv)
Men	18	0.09 – 0.6 Average = 0.32	25	2,250 – 15,000 8,100
Women	15	0.08 – 0.5 Average = 0.27	20	1,600 – 10,000 5,400
Total				13,500 (14,000)

coloring agent for glass (Emsley, 2003). In 1830 Josef Reidel set up a factory to make yellow uranium glass (Annagelb) and yellow-green uranium glass (Annagruen) named after his wife Anna Maria (Frame and Kolb, 2005). By the 1840s uranium dioxide (as bright yellow sodium diuranate) was commonly used with lead additives by glassmakers in Europe and the United States to produce a transparent, pale-yellow glass called canary glass. During and following the Civil War uranium dioxide was added to soda glass up to 2 % by weight to produce yellow to yellowish-green colors. In the early 1900s a new petroleum ointment [Vaseline© (Unilever PLC, London)] came on the market with the same coloration as uranium glass and the name Vaseline glass became popular. During the 1920s low-cost green glass was produced with uranium dioxide and iron additives which today is commonly called depression glass.

Uranium was very abundant in the period 1910 to 1940 and ~50 different companies in the United States used natural uranium oxides for glass coloring in tableware and decorative and ornamental items. Production of these items, however, came to an end around 1943. Very limited production began again around 1959 with the use of depleted uranium as a coloring agent. Currently about five to six companies in the United States and the Czech Republic continue to produce decorative uranium glass in jewelry items, perfume bottles, marbles, and decorative figurines. Uranium is no longer used in dinnerware. Buckley *et al.* (1980), based on data from 1958 to 1978, estimated that in the past ~200,000 pieces of uranium glassware were made per year. Current production figures are not known. However, most uranium glassware is considered a collector item and used only for displays in homes, shops and museums.

5.7.2 *Potential Radiation Exposures from Uranium in Glassware*

Current NRC regulations (in effect since January 1961) allow glassware to contain up to 10 % by weight of uranium as an exempt quantity (NRC, 2007c). Since uranium is blended with glass ingredients during smelting it becomes uniformly distributed throughout the glass. Thus, much of the radiation emitted by uranium is absorbed within the glass. Possible exposures include beta-particle irradiation from handling the glassware, beta-particle and gamma-ray irradiation while near the glassware, and ingestion of uranium that may be leached from the glass into water or food. Each of these potential exposures was evaluated by Schneider *et al.* (2001) as described below. The quantity effective dose equivalent (H_E) as formulated in ICRP (1977) was determined for different scenarios.

A person routinely handling glassware at home with 10 % uranium by weight for a year would receive an H_E estimated at 20 μSv. Other family members in the same home could receive an annual H_E of 10 μSv. For 500 families of four (each family using one set of uranium drinking glasses) the annual collective H_E would be 0.03 person-Sv. If 100 decorative pieces with 5 % by weight of uranium were on display in 1,000 public facilities, the annual collective H_E would be ~5 person-Sv. Schneider et al. (2001) estimated that the most exposed individual would likely be an express-delivery truck driver handling 20,000 cartons of decorative items (with 5 % uranium) a year. The calculated highest annual individual H_E for this person could be 0.04 mSv. The annual collective H_E for all distribution activities is estimated to be ~0.5 person-Sv.

Based on studies by Landa and Councell (1992), NRC estimated that ingestion of uranium leached from glassware by water and acids could result in an individual annual H_E of ~20 μSv. All of NRC H_E estimates were based on uranium glass at 5 to 10 % by weight, whereas most pieces of uranium glass contain only a few tenths of a percent of uranium.

5.7.3 Uranium as a Coloring Agent in Ceramics

During the late 1930s ~30 different companies in the United States used uranium oxide (sodium diuranate) as a coloring agent in the glaze on ceramic dinnerware, such as plates, dishes, bowls, cups and saucers. Uranium oxide when fired at high temperatures produces an orange or red coloring that became very popular. Perhaps the best known line of dinnerware using uranium oxide glaze, called Fiesta® (Fiesta Red®), was first produced in 1936 by the Homer Laughlin China Company of Newell, West Virginia. Fiesta Red® was produced with a natural uranium-oxide glaze from 1936 to 1943, the year the government confiscated all uranium supplies. Production of Fiesta Red® began again in 1959 using depleted uranium and continued as Mango Red® from 1969 until 1972. The use of uranium as a coloring agent was discontinued in the 1970s. Current regulations of NRC allow up to 20 % by weight of uranium in glazed ceramics (NRC, 2007c), although apparently ~14 % was the most ever used. Buckley et al. (1980) estimated that a plate could contain 4.5 g of uranium, and Piesch et al. (1986) reported a red-glaze thickness of 0.2 mm.

Buckley et al. (1980) estimated that ~200,000 pieces of uranium-glazed dinnerware were produced each year from 1959 to 1969. Although many of these pieces may still be in use, today they are considered antique collectibles and mostly displayed as such.

5.7.4   *Potential Radiation Exposures from Uranium Glaze on Ceramic Dinnerware*

Unlike the use of uranium oxides for coloring within glassware, uranium glaze is only on the surface of the ceramic and thus there is no inherent shielding of radiation. Persons handling or near uranium-glazed ceramics could be exposed to beta particles or gamma rays (external exposure). Moghissi *et al.* (1978) reported that contact with a typical dinner place setting of uranium-glazed dishes could result in an absorbed-dose rate of 130 µGy h^{-1}. Sitting at the table with these items could result in 30 µGy h^{-1} to the hands and arms, and 3 µGy h^{-1} to the main torso. Buckley *et al.* (1980) reported that absorbed-dose rates at the surface of glazed plates ranged from 4 to 130 µGy h^{-1}. The surface of a red-glazed teacup gave an absorbed-dose rate of 320 µGy h^{-1} according to Piesch *et al.* (1986). Measurements by McCormick (1992) on a variety of Fiesta Ware® items found absorbed-dose rates of 20 to 90 µGy h^{-1}. Schneider *et al.* (2001) estimated that a person handling a 25 cm glazed dinner plate containing 20 % by weight of 20 y old natural uranium would receive an absorbed dose to skin of 240 µGy h^{-1} from beta particles. Based on the range of these data and a w_T value of 0.01 for skin, the H_E rate at contact would be expected to vary from 0.04 to 3.2 µSv h^{-1}. The gamma-ray absorbed-dose rate from uranium-glazed plates is ~10 % of that for beta particles.

In addition, if a person consumes only liquids that have been in contact with uranium-glazed ceramics, this person could receive an annual H_E of 400 µSv from ingestion of leached uranium (Schneider *et al.*, 2001). A homemaker who stays at home, and spends much time in the kitchen washing and eating from uranium-glazed dinnerware could receive an annual H_E as much as 70 µSv. Others in the same household could receive an annual H_E up to 60 µSv (Schneider *et al.*, 2001).

The annual collective H_E for all handling of uranium-glazed dinnerware in distribution and sales is estimated to be about the same as for glassware, 0.5 person-Sv. Almost all uranium-glazed dinnerware is used only for display as antique collector's items. From the contact dose rates stated above, the dose at 1 m will range from 0.004 to 0.32 µSv h^{-1}. If the average person spends 15 min y^{-1} viewing the piece and 1 % of the U.S. population is exposed to this source, the annual collective H_E will range from 0.003 to 0.24 person-Sv. These dose estimates are based on use of uranium up to the exempt limit of 20 % by weight, whereas the highest concentration reported in actual pieces of tableware is only 14 %.

5.7.5 *Summary*

The annual H_E to an individual exposed to glassware or ceramic dinnerware containing uranium varies greatly according to use. Estimated values for annual collective H_E for various exposure scenarios are given below:

- glassware
  - home use: 0.03 person-Sv
  - public display: 5 person-Sv
  - distribution: 0.5 person-Sv
- ceramics
  - home use: 0.04 person-Sv (primarily from ingestion)
  - public display: 0.003 to 0.2 person-Sv
  - distribution: 0.5 person-Sv

The total is <10 person-Sv.

5.8 Building Materials

NCRP Report No. 95 (NCRP, 1987d) gave estimates of the radio-active-material concentrations in common building materials and estimates of the annual dose to individuals exposed to these materials. The information was summarized in Table 5.1 in NCRP Report No. 93 (NCRP 1987a). Radiation doses to individuals living and working in buildings constructed of these common materials have not changed since the previous reports. However, since those reports were published, coal combustion products (CCPs) which include both fly ash and bottom ash generated from coal-fired utilities, have become widely used in construction materials. The quantity of CCPs produced in 2002 in the United States was 128.7 million tons (76.5 million tons of fly ash, 19.8 million tons of bottom ash, 29.2 million tons of flue gas desulfurization materials, and 1.9 million tons of boiler ash) (ACAA, 2002). In 2002, 35.4 % of CCPs were used in cement, concrete, grout and other applications (ACAA, 2002). This percentage is expected to increase as research demonstrates the advantages of using these materials and the costs of depositing CCPs in landfills increases.

Coal contains numerous naturally-occurring radionuclides including uranium and thorium. Coal ash has concentrations of uranium, thorium and radium ~10 times higher than coal, due to burning off the organic content of the coal (UNSCEAR, 1993; USGS, 1997). Analysis of fly ash in the United States found ^{226}Ra within the range of 37 to 296 Bq kg^{-1} (EPA, 1983; Zielinski and Budahn, 1998). Analysis of fly ash from Wisconsin Electric Power Company and Wisconsin Gas LLC (We Energies) plants in 1993 and 2003 found ^{226}Ra concentrations in the range of 37 to 111 Bq kg^{-1} (Ramme and Tharaniyil, 2004), comparable to concentrations found in soil (7.4 to 111 Bq kg^{-1}). The annual individual dose to persons living in buildings in which ash was used in the building materials has been estimated to be 135 µSv, similar to calculations made for individuals living in a brick and masonry home (NCRP, 1987d; Smith *et al.*, 2001). Consequently, it is assumed that the use of CCP in building materials has not substantially increased the average dose to an individual in the population residing in a building constructed with brick or masonry materials. It is also assumed that approximately one-half the population of the United States resides in homes constructed of wood, which adds no additional radiation dose. The collective dose given in NCRP Report No. 93 (NCRP, 1987a) has been updated using the average H_E given there (70 µSv) and adjusting for the population of the United States in 2006 (*i.e.*, assumes a currently exposed population of 150 million) (Table 5.8). The use of zircon-glazed tiles and fixtures (tubs, toilets and sinks), granite countertops, desktops, wall and floor tiles, and marble in housing construction could add a small additional collective dose, which has not been included in the above estimate.

5.9 Other Minor Contributors

5.9.1 *Highway and Road Construction Materials*

Highway and road construction materials may contain aggregates made from granite and phosphates that have higher than average concentrations of uranium and thorium and now may also contain CCPs (Section 5.8). Although the maximum dose to individuals in some areas may be an order of magnitude greater than the average dose (EPA, 1990; Schneider *et al.*, 2001), it is assumed that the average dose to individuals traveling on highways has not changed since the previous report (NCRP, 1987a). The collective dose contained in that report has been updated considering the current population of the United States (*i.e.*, assuming a currently exposed population of six million) (Table 5.8).

5.9.2 *Mining and Agricultural Products*

Fertilizers containing phosphates and sulphates contain trace elements of several naturally-occurring radionuclides, principally

TABLE 5.8—*Summary of number of people exposed, average annual effective dose to an exposed individual (E_{Exp}), and annual collective effective dose (S) for consumer products and activities.*

Source	Number of People Exposed (millions)	E_{Exp} (μSv)	S (person-Sv)	Percent of Total S
Cigarette smoking	45	300	13,500	34.6
Building materials	150	70	10,500	27.0
Commercial air travel	—[a]		10,300	26.4
Mining and agriculture	250	10	2,500	6.4
Other sources[b]	—	—	1,000	2.6
Combustion of fossil fuels				
Natural gas cooking	155	4	620	1.6
Coal	300	1	300	0.8
Highway and road construction materials	6	40	240	0.6
Glass and ceramics	—	—	<10	<0.03
			Total = 38,970 (39,000)	

[a]Based on total number of passengers (Section 5.5); number of different individuals not available.

[b]Dental prostheses, opthalmic glass, luminous watches and clocks, gas and aerosol (smoke) detectors, electron tubes, and thorium products (including gas mantles and welding rods).

decay products of uranium and thorium, and ^{40}K. The use of these materials and the associated radiation exposure has not changed since the previous report (NCRP, 1987a). Other byproducts and waste products from phosphate mining were discussed in the previous report and there is no new information about radiation doses from these sources. The collective dose contained in that report has been updated considering the current population of the United States (Table 5.8) (*i.e.*, assuming a currently exposed population of 250 million).

5.9.3 *Combustion of Fossil Fuels*

Coal contains numerous naturally-occurring radionuclides including uranium and thorium. Coal ash (the noncombustible residue remaining when coal is burned) has concentrations of uranium, thorium and radium ~10 times higher than unburned coal, due to burning off the organic content of the coal (UNSCEAR, 1993; USGS, 1997).

NCRP (1987a; 1987d) reported that the estimated annual radiation dose to an individual exposed to the emissions from coal burning ranged from 0.3 to 3 µSv. Since then additional information has been published concerning the radionuclide content of CCPs and the potential radiation dose resulting from exposure to these products.

Analysis of fly ash in the United States found ^{226}Ra within the range of 37 to 296 Bq kg^{-1} (EPA, 1983; Zielinski and Budahn, 1998). Analysis of fly ash from We Energies plants in 1993 and 2003 found ^{226}Ra concentrations in the range of 37 to 111 Bq kg^{-1} (Ramme and Tharaniyil, 2004), comparable to concentrations found in soil (7.4 to 111 Bq kg^{-1}). The maximum annual dose determined from this evaluation was 1.5 µSv for a person living within 500 m of a plant stack releasing fly ash to the air, within the dose range reported in 1987. The collective dose contained in NCRP Report No. 93 (NCRP, 1987a) has been updated considering the current population (300 million) of the United States (Table 5.8) and assuming an annual average dose of 1 µSv.

Combustion of natural gas will release radioactive radon gas to the atmosphere. This additional source of radon can result in a small increment of exposure to people residing near gas-fired power plants or using natural gas for cooking or heating in their homes. NCRP (1987a) reported the average annual dose to an individual whose exposure resulted from cooking with gas as 4 µSv. Exposure from combustion of gas in power plants would be much less. There has been little additional information published on this source of exposure since NCRP (1987a; 1987d). The radiation dose estimates contained in those publications and summarized in Table 5.1 of NCRP (1987a) have been adjusted for the current dose conversion coefficients and weighting factors for radon dose estimation as described in Section 3 and for the current U.S. population and are given in Table 5.8 (*i.e.*, assuming a currently exposed population of 155 million).

5.10 Summary

As summarized in Table 5.8, the annual collective effective doses for the various consumer products and activities were: cigarette smoking, 13,500 person-Sv (35 %); building materials, 10,500 person-Sv (27 %); commercial air travel, 10,300 person-Sv (26 %); mining and agriculture, 2,500 person-Sv (6 %); other sources, 1,000 person-Sv (3 %); combustion of fossil fuels, 920 person-Sv; (2 %); highway and road construction materials, 240 person-Sv (0.6 %); and glass and ceramics, <10 person-Sv (<0.03 %). The distribution of the annual collective effective dose among these consumer products and activities is shown in Figure 5.1.

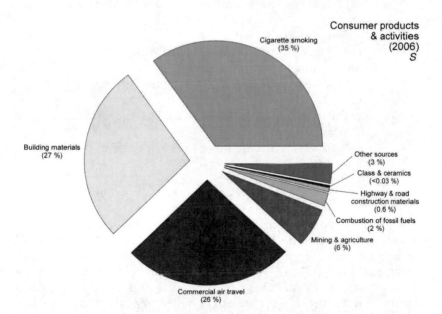

Fig. 5.1. Percent contribution of various sources of exposure to S for consumer products and activities (39,000 person-Sv) for 2006. Percent values have been rounded to the nearest 1 %, except for those <1 % [see Table 5.8 for the values of S (person-sievert)].

6. Industrial, Security, Medical, Educational and Research Activities

Thumbnail Sketch (for 2006) (rounded values):

- collective effective dose (S): 1,000 person-Sv
- effective dose per individual in the U.S. population (E_{US}): 0.003 mSv
  - percent of total S or E_{US} for the U.S. population (<0.1 %)
- subcategories included (percent of S and E_{US} for industrial, security, medical, educational and research activities)
  - exposure from nuclear-medicine patients (72 %)
  - nuclear-power generation (15 %)
  - industrial, medical, educational and research activities (13 %)
  - DOE installations («1 %)
  - decommissioning and radioactive waste («1 %)
  - security inspection systems («1 %)
- average effective dose for the exposed group (E_{Exp}): not determined
  - magnitude of E_{Exp} for the included categories: 1 to 10 µSv (0.001 to 0.01 mSv)
- group characteristics: members of the public in proximity to these activities

6.1 Introduction

For the purposes of this Report, industrial, security, medical, educational and research activities are those that use sources of radiation or radioactive material intentionally or produce sources as byproducts of these activities. Examples of such activities include: the nuclear fuel cycle; manufacture and use of radioactive sources and irradiators for sterilization, radiography, and materials processing; DOE facilities; radioactive waste transport and disposal; security inspection; and medical procedures such as in nuclear medicine and radiology. This section discusses exposure to members of the public from these sources. Exposure of the workers

171

employed in these activities is covered in Section 7. Exposure of patients in medicine is covered in Section 4.

There are no measured doses or dose rates for individuals or groups of individuals that can be used to estimate average or collective effective dose to the U.S. population from these sources. Consequently, one must rely primarily on measurements of activity or radionuclide concentrations associated with these sources and calculations of dose to the exposed population. The assumptions required for this purpose introduce significant uncertainties, but because the doses are quite low, the uncertainties do not alter the relative order of magnitude of the doses.

Two previous NCRP reports, Report No. 92 (NCRP, 1987c) and Report No. 93 (NCRP, 1987a) provide important background for population exposures from sources in this category.

6.2 Nuclear-Power Generation

6.2.1 *Introduction*

Operation of nuclear-power plants results in the irradiation of some members of the public from releases of radionuclides to the atmosphere and to bodies of water, and from direct gamma radiation emitted from those facilities. Various regulations promulgated by EPA and NRC require that releases of radionuclides and direct radiation exposure be controlled to very low levels. The goal is to limit radiation dose to an individual outside the boundary of the power plant to a small fraction of the dose received from naturally-occurring sources of radiation. The air- and water-borne radionuclides that are released deliver radiation doses by various pathways such as external exposure, intake from breathing or drinking, and intake of foods contaminated by these radionuclides. The most exposed persons are usually those in the immediate vicinity of a facility, and in the following discussion, the dose to the regional population within 80 km will be specified.

The entire fuel cycle must be considered in evaluating the radiation dose due to nuclear-power production. In the United States, the nuclear fuel cycle consists of uranium mining, uranium milling, uranium hexafluoride production, ^{235}U enrichment, uranium oxide fuel fabrication, power production, fuel reprocessing, and low- and high-level radioactive waste management. Some radiation exposure to members of the public occurs near facilities engaged in each of these fuel-cycle components, and also during transportation of radioactive material between the facilities. In the United States, the fuel cycle is focused almost entirely on the operation of light-water moderated reactors, specifically boiling water reactors (BWRs) and pressurized water reactors (PWRs). The fuel cycle for power generation in the United States is not complete because there is no commercial fuel reprocessing, and no permanent disposal for spent fuel yet in operation. Spent-fuel elements are now stored in special facilities (spent-fuel pools and dry casks) at nuclear-power plant sites.

Uranium is also mined, milled and enriched for purposes of the military along with any fuel reprocessing and high-level waste storage necessary to support the military fuel cycle.

Low-level radioactive waste from the nuclear industry and other sources (*e.g.*, medical applications) are shipped to designated sites for shallow land burial. There are two disposal facilities that accept a broad range of low-level waste. They are located in Barnwell, South Carolina, and Richland, Washington. In addition, Energy Solutions of Utah is licensed by NRC to operate a facility near Clive, Utah, for disposal of uranium and thorium mill tailings. The facility also accepts certain other radioactive waste under a State of Utah license.

Four former low-level radioactive waste-disposal sites are closed and no longer accept waste. They are located in or near Sheffield, Illinois; Morehead, Kentucky; Beatty, Nevada; and West Valley, New York.

6.2.2 *Sources of Data*

Nonoccupational radiation exposures from the nuclear fuel cycle are calculated for those persons judged to be exposed to the highest dose and for the population within 80 km of a facility. Beyond this distance, exposures are too small to warrant consideration. Data to calculate public exposures are obtained by facility operators in response to requirements by the regulatory agencies EPA and NRC, or by DOE, which are responsible for some of these facilities. A typical approach is to monitor or estimate annual radionuclide releases to air and to water, consider the various pathways by which persons may be exposed, and calculate the doses using selected computational models. Environmental radiological monitoring is performed, among other reasons, to ensure that regulatory limits are not exceeded. Direct exposure to radiation is monitored by detectors at the site boundary.

6.2.3 *Special Considerations*

In this section, the effective dose equivalent (H_E) is determined from the dose equivalent rates to various body organs resulting from the release of radionuclides to air, water and *via* the food chain (NCRP, 1987c). This permits comparison of maximum exposures and collective H_E among the various phases of the fuel cycle. However, the dose values were not derived by uniform methods for each phase of the fuel cycle. There were differences in the amount of effort expended in determining radionuclide release rates and radiation exposure rates, in the calculational models used to estimate individual and collective H_E, and in computation at the point of exposure of doses from calculated radionuclide concentrations. H_E is determined based on a dose commitment of 50 y.

6.2.4 *Estimates and Discussion*

Annual radiation dose estimates for public exposures from nuclear-power generation were presented in NCRP Report No. 92 (NCRP, 1987c). Sources of information were DOE, EPA and NRC compilations and selections of available effluent and dose reports by facility operators. In some instances, a range of values was given and a typical value selected. In other instances, a model facility was assumed, based on the range of operating characteristics and a model transportation network. Estimates were presented for annual doses to maximally-exposed individuals (MEIs) due to airborne effluents (doses due to liquid effluents were generally much lower), annual collective H_E, and annual collective H_E per nuclear-power plant (normalized to 1 GWe power production operating during 80 % of the year). The information for these estimates is given in Table 6.1.

The essence of the data in NCRP Report No. 92 (NCRP, 1987c) is that both maximum individual and collective H_E values from the nuclear fuel cycle are relatively low. Among the highest annual H_E values to MEIs (NCRP, 1987c) are:

- values up to 2.6 mSv for milling, but much smaller values apply to some mills;
- values up to 0.6 mSv due to uranium mining; and
- a value of 0.2 mSv due to transporting radioactive material, for which it was assumed that the amount of radionuclides and the exposure rates were at the maximum level within compliance, although, in practice, much lower exposures are usually experienced.

The annual collective H_E per model nuclear-power plant from the entire fuel cycle was estimated to be 1.36 person-Sv, with an estimated 69 % of this value from mining, and an additional 18 %

TABLE 6.1—*Summary of annual collective H_E to the regional population normalized to a 1 GWe reactor operating at full capacity 80 % of the time (i.e., 0.8 GWe).*

Facility	Annual Collective H_E (person-Sv)	Basis of Estimate
Mining	0.94	Weighted for 2 types of model mines [1/2 (open pit) + 3 (underground)]
Milling	0.25	0.4 (model mill)
Conversion	0.0003	Weighted for 2 plants (65 % wet)
Enrichment	0.0001	Paducah plus Oak Ridge
Fabrication	0.00004	Weighted for 7 plants
Nuclear-power plants	0.048	1980 data for 47 plants
Low-level waste storage	—	No estimate available
Transportation		
Incident-free	0.071	Excludes decommissioning waste
Accidents	0.054	
Total per 0.8 GWe	1.36	
Total for 90 GWe (estimated 2006 production)	153	

from milling (Table 6.1). This value was calculated based on information in the early 1980s, when there were a number of active uranium mines in the United States (Blanchard *et al.*, 1983). Mining for uranium was discontinued in the United States for a time. However, recent energy and economic conditions have changed such that uranium mining is again becoming active. Figure 6.1 shows the locations of uranium mines and mills in the United States as of the end of 2005 (EPA, 2007b). There is also renewed interest in uranium recovery using *in situ* leaching of ore bodies (NRC, 2008).

While an updated calculation of the collective effective dose from the uranium fuel cycle has not been performed, the previous calculation (NCRP, 1987c) can be considered a high estimate based

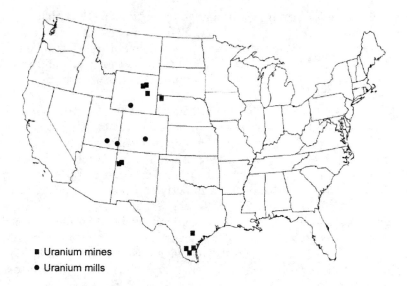

Fig. 6.1. Location of uranium mines and mills in the United States as of November 2005 (EPA. 2007b).

on the current substantially lower dose from mining and milling. In addition, changes in NRC regulations have made effluent controls more stringent, and the effective dose from reactor effluents is lower now than in the early 1980s.

In 2006, there were 104 operating nuclear-power plants in the United States, with an installed capacity of ~100 GWe. With an 89.6 % capacity factor in 2006, the generation was ~90 GWe (NEI, 2007). For nuclear-power plants operating in the United States in 2006, a conservative estimate of 1.36 person-Sv per 0.8 GWe generated (Table 6.1) yields a total collective effective dose of 153 person-Sv from nuclear electricity generation.

The reliability of the dose values differs for the various fuel-cycle components, and the individual values are not necessarily comparable because those who made the estimates used different pathway models and different approaches to dose calculations. For example, the doses estimated for nuclear-power plants are based on relatively detailed examinations of effluent data and pathways; those for conversion and fabrication are in some instances based on detailed concentration measurements at the points of maximum exposure; at mills, on the other hand, many values are predictions based on calculations (often maxima) reported in environmental impact statements.

Offsite doses arising from normal operations in the nuclear fuel cycle are evidently small. EPA (2007c) requires that the annual dose equivalent not exceed 0.25 mSv to the whole body or 0.75 mSv to the thyroid of any member of the public as the result of planned discharges of radioactive material and to direct radiation from operations.

The exposure of the U.S. population from accidental releases of radioactive material has been minor. The release that posed the greatest potential for exposure in the past three decades resulted from the accident at the Three Mile Island Nuclear Plant on March 28, 1979. Although that accident was a serious nuclear engineering event, the releases of radioactive material did not result in significant offsite doses. The collective H_E for the event estimated for the population within 80 km ranged from 16 to 53 person-Sv with a most probable value of 33 person-Sv. The maximum individual dose was <1 mSv while the average dose to individuals living within a 16 km radius was 0.8 mSv and within an 80 km radius it was 15 μSv (Behling and Hildebrand, 1986). These doses are small compared with the average annual H_E to members of the U.S. population from the other sources covered in this Report.

The accident at Chernobyl on April 26, 1986 in the former Soviet Union, although a much worse accident in every respect, had negligible impact on the population of the United States.

6.3 U.S. Department of Energy Installations

6.3.1 Introduction

DOE has a number of laboratories and other sites in the United States for research in science and energy and for cleanup of the nation's nuclear weapons complex. In addition, through the National Nuclear Security Agency, DOE is responsible for national security through the military application of nuclear science. The locations of the various sites and offices are shown in Figure 6.2 (DOE, 2006b).

6.3.2 Sources of Data and Estimates

Each year DOE facilities prepare annual site environmental reports to characterize site environmental-management performance (Andersen et al., 1998; DOE, 1991; 1994; 1995; 1996; 1997a; 1997b; 2000; 2001a; 2001b; 2002; 2003; 2004; 2005; Finley, 2004). These reports include estimates of radiological doses to members of the public.

Offsite radiation exposures from DOE nuclear and radiological sites are typically very low and cannot be determined by direct

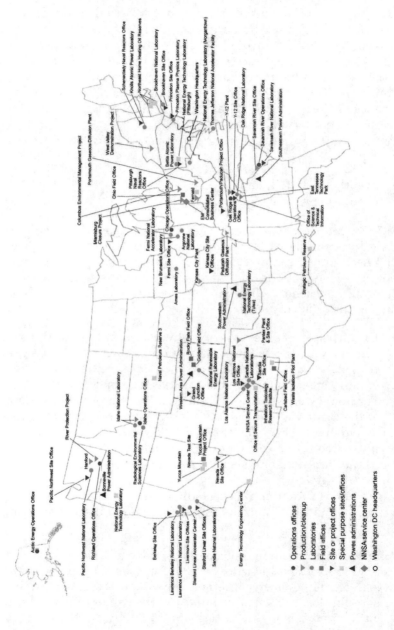

Fig. 6.2. Location of DOE sites (location within each state is not to scale) (DOE, 2006b).

measurement. As a result, these exposures are calculated based on measured effluent data and direct dose at the site boundary. Therefore, the maximum radiation doses reported in annual site environmental reports are potential doses and not actual doses to any individual or population. Radiation doses are estimated using the best available data. If adequate data are unavailable, then site-specific parameters are selected that would result in a high estimate of the maximum dose. For example, the assumed meat consumption rate of 80 kg y^{-1} is higher than the actual consumption rate for the majority of individuals in the United States. All parameter values are selected in this way.

Potential offsite doses from DOE sites are calculated for the following:

- hypothetical MEI; and
- population within a 80 km radius of the site.

6.3.2.1 *Estimated Doses to the Maximally-Exposed Individual.* When estimating doses to members of the public, the concept of MEI is used in environmental impact assessments for DOE sites. However, because of the lifestyle assumptions used in the dose models, this does not represent any specific individual. MEI is defined in the following ways:

- For airborne releases it is an individual that lives at the site boundary at the point of maximum deposition of airborne releases for 365 d y^{-1} and who consumes specified quantities of milk, meat and vegetables produced at that location.
- For liquid releases it is an individual that lives downstream of the facility at the point of highest concentration of radioactive material in the water for 365 d y^{-1}, drinks 2 L d^{-1} of untreated water, consumes a specified amount of fish caught at that location, and spends the majority of time on, near or in the water.
- For direct radiation it is an individual that lives at the fence line at the location of the highest measured direct radiation for 365 d y^{-1}.

Annual site environmental reports combine all three estimated doses to produce the all-pathway MEI dose, even though the three doses are calculated for hypothetical individuals residing at different geographic locations. The reliability of the values differs for the different laboratories and facilities, and the individual values are not necessarily comparable because those who made the estimates used different pathway models and different approaches to dose calculations. In some instances, detailed data were available for examination of effluent data and pathways, and in other instances, values are predictions based on calculations (often maxima) reported in environmental impact statements.

The range and the average MEI for each of the DOE facilities is given in Table F.1 of Appendix F for all reporting years from 1990 through 2004.

6.3.2.2 *Estimated Collective Doses.* The collective dose to the surrounding population is estimated for a region extending from the site for 80 km. This region is divided into concentric circles, each subdivided into 16 equally-spaced sectors. The dose to an individual is multiplied by the population for each sector to give a collective dose for that sector. The total collective dose represents the summation of the collective doses from all sectors.

Computer programs are used to predict both dispersion of airborne effluents and the dose to an individual at specific locations. The methods and parameters used are conservative in the following ways. The model assumes that:

- some portion of the food consumed by the individual was grown within the assessed area;
- the individual resided at this location continuously throughout the year; and
- all the radionuclides released were of the most hazardous form.

Consequently, this worst case is an upper-bound estimate and would estimate a dose that is not likely to be received by any single individual.

The collective H_E averaged over the reporting years from 1990 through 2004 and the most recently reported collective H_E for each DOE facility are given in Table F.1 of Appendix F. For all DOE facilities the total mean annual collective H_E is 1.6 person-Sv for the period 1990 through 2004.

6.3.2.3 *Estimated Doses to the Individual Member of the Public.* Members of the public residing >80 km from a DOE facility received negligible dose from DOE operations.

For members of the public residing within 80 km of a DOE facility, the reported collective dose for the facility was divided by the affected population to give an average H_E per individual. The average individual H_E for each facility over the reporting years from 1990 through 2004 is given in Table F.1 of Appendix F. The range of the average annual values for all DOE sites is <0.001 to 0.6 μSv with almost all <0.05 μSv.

6.4 Decommissioning and Radioactive Waste

6.4.1 *Introduction*

Decommissioning is defined by NRC as the removal of a site or facility safely from service and reduction of residual radiation and radioactive material to a level that permits release of the property for unrestricted use, or release of the property under restricted conditions, and termination of the license (NRC, 1988). This activity may result in the removal and shipment of material containing radionuclides to a licensed disposal site. Currently three such sites operate in the United States. These sites, licensed by Agreement States, also receive radioactive waste from operating nuclear facilities, both commercial and those under the authority of DOE. In addition, large quantities of waste containing varying amounts of NORM are produced in the United States through a variety of mining, energy production and industrial processes. In some cases these radionuclides are either concentrated in waste streams or made more accessible to the human environment in which case material is commonly referred to as TENORM (technologically-enhanced NORM) (Gesell and Prichard, 1975). NCRP has reported some limited dose estimates from waste discharges and recycling of TENORM waste into consumer products (NCRP, 1987d; 1993b).

6.4.2 *Sources of Data*

Sources of data are varied. Some data are found in peer-reviewed scientific journals but most of the information appears in reports prepared by and for government agencies. Some data appear in reports prepared for trade associations whose members are involved in TENORM activities. NRC issues Environmental Impact Statements, both generic and specific, to support rulemaking and specific licensing for decommissioning of major nuclear facilities and license termination. NRC also issues annual reports on decommissioning activities. EPA has issued a very large number of reports on NORM and TENORM and other U.S. government agencies have issued reports on the same topic.

6.4.3 *Special Considerations*

Most of the studies regarding exposure to radioactive waste have not been directed to the study of dose to either the U.S. population or even a specific group within that population. They were designed to determine if additional regulation was needed or to meet other regulatory requirements. The modeling is generally based on hypothetical scenarios and dose assessments are somewhat conservative in that they estimate a dose that is greater than any individual or population is expected to receive.

In the case of decommissioning of licensed nuclear facilities, regulatory requirements for residual dose must be met, and for NRC licensees the annual limit is 0.25 mSv to the average member of the critical group (NRC, 2007d). In actual practice, much lower residual doses are achieved over most if not all the sites. Many licensees use a method that involves conservative screening criteria. With this method, if the residual concentrations are below certain low levels of contamination (screening criteria), the site can be released without developing detailed site specific models and performing dose calculations (Smith *et al.*, 2003).

Finally, many of the studies on NORM and TENORM are based on specific geographic areas. Concentrations of NORM in similar mineral formations in different parts of the United States (USGS, 1997; 1999) and the world vary significantly (IAEA, 2004). This makes it very difficult even to determine the source term that should be used in any dose assessment. Data do not exist to approximate the dose to the U.S. population from TENORM waste.

6.4.4 *Estimates of Dose*

6.4.4.1 *Waste Sites.* Of the three operating commercial waste sites in the United States, the one in Utah, located in a remote area of the Mohave Desert, accepts only the least concentrated levels of radioactive waste. The waste usually consists of very large volumes of slightly contaminated soil. A second site is located well inside the DOE Hanford Site and is remote from any member of the public. The third site, located in South Carolina, does have liquid releases but there are no consumers of surface water in the down gradient direction.

Release of radioactive material from such sites must be controlled to meet the annual dose limits specified by NRC. These annual limits require that the whole-body dose to any individual outside the site boundary not exceed 0.25 mSv, the dose to the thyroid not exceed 0.75 mSv, and the dose to any other organ not exceed 0.25 mSv (NRC, 2007e). Because the sites are remote, no individual is likely to receive a dose that is more than a fraction of these dose limits. As an example, the environmental assessment for the site in South Carolina shows a maximum annual individual dose of 0.13 mSv from surface water at the point of compliance if the water were used (CNS, 2003).

In summary, the annual dose to the highest exposed offsite member of the public from waste-disposal site activities is likely to be on the order of 0.1 mSv and the collective effective dose is negligible for the purpose of this Report.

6.4.4.2 *Decommissioning*. NRC (2007d) addresses requirements for decommissioning of commercial nuclear facilities for unrestricted or restricted release and requires that the annual dose not exceed 0.25 mSv TEDE from all pathways to the average member of a critical group. Smith *et al.* (2003) provides guidance on the assessment necessary to demonstrate compliance with this dose limit. Generally the average member of the critical group is a resident farmer. In addition, conservative screening criteria are provided for licensees not wishing to characterize the site for specific modeling. NRC has described the status of decommissioning in its NUREG reports (Buckley, 2005; 2007). However, these reports provide no estimate of final doses received by individuals occupying facilities or sites after they have been released for unrestricted use. This is, in part, because the actual use results in a much lower dose than would be permitted by criteria used in establishing residual contamination limits. For example, sites are usually not occupied by resident farmers but may be used for an industrial or other purpose.

6.4.4.3 *Technologically-Enhanced Naturally-Occurring Radioactive Material Waste Disposal*. EPA (2000a) estimates the total amount of TENORM waste produced in the United States may exceed one billion tons annually. There is no generally-accepted estimate of the total dose to members of the public from TENORM exposure. Table 6.2 presents the principal sources of TENORM in the United States, based on EPA (2000a), supplemented by additional data sources.

A comprehensive draft report (EPA, 1993b) including sources, concentrations, waste volumes, and dose assessment based on modeling has not been publicly released although data from the report have been frequently used in later reports.

Some modeling has been performed to estimate doses to individuals from various types of TENORM waste and disposal methods. Landspreading is a method in actual use for disposing of petroleum industry NORM (Andersen *et al.*, 1998) and municipal sewage sludge (ISCORS, 2005a). For landspreading of municipal waste, the ISCORS modeling shows the highest doses to persons occupying the land after repeated spreading of waste. After a period of 20 y of applications the onsite annual dose is 0.09 mSv TEDE (Table 5.2,

TABLE 6.2—Sources of TENORM (EPA, 2000a; ISCORS, 2003).

TENORM Sources	Radioactive Concentrations [^{226}Ra (Bq kg^{-1}) unless otherwise specified]			Comments and Additional Data
	Low	Average	High	
Soils of the United States (natural background levels)	7.4	41	155	^{232}Th 3.7 – 126 (range), 36 (average) ^{238}U 4.4 – 141 (range), 37 (average) (Myrick et al., 1983)
Geothermal energy waste (scales)	370	4,900	9,400	^{228}Ra <37 – 6,800 (range), 3,400 (average) ^{228}Th 925 (average) (EPA, 1993b)
Oil and gas production waste				
Produced water	3.7 Bq m^{-3}	NA^a	0.3 MBq m^{-3}	^{228}Ra and ^{228}Th also reported
Pipe/tank scale	<0.93	<7,400	>3.7 MBq kg^{-1}	(Swann et al., 2004; Wilson and Scott, 1992)
Water treatment waste				
Treatment sludge	48 Bq m^{-3}	410 Bq m^{-3}	0.4 MBq m^{-3}	
Plant filters	NA	1.5 MBq m^{-3}	NA	
Waste water treatment waste				
Treatment sludge (dry)	ND^b	74 (median)	480 (95th %) 1,700 high	^{228}Th 2.6 – 330 (range), 22 (median) ^{238}U 0.7 – 960 (range), 52 (median)
Treatment plant ash		110 (median)	670 (95th %) 810 high	^{228}Th ND – 1,100 (range), 93 (median) ^{238}U 30 – 2,700 (range), 120 (median)
Aluminum production waste				
Bauxite ores	160	NA	270	
Product	NA	8.5	NA	
Production waste	NA	140 – 210	NA	

TABLE 6.2—(continued).

TENORM Sources	Radioactive Concentrations [^{226}Ra (Bq kg^{-1}) unless otherwise specified]			Comments and Additional Data
	Low	Average	High	
Coal and coal ash				
Bottom ash	59	130 – 154	280	
Fly ash	74	210	360	
Copper production waste	26	440	3,100	
Phosphate production				
Ore	260	640 – 1,500	230 – 2,000	^{238}U 300 – 1,400 (range)
Phosphogypsum	NA	430 – 910	1,400	
Phosphate fertilizer	NA	210	780	^{238}U 1,480 – 3,000 (range) (Roessler et al., 1979)
Rare earths (monazite, xenotime, astnsite)	210	NA	120,000	
Titanium ores	140	30	910	
Rutile	NA	730	NA	
Ilmenite	NA	210	NA	
Waste	NA	440	NA	
Uranium mining overburden	110	110	~4,000	
Uranium in situ leach (evaporation pond solids)	11,000	NA	110,000	
Zircon	NA	2,500	NA	
Waste	3,200	NA	48,000	

[a]NA = not available.
[b]ND = not detectable.

Section 5.3). Note that TENORM in sewage sludge is not associated with decommissioning of TENORM sites, but is incidental from naturally-occurring radionuclides in groundwater.

6.4.5 *Comments*

The effective dose to the U.S. population from TENORM waste cannot be estimated with confidence because the distribution of the radioactive waste in the environment, its radionuclide composition, the distribution of population around it, and the contributions of the various exposure pathways are not well known. However, certain conclusions can be made. The concentrations of TENORM that are placed in the environment, especially at inactive uranium processing sites, can lead to doses higher than that permitted in the case of Atomic Energy Act (AEA, 1954) waste and decommissioning activities regulated by either DOE, NRC or Agreement States. The amount of TENORM waste material is much greater than that generated in decommissioning activities or other uses of AEA regulated material. Finally, there are many more TENORM waste-disposal sites than those available for AEA and decommissioning waste. Therefore, it is very likely that the U.S. population dose is higher from TENORM waste than from AEA waste sources.

The annual collective effective dose (S) from TENORM is only a very small fraction of that from natural background. However, there are likely to be critical groups with annual individual doses >0.25 mSv, and possibly >10 mSv in the case of inactive uranium processing sites.

6.5 Industrial, Medical, Educational and Research Activities

6.5.1 *Methodology and Discussion*

Radioactive material, x-ray equipment and accelerators are used for various purposes in medicine, industry and commerce, and education and research. These purposes include diagnosis, therapy, sterilization, materials processing, transportation and labeling of research material. All of these operations are controlled by federal or state regulations that require licensing or permitting. The operators of these facilities are required to measure the radiation doses received by their exposed employees, and although the annual occupational limit is 50 mSv, typical annual occupational doses are <1 mSv (Section 7). They are required to maintain the potential annual dose to any member of the public who might be exposed to their radiation sources to not exceed 1 mSv. To estimate the population dose from these sources a number of assumptions were made, and these assumptions are shown in Table 6.3.

TABLE 6.3—*Derivation of estimates of annual collective effective dose to members of the public from medical, industry and commerce, and education and research activities.*

Source	Estimate of Exposed Population	Average Dose per Person (mSv)	Collective Effective Dose (person-Sv)	Comments
Medical: occupational	740,000	0.8	550	Estimate of exposed population and average dose per person taken from Section 7.1.3, Table 7.3 for 2006.
Medical: public	74,000,000	0.0016	120	A large number of members of the public (~100 times the occupational workforce) are estimated to spend some time each year near medical sources. Average dose per member of the public is based on 1 week y^{-1} at medical facility (1/50 of occupational) and 1/10 of dose rate, because members of the public are kept outside of radiation areas and generally away from sources. Total reduction in average dose is 1/500.
Industry and commerce: occupational	130,000	0.8	110	Estimate of exposed population and average dose per person taken from Section 7.1.3, Table 7.3.

Industry and commerce: public	1,300,000	0.002	3	The number of members of the public that might be exposed to industrial and commerce sources, including transportation of sources, is estimated to be ~10 times the occupational workforce. Average dose per member of the public is based on 0.25 y near industrial sources (1/4 of occupational) and 1/100 of dose rate, because members of the public are kept well outside of radiation areas and generally away from sources. Total reduction in average dose is 1/400.
Education and research: occupational	84,000	0.7	60	Estimate of exposed population and average dose per person taken from Section 7.1.3, Table 7.3.
Education and research: public	840,000	0.0018	2	The number of members of the public that might be exposed to educational and research sources is estimated to be ~10 times the occupational workforce. Average dose per member of the public is based on 0.25 y near educational and research sources (1/4 of occupational) and 1/100 of dose rate, because members of the public are kept well outside of radiation areas and generally away from sources. Total reduction in average dose is 1/400.
Total S for members of the public			125	

The general methodology for dose estimation for members of the public from these sources used the known exposures to the monitored occupational workforce (Section 7), and then estimated the dose to members of the public. The potentially exposed number of members of the public is uncertain, but for this purpose is estimated to be larger than the occupational group (10 times larger for industrial, educational and research sources, and 100 times larger for the medical sources). However, the dose to members of the public is expected to be significantly lower due to the regulatory controls on these sources. The occupational workforce is exposed on a regular basis. However, individuals outside the workforce are exposed only when visiting a facility containing sources or when in the close vicinity of such a facility. Such individuals do not come in contact with these sources of radiation because of restrictions on entry into radioactive-material and radiation areas. For transportation of radioactive source material DOT regulations for packaging and shipping limit the dose rates on packages and on the vehicles themselves. The collective effective dose estimate for exposure to the population from transportation is treated as part of the estimate for industry and commerce given in Table 6.3. In all cases, the exposure to the members of the public will be much smaller than that for potentially exposed workers.

The annual collective effective dose to the population from these sources of radiation is estimated to be 125 person-Sv.

6.5.2 *Exposure to Members of the Public from Diagnostic Nuclear-Medicine Patients*

Nuclear-medicine procedures may result in radiation exposure of family members and coworkers that would add to the collective effective dose listed in Table 6.3. For diagnostic procedures, NCRP Report No. 124 (NCRP, 1996) provided a conservative estimate of dose to a member of the public of 10 µGy per procedure. It is assumed that this is an appropriate value for effective dose per procedure (10 µSv). Table 4.16 projects that there were 18 million procedures performed in 2006. If it is assumed that four persons (family and coworkers) are exposed during each procedure, the annual collective effective dose to the exposed population is 720 person-Sv.

6.6 Security Inspection Systems

Since NCRP Report No. 93 (NCRP, 1987a) was published, there has been an increase in the use of security inspection systems for detection of contraband, such as drugs, explosives or flammable material, both for screening of cargo and individuals. For example, inspection systems for checked luggage and carry-on items are now widely used at airports.

These security inspection systems employ x-ray technologies or a variety of radioactive sources, and include scanners capable of imaging cargo in trucks, trains and boats, as well as personnel security systems that can image items hidden on and in the body of an individual.

6.6.1 *Cabinet X-Ray Systems*

Baggage inspection systems are classified as cabinet x-ray systems because the x rays are contained within a shielded enclosure. These systems are subject to a federal cabinet x-ray system standard (FDA, 2007d), for all systems manufactured after April 10, 1975, that limits exposure to ≤ 0.17 C kg^{-1} (5 µGy air kerma) in 1 h at any point 5 cm outside the external surface of the system. Since the previous NCRP (1987a) report on exposure of the U.S. population, cabinet x-ray systems have increased in number and are no longer limited to airports. They are currently used widely in office buildings and anywhere security is a concern. In addition, a new type of cabinet system, designed to detect explosives, utilizes CT to inspect checked luggage at airports. However, the dose rate at any point outside all cabinet systems is essentially zero.

6.6.2 *Nonintrusive Inspection Equipment (Cargo Scanners)*

A number of types of nonintrusive inspection (NII) equipment based on technologies using low-energy x or gamma rays have been deployed at 301 air, sea and land ports-of-entry throughout the United States and Puerto Rico (CBP, 2004). A linear-accelerator system is also available. These imaging systems enable the user to perform effective and efficient NII of cargo vehicles including tanker and trailer trucks, trailer mounted cargo containers, and railroad cars for contraband such as illicit drugs, currency and guns. In very limited applications, this technology has also been used for the detection of contraband and illegal aliens. The detection is based on the size, shape, density of the materials identified in the radiographic image as produced by the NII systems. An NII prototype using pulsed fast-neutron analysis (PFNA) which uses neutrons for interrogation of cargo and identification of contraband is being developed.

Khan *et al.* (2004) reported that an individual hidden in a cargo container that is inadvertently exposed could receive a dose equivalent from various NII systems as noted below (Table 6.4 for additional information for these systems):

TABLE 6.4—*Typical screening devices, radiation types, and dose rates for NII systems (Khan et al., 2004).*

Device Type	Radiation	Source Strength	Dose Rate at 1 m	Average Dose Equivalent
Truck x ray	Two x-ray sources	450 kVp; 10 mA each	0.30 Gy min^{-1}	0.40 μSv
Mobile truck x ray: wide eye	One x-ray source	450 kVp; 6.6 mA	0.20 Gy min^{-1}	0.53 μSv
Mobile truck x ray: low under carriage[a]	One x-ray source	420 kVp; 10 mA	0.21 Gy min^{-1}	2.3 μSv
VACIS® II[b]	^{137}Cs or ^{60}Co	37 GBq / 18.5 – 37 GBq	53 μGy min^{-1} / 107 μGy min^{-1}	0.05 μSv / —
Mobile truck VACIS®	^{137}Cs or ^{60}Co	59.2 GBq / 37 GBq	85 μGy min^{-1} / 213 μGy min^{-1}	0.04 μSv / —
Pallet VACIS®[c]	^{137}Cs or ^{60}Co	18.5 GBq / 9.25 GBq	26 μGy min^{-1} / 53 μGy min^{-1}	— / —
Railroad inspection (RailVACIS®)	^{137}Cs or ^{60}Co	74 GBq / 37 GBq	107 μGy min^{-1} / 213 μGy min^{-1}	0.025 μSv / —
Mobile x ray (LINAC)[b]	Electron beam	2 MeV / 6 MeV	8.3 mGy min^{-1} / 16.7 mGy min^{-1}	115 μSv / —
PFNA	Neutron generator	8 MeV neutrons; gamma rays	Neutron flux = 10^7 n cm^{-2} s^{-1}	315 μSv / —

[a]Use of the mobile truck x ray for low under carriage use has been discontinued.
[b] VACIS = Vehicle and Cargo Inspection System (Science Applications International Corporation, San Diego, California)
LINAC = linear electron accelerator
[c]CBP (2004). Table I, source variants offered for VACIS®.

- range of 0.025 to 0.53 μSv for x- and gamma-ray systems;
- 115 μSv for a linear-accelerator (electron-beam) system; and
- 315 μSv for the PFNA system.

However, the number of individuals inadvertently exposed as a result of searches at U.S. points of entry is low and any exposure is estimated to be within the dose estimates provided here.

NCRP has also performed an analysis of the PFNA system and concluded that such a system should be designed and operated in a manner to ensure that, under normal circumstances, an inadvertently-exposed individual will not receive an effective dose >1 mSv (or >5 mSv, if necessary to achieve national security objectives) (NCRP, 2003a).

As the largest user of gamma-based NII screening systems, the U.S. Customs and Borders Protection has established a maximum dose rate of 0.5 μSv h^{-1} and 2,000 h y^{-1} as the maximum time of exposure, so that neither the Customs inspectors nor members of the public will experience an annual dose >1 mSv from this radiation source (CBP, 2004).

NCRP has also evaluated a proposed Cargo Advanced Automated Radiography System (CAARS), which is an electron accelerator-based high-energy photon scanning system, and recommended it be designed and operated such that:

- effective dose to inadvertently-exposed individuals not exceed 5 mSv;
- effective dose to individuals inside the CAARS facility perimeter not exceed 0.5 μSv in an hour; and
- annual effective dose to individuals outside the CAARS perimeter not exceed 0.25 mSv (NCRP, 2007).

Portal systems designed to inspect passenger vehicles passing through a border checkpoint are also being evaluated. Because the passengers would be scanned along with the vehicle, these systems are designed to comply with the recommendations and standards listed in Section 6.6.3 for personnel security systems.

6.6.3 *Personnel Security Systems*

X rays are used to screen people directly for security purposes in some countries and industries, such as the diamond industry. These systems have been used in the United States on an extremely-limited basis to date, primarily by prisons, but only to screen prisoners. However, the Transportation Security Administration is evaluating the use of such systems for general passenger screening at airports. Although some state governments prohibit the use of x-ray screening for nonmedical purposes, there is no similar federal prohibition.

NCRP published a commentary on this subject (NCRP, 2003b) and recommended classifying these systems into two categories: general- and limited-use systems. General use systems should adhere to an effective dose of 0.1 μSv or less per scan, and typically utilize a backscatter technology, for which the effective dose is ~0.03 μSv per scan. Limited-use systems deliver an effective dose >0.1 μSv but are limited to ≤10 μSv per scan, and typically utilize a transmission type x-ray system, for which the effective doses are in the range of 0.5 to 6 μSv per scan. ANSI (2002) provides a voluntary standard for personnel screening security systems of 0.1 μSv per scan and NCRP (2003b) is consistent with that standard for the general use systems that utilize backscatter technology. At present, these systems are only used to screen prisoners, and because of the very low doses contribute a negligible collective effective dose to the U.S. population.

6.7 Summary

The annual collective effective dose (S) for this category of exposures is quite low [~1,000 (998) person-Sv for 2006] and minor relative to that for other exposure categories. It is based mostly on best estimates from very limited information on numbers of individuals exposed and the associated effective doses. An estimated 72 % of the collective dose from industrial, security, medical, educational and research activities results from exposure to members of the public who have come in contact with patients who have received radionuclides for a nuclear-medicine procedure. The effective dose to an individual in this situation is low, 10 μSv, but the number of people exposed may be quite large. The estimated S is 720 person-Sv for 2006. Exposures to other industries are minor. Nuclear power is estimated to deliver 153 person-Sv and the estimated sum for medical, industrial and commerce, educational and research activities is 125 person-Sv (*i.e.*, 120 person-Sv for medical, 3 person-Sv for industry and commerce, 2 person-Sv for education and research).

The distribution of the collective effective dose among the industrial, security, medical, educational and research sources is shown in Figure 6.3.

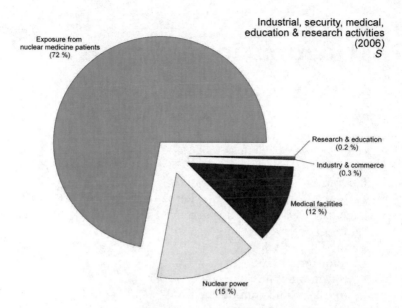

Fig. 6.3. Percent contribution of various sources of exposure to S for industrial, security, medical, educational and research activities (1,000 person-Sv) for 2006. Percent values have been rounded to the nearest 1 %, except those <1 % [see Section 6.7 for the values of S (person-sievert)].

7. Occupational Exposure

Thumbnail Sketch (for 2006) (rounded values):

- collective effective dose (S): 1,400 person-Sv
- effective dose per individual in the U.S. population (E_{US}): 0.005 mSv
  - percent of total S or E_{US} for the U.S. population (<0.1 %)
- subcategories included (percent of total S or E_{US} for occupational exposure)
  - medical (39 %)
  - aviation (38 %)
  - commercial nuclear power (8 %)
  - industry and commerce (8 %)
  - education and research (4 %)
  - government, DOE, military (3 %)
- average effective dose for the exposed group (E_{Exp}): 1.1 mSv
  - variation in E_{Exp} among the included categories: 0.6 to 3.1 mSv
- group characteristics: all adults

7.1 Introduction

Available data have been collected and evaluated for occupationally-exposed workers in various groups. Personal monitoring data were obtained from currently available sources, including the U.S. military, DOE, NRC and two major dosimeter providers (Global Dosimetry Solutions, Inc. and Landauer, Inc.). Personal monitoring programs cited in this Report are accredited by either the National Voluntary Laboratory Accreditation Program (NIST, 2008) or the DOE Laboratory Accreditation Program (DOE, 2007). Airline crews are not personally monitored. Therefore, doses for airline crews were calculated based on other available information.

7.1.1 *Exposure Categories and Dose Quantities*

The data are grouped by occupational category and, when appropriate, by additional subcategories. The following occupational categories were used:

- medical (including dental and veterinary medicine)
- aviation
- commercial nuclear power
- industry and commerce
- education and research
- government, DOE, military

Data are presented for the years 2003 through 2006 for the number of individuals monitored, the number receiving a recordable dose,[25] and, for those with a recordable dose, the collective dose, the average dose, and the dose distributions. The data are presented as effective doses, without adjustments made to the actual surrogate quantities reported. The categories are presented in the order listed above starting with the highest collective effective dose category and ending with the lowest.

Table 7.1 summarizes the occupational categories, subcategories, and data sources. Table 7.2 provides the associated references, data types, and dosimetry methods.

7.1.2 *Limitations and Sources of Uncertainty*

Most of the data reported for external doses are measurements from dosimeters [*e.g.*, thermoluminescent dosimeters (TLDs), film, optically-stimulated luminescent dosimeters] purportedly worn in the exposure environment. These data, while perhaps the best estimates of occupational doses in most circumstances, have uncertainties due to the many variables that can impact the accuracy of the exposure assessment and determination of delivered dose. For the data presented, no attempt has been made to correct for any of the variables discussed below.

- Not every supplier of personal monitoring systems was included. As a result, although average doses, dose distributions, and the relative fraction of collective dose in different occupations are likely to be relatively accurate, the collective doses are likely to be underestimated.

---

[25]Each organization establishes a "minimum recordable dose" based on a number of factors. Recordable dose in the context of this Report refers to values greater than a minimum detectable level. Minimum detectable levels vary, but are on the order of 0.1 to 0.15 mSv for film and thermoluminescent dosimeters (TLDs), and 0.01 mSv for optically-stimulated luminescent dosimeters.

TABLE 7.1—*Summary of occupational categories, subcategories, and data sources.*

Category/Subcategory	Data Source
Medical	
Dental practices	Global Dosimetry Solutions, Inc.[a]
	Landauer, Inc.
Hospitals/medical centers	Global Dosimetry Solutions, Inc.
	Landauer, Inc.
Medically-related schools	Landauer, Inc.
Other medical practices	Global Dosimetry Solutions, Inc.
	Landauer, Inc.
VA hospitals	Global Dosimetry Solutions, Inc.
	Landauer, Inc.
Veterinary medicine/practice	Global Dosimetry Solutions, Inc.
	Landauer, Inc.
Aviation	U.S. Department of Labor
	U.S. Department of Transportation
Commercial nuclear power	U.S. Nuclear Regulatory Commission
Industry and commerce	
General manufacturing	Landauer, Inc.
Other fuel cycle, uranium mining	Landauer, Inc.
Other industrial uses	Global Dosimetry Solutions, Inc.
	Landauer, Inc.
Source production	Global Dosimetry Solutions, Inc.
	Landauer, Inc.
Testing and inspection	Landauer, Inc.
Education and research	
Research laboratories	Global Dosimetry Solutions, Inc.
Universities, colleges	Global Dosimetry Solutions, Inc.
	Landauer, Inc.
Government, DOE, military	
Air Force	U.S. Department of the Air Force
Army	U.S. Department of the Army
DOE/DOE contractors	U.S. Department of Energy
Government	Global Dosimetry Solutions, Inc.
	Landauer, Inc.
Naval nuclear propulsion	U.S. Department of the Navy
Navy/Marines	U.S. Department of the Navy

[a]A division of Mirion Technologies.

TABLE 7.2—*Summary of data sources, references, data types and dosimetry methods.*

Data Source	Reference	Data Type	Dosimetry Method
U.S. Department of Labor	DOL (2008)	Number of airline crew members	—
U.S. Department of Transportation	Friedberg and Copeland (2003)	Effective dose	Computer code
U.S. Navy (nuclear propulsion)	Mueller et al. (2007)	Monitored workers Deep dose equivalent	TLD[a]
U.S. Army U.S. Air Force U.S. Navy	Personal communications[b,c,d]	Monitored workers Deep dose equivalent	TLD
Landauer, Inc.	Personal communication[e]	Monitored workers Deep dose equivalent	TLD, optically-stimulated luminescent dosimeter, film
U.S. Department of Energy	DOE (2006a)	Monitored workers TEDE[a]	TLD, bioassay
U.S. Nuclear Regulatory Commission	Dickson et al. (2007)	Monitored workers TEDE	TLD, bioassay
Global Dosimetry Solutions, Inc.	Personal communications[f,g]	Monitored workers Deep dose equivalent	TLD, film

[a] TLD = thermoluminescent dosimeter
TEDE = total effective dose equivalent
[b] Harris, W. (2007). Personal communication (U.S. Army Dosimetry Center, Huntsville, Alabama).
[c] Nichelson, S.M. (2008). Personal communication (U.S. Air Force Office of the Surgeon General, Washington).
[d] Benevides, L. (2003). Personal communication (Naval Dosimetry Center, Bethesda, Maryland).
[e] Yoder, C. (2007). Personal communication (Landauer, Inc., Glenwood, Illinois).
[f] Perle, S.C. (2006). Personal communication (Global Dosimetry Solutions, Inc, Irvine, California).
[g] Cords, R. (2007). Personal communication (Global Dosimetry Solutions, Inc, Irvine, California).

- Workers may change employment during the year. As a result, they may be monitored at more than one location and by more than one monitoring program. Therefore, the entries for the number of monitored workers and those with recordable dose overestimate the actual number of individuals monitored. This does not affect S, but would underestimate E_{Exp}. This has been corrected for the commercial nuclear-power data and does not apply to the aviation data because the number of airline crew members comes from employment statistics.

- Workers may not wear their personal monitors at all times. Consequently some exposures may be missed. This would lead to an underestimate of average individual and collective doses.

- Monitoring programs do not exist for some occupationally-exposed work groups (in particular, airline crews). In that case, doses were estimated from calculations of dose rate distributions and estimated exposure time.

- Occupational doses that are below each organization's recordable dose (minimum detectable level) are not included; therefore, the collective doses are likely to be underestimated. Recordable doses vary depending on dosimeter type and the policies and practices of the organization.

- Administrative variability, that is, when dosimetry is or is not issued or audited when radiation levels are expected to be low (e.g., use of fluoroscopy in operating rooms, use of conventional radiography or fluoroscopy in morgues, presence of unregulated radioactive material at industrial facilities) alters the ability to develop a precise assessment of occupational exposure.

- There is no direct way to measure effective dose from exposure received in occupational settings. Algorithms that make adjustments to monitored doses can often provide closer estimates of effective dose (Faulkner et al., 1996; Huda et al., 1997; Kocher and Eckerman, 1988; Meinhold, 1989; NCRP, 1995b; Niklason et al., 1994; Rosenstein and Webster, 1994; Sherbini and DeCicco, 2002; Webster, 1989). Typically, the effective dose computed from an algorithm is numerically less than the monitored dose. In most cases the doses reported from personal monitoring are assumed to be adequate indicators of the actual effective dose received by the monitored individuals.

- Methods and practices for calculating and assigning internal doses are used for those occupations where internal exposure is of concern. However, in most occupational categories, effective doses from internally-deposited radioactive material are either not present or small compared with effective doses from the external contribution, and are therefore not monitored.

- Statistical errors associated with the dose measurement and data analysis are rarely documented.
- Organizations may use different conversion coefficients to convert various types of exposure to effective dose.
- The orientation of the worker and the dosimeter in relation to the radiation source is not known.
- In some occupational settings, particularly in medical facilities, workers wearing dosimeters might also be wearing protective devices such as leaded aprons, thyroid collars, or leaded glasses. Thus, reported doses may overestimate the actual doses.[26]

7.1.3 *Overview of Occupational Doses*

Table 7.3 provides the total number of monitored individuals in each occupational category, the number of monitored individuals who received recordable doses, the collective effective dose, and the average effective dose, which is based on the number of workers receiving a recordable dose. Figures 7.1 through 7.4 provide graphical representations of these data.

- Figure 7.1 shows the number of workers with a recordable occupational dose for 2003 to 2006.
- Figure 7.2 shows the occupational collective effective dose for 2003 to 2006.
- Figure 7.3 shows the 2006 occupational collective effective dose in pie-chart format (percent of total).
- Figure 7.4 shows the average annual effective dose for those with a recordable dose for the years 2003 to 2006.

Figures 7.1 through 7.4 show that, for 2006, the medical category contains the largest number of monitored workers, workers with

---

[26]For example, use of a single monitor worn outside and above a protective apron will overestimate E by a factor of 21 and H_E by a factor of 5.6 (NCRP, 1995b). Use of two monitors, the aforementioned one and one worn under the protective apron at the waist or chest, along with appropriate weighting of the two values, yields much improved estimates of E and H_E (NCRP, 1995b).

TABLE 7.3—Summary of occupational doses for U.S. workers.

Category	Numbers of Workers and Doses	2003	2004	2005	2006
Medical	Monitored workers	1,957,088	2,220,861	2,352,976	2,519,693
	Workers with recordable dose	690,661	735,400	693,941	735,347
	Collective effective dose (person-Sv)	508	559	546	549
	Average effective dose[a] (mSv)	0.74	0.76	0.79	0.75
Aviation	Monitored airline crew	0	0	0	0
	Number of airline crew	177,000	180,000	176,000	173,000
	Collective effective dose (person-Sv)	543	553	540	531
	Average effective dose[b] (mSv)	3.07	3.07	3.07	3.07
Commercial nuclear power	Monitored workers	109,990	110,290	114,344	116,354
	Workers with recordable dose	55,967	52,873	57,566	58,788
	Collective effective dose (person-Sv)	120	104	115	110
	Average effective dose[a] (mSv)	2.14	1.97	2.00	1.87
Industry and commerce	Monitored workers	360,069	556,325	579,864	505,369
	Workers with recordable dose	112,671	133,926	125,257	134,105
	Collective effective dose (person-Sv)	98	114	117	109
	Average effective dose[a] (mSv)	0.87	0.85	0.93	0.81

Education and research	Monitored workers	351,309	504,948	514,267	437,007
	Workers with recordable dose	79,901	88,125	81,732	83,700
	Collective effective dose (person-Sv)	43	73	51	60
	Average effective dose[a] (mSv)	0.54	0.83	0.62	0.72
Government, DOE, military[c]	Monitored workers	265,870	289,979	301,498	284,192
	Workers with recordable dose	36,559	36,788	33,934	30,591
	Collective effective dose (person-Sv)	44 (24)[d]	49 (27)[d]	38 (17)[d]	39 (18)[d]
	Average effective dose[a] (mSv)	0.66	0.73	0.50	0.59
Total monitored workers		3,044,326	3,682,403	3,862,949	3,862,615
Total workers with recordable or estimated dose		1,152,759	1,227,112	1,168,430	1,215,531
Total collective effective dose (person-Sv)		1,356	1,452	1,407	1,399
Average effective dose[e] (mSv)		1.16	1.17	1.19	1.13

[a]The average annual effective dose for those with recordable dose for the respective year.

[b]The average annual effective dose for airline crew, based on estimate for 2006.

[c]Data from 2004 were used for 2005 and 2006 for three military subcategories (Section 7.7.3) as it was the latest available. This has only a small effect on the values given for this category for 2005 and 2006.

[d]Values in parenthesis exclude the portion of collective effective dose for which information on the number of workers in the government, DOE, military category with recordable dose was not available (Table 7.8) [e.g., for 2006: 21 (39 − 18) person-Sv is excluded]. The average effective dose listed for this category (for 2006) (0.59 mSv) is therefore computed as 18 person-Sv divided by 30,591 workers with recordable dose.

[e]Based on the number of workers for which recordable dose was available (see footnote d) [e.g., for 2006: 1,378 (1,399 − 21) person-Sv divided by 1,215,531 workers with recordable dose)].

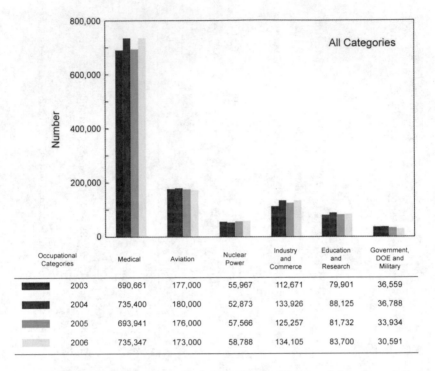

Occupational Categories	Medical	Aviation	Nuclear Power	Industry and Commerce	Education and Research	Government, DOE and Military
2003	690,661	177,000	55,967	112,671	79,901	36,559
2004	735,400	180,000	52,873	133,926	88,125	36,788
2005	693,941	176,000	57,566	125,257	81,732	33,934
2006	735,347	173,000	58,788	134,105	83,700	30,591

Fig. 7.1. Number of monitored workers with recordable dose and number of airline crew members for the occupational categories, 2003 to 2006.

recordable dose, and collective effective dose. However, the largest average effective dose (3.07 mSv) occurs in aviation. The average effective dose in 2006 for the medical (0.75 mSv), industry and commerce (0.81 mSv), education and research (0.72 mSv), and government, DOE, military (0.49 mSv) categories are fairly similar while the average effective dose for commercial nuclear power was 1.87 mSv. All average annual effective doses are much less than the 50 mSv occupational limit recommended by NCRP (1993a).

7.2 Occupational Exposures from Medical Practice

The previous report (NCRP, 1989b) relied heavily on the compilations of Kumazawa *et al.* (1984) for the characterization of exposures for medical personnel. For occupational exposures in the medical category,[27] this Report utilizes the results of personal monitoring dosimetry information accumulated from Global Dosimetry Solutions, Inc. and Landauer, Inc. to produce estimates for the

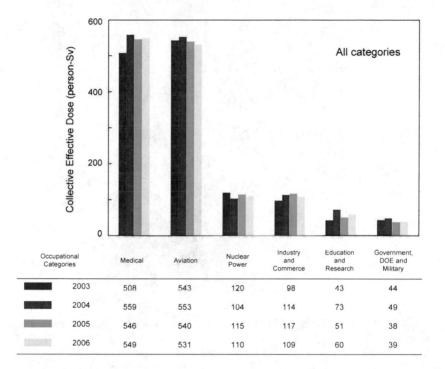

Fig. 7.2. Annual collective effective dose for the occupational categories, 2003 to 2006.

period 2003 to 2006 in the United States. In these personal monitoring programs, the medical category is divided into subcategories according to type of facility, as opposed to the specific discipline. Additional brief perspectives for workers in the disciplines of diagnostic radiology, nuclear medicine, radiation oncology, chiropractic practice, podiatry, osteopathic practice, dental practice, and veterinary medicine are also given, using information provided in UNSCEAR (2000) and the more recent literature.

7.2.1 *Summary of Personal Monitoring Information*

The medical category has the largest number of occupationally-exposed individuals and the highest collective effective dose (Table 7.3). The dose distribution for this category (Figure 7.5)

---

[27]For purposes of this Report, chiropractic practice, podiatry, osteopathic practice, dental practice, and veterinary practice are included in this occupational category.

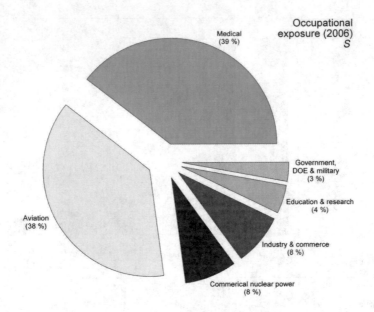

Fig. 7.3. Percent contribution of various sources to S for occupational exposure (1,400 person-Sv) for 2006. Percent values have been rounded to the nearest 1 % [see Table 7.3 for the values of S (person-sievert)].

shows that the vast majority of workers with recordable dose (81 %) received annual doses <1 mSv and 96 % received <5 mSv. The average annual effective dose was 0.75 mSv (Table 7.3)

Figure 7.6 shows the collective effective doses (person-sievert and percent of total) for 2006 for the medical subcategories. The greatest percentage of collective effective dose (70 %) was accrued in hospitals and medical centers where procedures are done that have the highest potential for occupational exposure (*e.g.*, cardiac catheterization, nuclear-medicine procedures). The "other medical practices" subcategory resulted in 23 % of the collective effective dose; VA hospitals, medically-related schools, dental practices, and veterinary medicine each constituted on the order of 1 to 2 % of the collective effective dose. The "other medical practices" subcategory included chiropractic practices, osteopathic practices, radiology, podiatry, general medical doctors and medical clinics, medical laboratories, orthopedic surgeons, and sports medicine. Table 7.4 provides the available personal monitoring data for the chiropractic, podiatry, osteopathic, dental and veterinary practices, showing relatively low contributions to the collective effective dose for this occupational category.

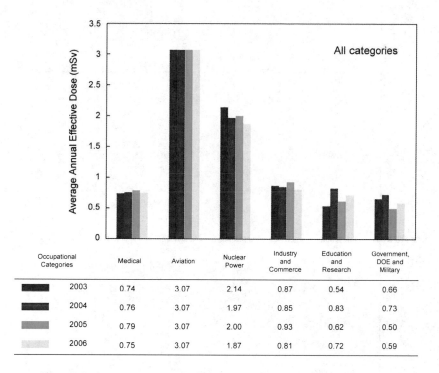

Occupational Categories		Medical	Aviation	Nuclear Power	Industry and Commerce	Education and Research	Government, DOE and Military
	2003	0.74	3.07	2.14	0.87	0.54	0.66
	2004	0.76	3.07	1.97	0.85	0.83	0.73
	2005	0.79	3.07	2.00	0.93	0.62	0.50
	2006	0.75	3.07	1.87	0.81	0.72	0.59

Fig. 7.4. Average annual effective dose for workers with record-able dose (E_{Exp}) for the occupational categories, 2003 to 2006.

7.2.2 *Supplemental Information on Medical Specialties*

Occupational doses to interventional radiologists and cardiologists can be estimated because of the wealth of literature available. For example, for cardiologists, Kim *et al.* (2008) evaluated the published data from the early 1970s through 2007 and discovered variations of several orders of magnitude in radiation doses per procedure to operators performing the various cardiology procedures. The widest range of doses (0.02 to 38 µSv per procedure) was found for diagnostic catheterizations.

Several reports in the literature (Chiesa, *et al.*, 1997; Dignum and van Lingen, 1997; Guillet *et al.*, 2005; Robinson *et al.*, 2005; Schleipman *et al.*, 2006; Seierstad *et al.*, 2007) review occupational doses for those staff working primarily or solely with radionuclides used in PET. Effective doses were reported to range from 9 to 25 nSv MBq^{-1}. Schleipman *et al.* (2006) and Robinson *et al.* (2005) also reported doses for typical nuclear-medicine procedures. The range of doses per procedure was consistently between 0.14 and

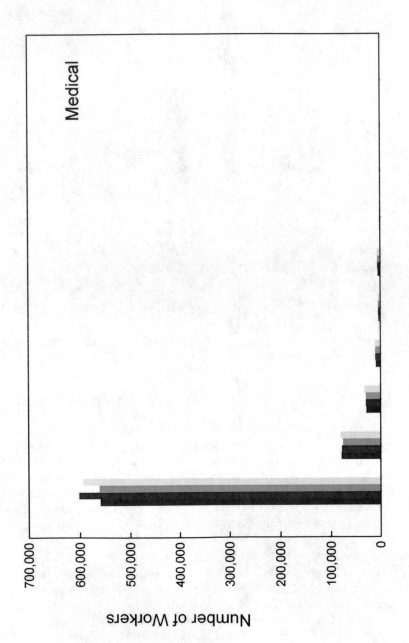

Dose (mSv)	>0 – <1	1 – 2.5	2.5 – 5	5 – 7.5	7.5 – 10	10 – 20	20 – 30	30 – 40	40 – 50	>50
2003	560,203	79,768	28,889	9,764	4,278	5,245	1,343	527	246	398
2004	602,153	78,944	30,076	10,495	4,834	6,032	1,504	612	289	461
2005	562,323	76,247	30,251	10,737	4,970	6,254	1,630	678	320	531
2006	594,394	81,758	32,782	11,536	5,242	6,506	1,631	646	328	524

Fig. 7.5. Dose distribution for workers with recordable dose for the medical category, 2003 to 2006.

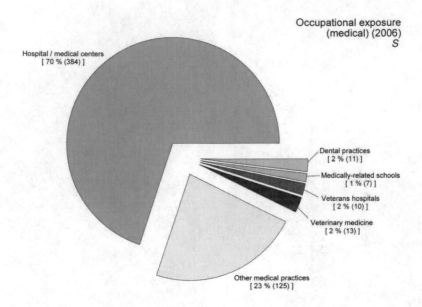

Fig. 7.6. Contribution of the various subcategories to S (percent and person-sievert) for the medical category of occupational exposure for 2006. Total for S is 550 person-Sv. Percent values have been rounded to the nearest 1 %.

0.4 µSv for all procedures except ^{99m}Tc sestimibi myocardial scans and RBC angiograms. Doses per procedure for those were 0.67 to 1.26 µSv and 1.19 to 2.5 µSv, respectively.

Achey *et al.* (2004) estimated technologist doses from ^{99m}Tc DTPA aerosol studies by measuring air concentration during 190 consecutive procedures. They concluded that one technologist performing all 190 procedures could receive a whole-body dose of 0.1 mSv and a lung dose of 1 mSv.

For the years 1990 to 1994, UNSCEAR (2000) indicated a worldwide average dose for measurably exposed workers in nuclear medicine of 0.8 mSv. However, for individuals doing radiopharmaceutical preparation and assay the whole-body annual doses could be 5 mSv and 500 mSv for the hands.

Individuals working solely with linear accelerators, high dose-rate afterloaders, gamma-ray stereotactic units, or teletherapy units in appropriately shielded radiation oncology facilities should receive no measurable radiation exposure.

Brachytherapy is performed manually using gamma-emitting sealed sources, typically ^{103}Pd or ^{125}I for prostate, ^{192}Ir for interstitial and intravascular, ^{137}Cs for intracavitary treatment, and occasionally [131]Cs, ^{125}I and [198]Au for other procedures. This may result in individuals receiving some whole-body radiation exposure. Schwartz *et al.* (2003) reporting on 155 prostate brachytherapy cases (both [103]Pd and ^{125}I) indicated that the average monitored dose is between 0.07 and 0.15 mSv per procedure. However, most, or all, of that dose is likely due to the fluoroscopy used in the procedure. Balter *et al.* (2000), Bohan *et al.* (2001), and Kirisits *et al.* (2004) indicate that doses to the radiation oncologist, physicist, cardiologist, and cardiology technologist are <10 μSv per procedure for intravascular brachytherapy with [192]Ir.

A majority of x-ray procedures in chiropractic medicine, podiatry, and dental practice use plain-film or digital radiography. The use of shielded control booths, control panels, or distance is usually sufficient to minimize occupational exposures. UNSCEAR (2000) estimated the annual effective dose to monitored workers in dental radiography at 0.32 mSv in 1990 and 0.06 mSv in 1994.

In routine practice, the occupational exposure in veterinary medicine would come from conventional radiography and fluoroscopy. In specialty practices, the occupational exposure would include the use of radiopharmaceuticals for diagnostic and therapeutic purposes. The most commonly used radionuclides include those most often used for human nuclear-medicine procedures: [99m]Tc and [131]I (Berg *et al.*, 1990; Ehrlich *et al.*, 1999; Koblik *et al.*, 1988; NCRP, 2004b). The use of positron emitters (*e.g.*, ^{18}F) is beginning to expand in the animal sciences area though they still are not common. UNSCEAR (2000) estimated a total of 85,000 monitored workers in veterinary medicine in the United States with the 38,000 receiving measurable dose having an annual average of 0.95 mSv.

7.3 Commercial Aviation

Commercial aviation is an occupational group that has a collective effective dose almost equal to the medical group and the highest average annual individual dose (Figures 7.1 to 7.4). Unlike other occupationally-exposed workers, commercial airline crews and pilots of corporate and cargo aircraft are not monitored. Consequently, doses are estimated based on calculations of galactic cosmic-ray doses for various flight routes and altitudes. The data used for the dose estimates in this Report are 45 y average effective doses for the flights and are listed in Table 7.5. The variation from these average doses over the 11 y solar cycle is estimated to be about ±10 %.

NCRP (1989b) noted that cosmic and solar particles were major sources of radiation exposure to airline crews during commercial aviation. These high-energy particles interact with nitrogen, oxygen

TABLE 7.4—*Personal monitoring information for chiropractic practices, podiatry, osteopathic medicine, dental practices, and veterinary medicine.*

Subcategory	2003	2004	2005	2006
Chiropractic practices				
Monitored workers	9,196	9,519	9,317	9,386
Workers with recordable dose	1,355	1,322	994	1,084
Collective effective dose (person-Sv)	0.3	0.3	0.3	0.4
Average effective dose (mSv)	0.22	0.23	0.30	0.42
Podiatry				
Monitored workers	7,782	8,674	9,026	8,704
Workers with recordable dose	84	145	124	141
Collective effective dose (person-Sv)	0.02	0.04	0.04	0.04
Average effective dose (mSv)	0.24	0.28	0.32	0.28
Osteopathic medicine				
Monitored workers	1,280	1,461	1,417	1,257
Workers with recordable dose	542	491	425	378
Collective effective dose (person-Sv)	0.1	0.3	0.1	0.1
Average effective dose (mSv)	0.18	0.61	0.24	0.26

Dental practices

Monitored workers	158,909	171,369	215,136	329,856
Workers with recordable dose	14,478	16,636	17,506	28,231
Collective effective dose (person-Sv)	2.3	3.1	4.5	10.5
Average effective dose (mSv)	0.16	0.19	0.26	0.37

Veterinary medicine

Monitored workers	221,554	271,722	296,341	294,789
Workers with recordable dose	42,381	49,347	44,484	46,998
Collective effective dose (person-Sv)	21.6	13.7	11.4	13.1
Average effective dose (mSv)	0.51	0.28	0.26	0.28

TABLE 7.5—*Effective dose of galactic cosmic radiation received by airline crews on flights as calculated by the computer code CARI-6 (adapted from Friedberg and Copeland, 2003).*

Origin – Destination	Highest Altitude [feet (thousands)][a]	Distance (statute miles)[b]	Air Time (h)	Block Hours[c]	Effective Dose[d] (µSv)	Effective Dose Rate (µSv per air hour)	Effective Dose Rate (µSv per block hour)
Domestic							
Seattle, WA – Portland, OR	21	150	0.4	0.6	0.17	0.43	0.28
Houston, TX – Austin, TX	20	140	0.5	0.6	0.17	0.34	0.28
Miami, FL – Tampa, FL	24	200	0.6	0.8	0.39	0.65	0.49
St. Louis, MO – Tulsa, OK	35	340	0.9	1.1	1.71	1.90	1.55
Tampa, FL – St. Louis, MO	31	870	2.0	2.2	4.71	2.36	2.14
New Orleans, LA – San Antonio, TX	39	480	1.2	1.3	3.27	2.73	2.52
Los Angeles, CA – Honolulu, HI	35	2,550	5.2	5.6	14.7	2.83	2.63
Honolulu, HI – Los Angeles, CA	40	2,550	5.1	5.5	16.4	3.22	2.98
New York, NY – San Juan, PR	37	1,600	3.0	3.4	10.1	3.37	2.97
Washington, DC – Los Angeles, CA	35	2,290	4.7	4.9	19.1	4.06	3.90
New York, NY – Chicago, IL	39	720	1.8	2.3	8.92	4.96	3.88
San Francisco, CA – Chicago, IL	41	1,870	3.8	4.3	20.7	5.45	4.81
Chicago, IL – San Francisco, CA	39	1,870	3.8	4.3	19.4	5.11	4.51
Seattle, WA – Anchorage, AK	35	1,430	3.4	3.7	16.9	4.97	4.57
Seattle, WA – Washington, DC	37	2,340	4.1	4.4	19.2	4.68	4.36
New York, NY – Seattle, WA	39	2,440	4.9	5.6	28.0	5.71	5.00
Average		1,365	2.84			3.30	2.93
Standard deviation						1.81	1.63

International

Los Angeles, CA – Tokyo	40	5,510	11.7	12.0	43.4	3.71	3.62
Tokyo – Los Angeles, CA	37	5,510	8.8	9.3	33.4	3.80	3.59
Lisbon – New York, NY	39	3,330	6.5	6.9	28.9	4.45	4.19
London – Dallas/Fort Worth, TX	39	4,750	9.7	10.2	43.7	4.51	4.28
Dallas/Fort Worth, TX – London	37	4,750	8.5	9.0	39.6	4.66	4.40
London – New York NY	37	3,450	6.8	7.3	37.4	5.50	5.12
New York, NY – Tokyo	43	6,800	13.0	13.6	75.4	5.80	5.54
Tokyo – New York, NY	41	6,800	12.2	12.5	69.6	5.70	5.57
London – Los Angeles, CA	39	5,440	10.5	11.0	61.6	5.87	5.60
Chicago, IL – London	37	3,950	7.3	7.7	43.0	5.89	5.58
London – Chicago, IL	39	3,950	7.8	8.3	47.5	6.09	5.72
Athens – New York, NY	41	4,920	9.4	9.7	61.3	6.52	6.32
Average		4,930	9.35			5.21	4.96
Standard deviation						0.94	0.91

[a] To convert to meters (approximately), divide by 3.28.

[b] To convert to kilometers (approximately), divide by 0.62.

[c] Block hours are measured from the time the aircraft parking brake is first released after the door is closed (prior to take-off) until the last time the aircraft parking brake is set before the door is opened (after landing).

[d] 45 y average effective dose for the flight, January 1958 through December 2002.

and argon nuclei in the upper atmosphere. Once a primary cosmic or solar particle interacts with an atmospheric gas nucleus, a cascade of secondary particles is produced. Though the ratio of secondary particles will vary with latitude, at 9,100 m this radiation field includes neutrons (42 to 52 %), electrons and photons (18 to 31 %), protons (~24 %), and muons (<5 %) (Friedberg *et al.*, 2000). Airline crews are exposed to this complex secondary particle and photon radiation field while at altitude. Typical flight altitudes for commercial aviation in the United States are between 6,100 and 12,200 m. Private passenger jet aircraft routinely fly at 15,000 to 17,000 m. At the equator, the mean effective dose from galactic cosmic rays varies from 0.54 to 3.89 μSv h^{-1} between 6,100 and 18,300 m, and at high latitudes, the dose varies from 1.05 to 14.5 μSv h^{-1} for the same altitudes (Friedberg *et al.*, 2000).

The Bureau of Labor Statistics reports employment data for airline pilots, copilots, flight engineers, and flight attendants by year (DOL, 2008). The information for 2003 to 2006 is shown in Table 7.3 and Figure 7.1. For 2006 there were ~76,000 aircraft pilots, copilots and flight engineers, and 97,000 flight attendants for a total number of 173,000 airline crew members.

UNSCEAR (2000) reviewed the potential for exposure to airline crews from cosmic rays and solar particles and found that during normal solar activity at the highest altitudes flown (typically 12,200 m) the dose rate averages 5.8 μSv h^{-1}. UNSCEAR (2000) further indicates:

- location within an aircraft does not affect the exposure by more than ±10 %;
- in going from the equator to either pole, the dose rate increases up to a geomagnetic latitude of ~58 degrees and remains approximately constant at higher latitudes with the increase for the high linear energy transfer component being about double that for the low linear energy transfer component; and
- the total dose equivalent rate increases with altitude for all latitudes.

Total annual doses depend on the flight route patterns and the total number of flying hours per year. O'Brien and Friedberg (1994) estimated that the annual doses ranged from 0.2 to 5 mSv. Actual data are difficult to obtain, but NCRP (1995c) noted flight time for members of U.S. airline crew may not exceed 1,000 h, assuming the crew members are not part of a second onboard relief crew for long duration flights. Currently members of the cockpit crew are limited to 1,000 h y^{-1}, but flight attendants have no yearly limit and may fly 1,000 to 1,200 h y^{-1} on average.[28] Note that hours, termed block hours, are measured from the time the aircraft parking brake is first released after the door is closed (prior to take-off) until the last time the aircraft parking brake is set before the door is opened (after landing).

UNSCEAR (2000) estimated that airline crews who make long-haul runs may be airborne for 600 h y^{-1} and experience annual effective doses of 3 mSv; whereas, short-haul flight (lower altitude) crews typically accrue 2 mSv during average annual times aloft of 500 h. Friedberg *et al.* (2000) calculated an annual dose to members of airline crew who make long-haul runs of 4.4 mSv using 700 block hours per year. Boice *et al.* (2000) estimated that a member of an airline crew flying between Los Angeles and Frankfurt for 700 block hours would receive an estimated yearly average dose of 4.1 mSv (range between 3.5 to 4.7 mSv depending on solar activity). Waters *et al.* (2000) indicated that the annual dose equivalent to flight attendants using 900 block hours can range from 0.82 to 5.4 mSv. From Table 7.5 (Friedberg and Copeland, 2003), a range in average annual effective dose of 0.2 to 4.4 mSv can be calculated using 700 block hours per year. However, for 1,000 block hours per year, the annual dose could be as high as 6.3 mSv. The range in average annual effective dose arises because of the variations in dose rate with altitude and latitude.

Using 700 block hours and the average dose rate for domestic flights (2.93 µSv per block hour) results in an average annual individual effective dose of 2.05 mSv for the cockpit crew. For 700 block hours on international flights (dose rate is 4.96 µSv per block hour) the average annual individual effective dose would be 3.47 mSv. Flight attendants flying an average of 1,000 to 1,200 block hours per year on domestic flights would receive an average annual individual effective dose of 2.93 to 3.52 mSv, and 4.96 to 5.95 mSv for the same times on international flights. In 2006, 89 % of travelers in the United States embarked on domestic flights and 93 % of all departures were domestic flights (BTS, 2008). To estimate an average annual dose for all airline crew, the average effective doses were weighted 90 % for domestic and 10 % for international flights. This results in an annual effective dose for cockpit crews of 2.19 mSv and for flight attendants a range of 3.13 to 3.76 mSv. A weighted average using 2.19 mSv for 76,000 cockpit crew members and the higher value of 3.76 mSv for 97,000 flight attendants

[28]Holland, M. (2008). Personal communication (American Airlines and Allied Pilots Association, Fort Worth, Texas).

results in an average individual effective dose for 2006 of 3.07 mSv for members of U.S. airline crew. This average value was used to calculate the collective effective dose for each year (Table 7.3).

The collective effective dose for pilots is probably underestimated because pilots of corporate and cargo aircraft were not included. Current trends indicate that airline crew staffing may be increasing again, which would increase the collective dose (S) for this employment category. More importantly, individual doses may be higher than estimated for several reasons. For fuel economy, flight routes may be at higher altitudes than were used in the dose calculations given in Table 7.5. International flights typically have a larger crew than domestic flights and therefore >10 % of crew flights may be international. Finally, airline crews may fly more hours than were estimated. These various factors could increase the estimate of the annual average effective dose (E_{Exp}) for members of airline crew by 10 to 20 %.

7.4 Industry and Commerce

7.4.1 General Trends

The industry and commerce exposure category includes a wide variety of industries:

- general manufacturing (*e.g.*, x-ray equipment manufacturing);
- various industrial uses (*e.g.*, construction, metal processing, petroleum refineries, petrochemical companies, mining, transportation/security, well loggers, highway construction);
- other fuel cycle (uranium);
- source production (*e.g.*, any industrial company, pharmaceutical companies, manufacturing companies); and
- testing and inspection (*e.g.*, industrial radiography, nuclear component construction).

Sources of radiation exposure include those used for industrial radiography, well logging, thickness and density measurement, static elimination, materials processing, sterilization, and production and distribution of radioactive material for nonmedical uses. Some workers in these industries may not be routinely monitored and for that reason their numbers and doses are not known. The uses most likely to result in the greatest exposure to an individual include radiography, and radiation-source manufacture and distribution (including x-ray machines). While the maximum dose to an individual working in one of these occupations may be higher than for other industrial uses, the number of persons potentially exposed is small.

Industry and commerce accounts for ~8 % of the occupational collective effective dose; as shown in Figure 7.2, there is a relatively flat collective dose trend over the 2003 to 2006 period. As shown in Figure 7.7, the dose distribution is similar to other occupational groups; the majority of workers with recordable doses (82 %) received annual doses <1 mSv and 96 % received <5 mSv. The average annual effective dose for those with recordable dose was 0.81 mSv (Table 7.3).

Figure 7.8 shows the distribution of doses within the industry and commerce subcategories. Source production and general manufacturing, including x-ray equipment manufacturing, contribute nearly 71 % of the annual collective effective dose in this category.

7.4.2 *Naturally-Occurring Radioactive Material and Technologically-Enhanced Naturally-Occurring Radioactive Material*

In recent years it has been recognized that certain materials used or generated in certain industry sectors have higher than average levels of NORM, or may concentrate NORM into TENORM. TENORM is usually defined as any NORM whose radionuclide concentrations or potential for human exposure have been increased by any human activities. Examples of industry sectors where such occupational exposures may occur are mining (uranium and other metal), metal works (ore processing, welding and fabrication, casting, grinding or sand-blasting), material production (phosphate fertilizer, phosphorus, paper and pulp, decorative or optical glass), energy production (oil and gas, geothermal, coal combustion), water treatment (drinking water, waste water), the building industry (stone cutting and polishing, building materials), and the chemical industry.

To the extent that monitored workers in the five subcategories of industry and commerce (Section 7.4.1) are exposed to TENORM sources, the doses from TENORM sources are included in the doses shown in Figure 7.8.

7.5 Commercial Nuclear-Power Industry

As shown in Table 7.3 and Figure 7.3, the commercial nuclear-power industry accounts for ~8 % of the occupational collective effective dose in the United States. Table 7.3 gives the average

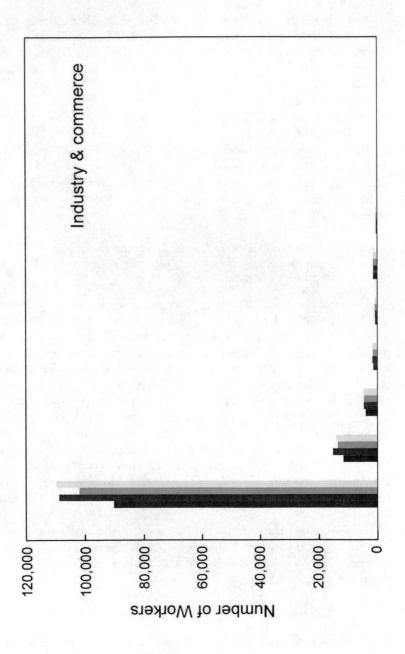

Dose (mSv)	>0 – <1	1 – 2.5	2.5 – 5	5 – 7.5	7.5 – 10	10 – 20	20 – 30	30 – 40	40 – 50	>50
2003	90,337	11,736	4,105	1,470	821	1,443	472	188	73	81
2004	108,843	15,385	4,756	1,748	905	1,459	477	199	66	88
2005	101,953	13,648	4,624	1,673	945	1,503	509	220	68	114
2006	109,849	14,288	4,780	1,723	938	1,597	515	207	80	128

Fig. 7.7. Dose distribution for workers with recordable dose for the industry and commerce category, 2003 to 2006.

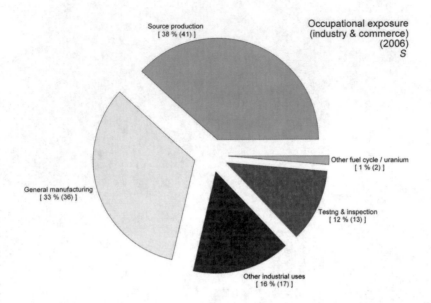

Fig. 7.8. Contribution of the various subcategories to S (percent and person-sievert) for the industry and commerce category of occupational exposure for 2006. Total for S is 110 person-Sv. Percent values have been rounded to the nearest 1 %.

annual dose in the nuclear-power industry as 1.9 mSv, which is second only to aviation (3.1 mSv); all other occupational groups have average annual doses <1 mSv.

Figure 7.9 indicates that the nuclear-power industry has relatively more workers than other industry sectors receiving doses >1 mSv. For perspective, 3.5 % of workers with recordable doses in the medical category received annual doses >5 mSv while 5 % of those in the commercial nuclear-power category received doses >5 mSv.

Information regarding radiation dose and dose trends for the light water reactors (the only type of power reactor in use in the United States) and their subsets, BWRs and PWRs, is available in NUREG-0713 (Dickson *et al.*, 2007), which provides graphs that show a rather steady increase in the number of operating nuclear-power plants in the United States from 1973 to 1988. A few plants have been decommissioned since the late 1970s and the total number of operating nuclear-power plants has remained at just over 100 for the past decade.

The annual collective dose for nuclear-power operation peaked in the early 1980s reaching a maximum of 565 person-Sv. Since then, there has been a steady decrease in both the number of individuals with recordable doses and the annual collective dose. The data for 2006 indicate that 58,788 individuals had a recordable dose and that the collective effective dose for that year was 110 person-Sv. While considerably more individuals are monitored in the PWR community than in the BWR community, the number of individuals with recordable dose in each and their respective contributions to the annual collective effective doses are about the same.

The decrease in annual collective effective dose for U.S. power plant workers occurred during a period in which the electricity generated by this industry increased. This can be accounted for because the efficiency of reactor operation increased with fewer and shorter outages, improved reactor coolant chemistries and materials, careful planning for outages, increased emphasis on the as low as reasonably achievable principle and radiation safety, improved tools and procedures, and a renewed emphasis on cleanliness of the work environment.

7.6 Academic Institutions

Academic institutions (education and research category) include colleges, universities and research institutes, and as shown in Figure 7.3, contribute ~4 % of the occupational dose in the United States. The majority of workers with recordable doses (88 %) received annual doses <1 mSv; 98 % received <5 mSv (Figure 7.10), and the average annual effective dose for those with recordable dose was 0.72 mSv (Table 7.3). The data do not include doses at academic institutions from work around research reactors or research on the nuclear fuel cycle.

Some of the more commonly used radionuclides in education and research environments include ^{3}H, ^{14}C, ^{32}P, ^{33}P, ^{35}S, ^{45}Ca, ^{51}Cr, ^{111}In, and ^{125}I. The data from Landauer, Inc. show that while the number of individuals monitored in academic and research organizations increased over the years 2003 to 2006, the average annual dose for those with recordable dose remained about the same.

These indications compare favorably with the UNSCEAR (2000) data for the United States for 1985 to 1989 showing an average annual dose per person with measurable exposure to be 0.86 mSv.

7.7 Government, DOE and Military

Government includes city and county agencies, DOT, FDA, the Federal Emergency Management Agency, federal and state prisons; DOE includes DOE and its contractors and subcontractors;

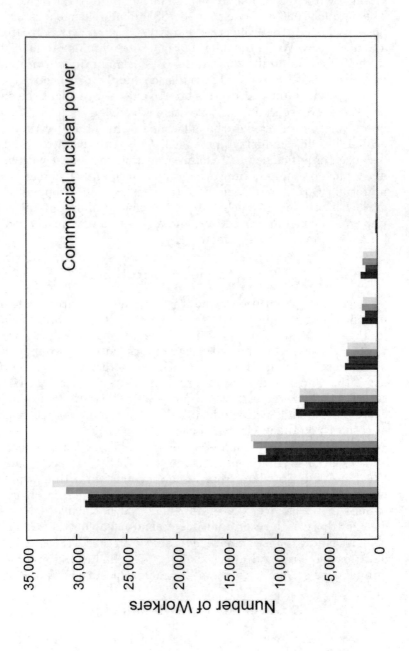

Dose (mSv)	>0 – <1	1 – 2.5	2.5 – 5	5 – 7.5	7.5 – 10	10 – 20	20 – 30	30 – 40	40 – 50	>50
2003	29,164	11,978	8,199	3,249	1,524	1,651	184	18	0	0
2004	28,863	11,179	7,334	2,873	1,233	1,190	188	13	0	0
2005	31,043	12,427	7,815	3,104	1,537	1,490	147	3	0	0
2006	32,426	12,685	7,796	2,975	1,416	1,406	147	2	0	0

Fig. 7.9. Dose distribution for workers with recordable dose for the commercial nuclear-power category, 2003 to 2006.

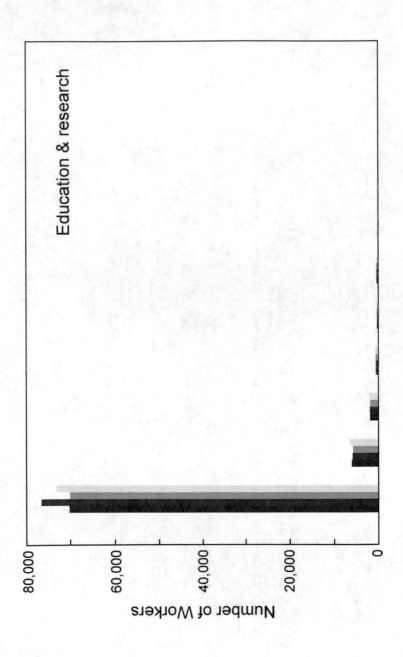

Dose (mSv)	>0 – <1	1 – 2.5	2.5 – 5	5 – 7.5	7.5 – 10	10 – 20	20 – 30	30 – 40	40 – 50	>50
2003	70,222	6,125	1,921	617	319	372	118	48	23	136
2004	76,672	5,923	1,972	617	316	400	118	56	30	84
2C05	70,067	5,825	1,879	633	351	442	117	49	29	75
2006	73,222	6,544	2,091	723	377	480	130	42	26	65

Fig. 7.10. Dose distribution for workers with recordable dose for the education and research category, 2003 to 2005.

military includes Army, Air Force, Navy/Marines, and the Naval Nuclear Propulsion Program.

As shown in Figure 7.3, the government, DOE, and military category contributes ~3 % of the occupational dose in the United States; the average annual dose varied between 0.5 and 0.7 mSv during 2003 to 2006 (Table 7.3). As shown in Figure 7.11, the majority of those with recordable doses (87 %) received <1 mSv; 98 % received <5 mSv. The average annual effective dose for those with recordable dose was 0.59 mSv (Table 7.3).

The percent of dose accrued in 2006 in various subcategories is shown in Figure 7.12. The Naval Nuclear Propulsion Program contributed 51 % of the government, DOE, military dose in 2006.

7.7.1 *Government*

Combined data from Global Dosimetry Solutions, Inc. and Landauer, Inc. for workers in government (Table 7.6) show significant variation for the years 2003 to 2006; the number of individuals monitored varied by ~50 %, the annual collective effective dose and the average annual effective dose for those with recordable dose were low but varied by more than a factor of two.

Because it was not possible to segregate doses received in connection with DOE activities from other government agencies using the Global Dosimetry Solutions, Inc. and Landauer, Inc. data, there may be minor duplication of data shown in the DOE category (Section 7.7.2). However, this duplication does not introduce a significant error. Also, an agency may appear in more than one subcategory because Global Dosimetry Solutions, Inc. and Landauer, Inc. grouped them differently; this is not a duplication of data.

7.7.2 *U.S. Department of Energy and U.S. Department of Energy Contractors*

DOE data include DOE employees, contractors and subcontractors (including "transient" workers). Detailed dose information is available in *DOE Occupational Radiation Exposure* (DOE, 2006a) report.

Over the time period 2003 to 2006, the number of monitored workers decreased each year, from 102,509 in 2003 to 91,280 in 2006 (a decrease of 11 %) (Table 7.7). The average dose is also on a decreasing trend, from 0.83 mSv in 2003 to 0.63 mSv (down ~25 %) in 2006. Similarly, the collective effective dose decreased from 14.4 person-Sv in 2003 to 8.1 person-Sv (down ~40 %) in 2006. From 2003 to 2006, all annual doses in excess of 30 mSv (none exceeded 50 mSv) resulted from internally-deposited radionuclides.

Due to the nature of work it carries out, DOE workers are more likely than others to receive neutron and internal doses. During the years 2003 to 2006, neutron dose contributed between 15 and 21 % of the collective TEDE, internal dose contributed between 6 and 7 %, and photon dose contributed between 73 and 79 %.

While weapons-related activities are declining at DOE facilities, other types of basic research continue, and new facilities are being built and staffed at some locations. As facilities are closed and decommissioned, the potential for exposure at many of the remaining facilities is changing. The increases and decreases in average doses reflect both the decommissioning activities as well as the initiation of new programs.

7.7.3   *Military*

The Naval Nuclear Propulsion Program contributes 87 % of the collective effective dose in the military group (Table 7.8). This includes doses to crews on ships and submarines (*i.e.*, the "fleet"), shipyard workers, laboratory workers, and prototype reactor workers. The dominant contribution to radiation exposure in the Naval Nuclear Propulsion Program is from the fleet and shipyard workers.

For the U.S. Army, the number of individuals receiving a recordable dose has remained fairly constant from 2003 through 2006, as has the average annual dose (0.62 to 0.7 mSv) (Table 7.8). The average annual collective effective dose of 1 to 1.2 person-Sv is low in comparison to the annual collective effective dose within other occupations such as medicine, industry or education.

For the U.S. Air Force, the average annual dose (0.5 to 0.9 mSv) and annual collective effective dose (0.5 to 1.1 person-Sv) for the years 2003 through 2006 (Table 7.8) are low and comparable to that for the Army.

For the U.S. Navy/Marines, the annual collective effective doses (1.3 to 1.4 person-Sv) are also similar to that for the Army (Table 7.8).

The data do not include for any of the military services exposure of pilots from cosmic rays and solar particles during flight operations, nor potential dose from internally-deposited depleted uranium for combat soldiers.

7.8 Summary

For occupationally-exposed workers, the medical category constitutes the largest number of individuals and shares the highest collective effective dose with the aviation category. Together these

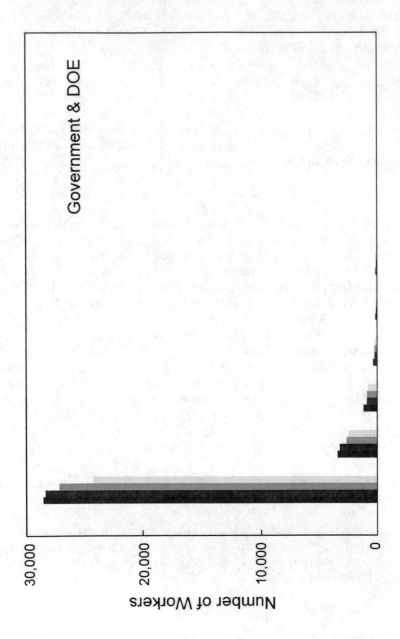

Dose (mSv)	>0 – <1	1 – 2.5	2.5 – 5	5 – 7.5	7.5 – 10	10 – 20	20 – 30	30 – 40	40 – 50	>50
2003	28,580	3,408	1,184	365	164	150	28	10	8	20
2004	28,417	3,224	911	232	114	86	32	7	4	19
2005	27,231	2,648	894	247	88	94	27	17	4	14
2006	24,327	2,455	803	210	83	90	20	6	6	8

Fig. 7.11. Dose distribution for workers with recordable dose in the government and DOE, 2003 to 2006. Data on dose distribution are not available for the military (Army, Air Force, Navy Nuclear Propulsion, and Navy/Marines); therefore, the number of workers represented in Figure 7.11 are less than the those represented in Table 7.3 and Figure 7.1 for the overall government, DOE and military subcategory.

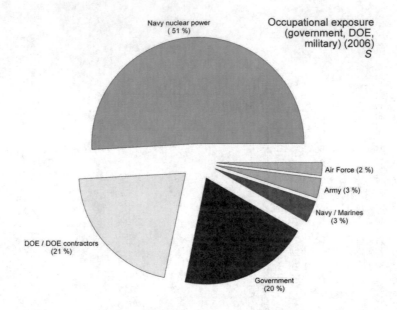

Fig. 7.12. Contribution of the various subcategories to S (percent) for the government, DOE and military category of occupational exposure for 2006. Total for S is 39 person-Sv. Percent values have been rounded to the nearest 1 % [see Tables 7.6, 7.7, and 7.8 for the individual values of S (person-sievert)].

two categories account for 77 % of the collective effective dose for occupational exposures. Medical, industrial and commerce, education and research, and government (including DOE and military) all have average annual effective doses <1 mSv. The commercial nuclear-power industry has a somewhat higher average annual effective dose (1.9 mSv), and aviation has the highest average annual effective dose (3.1 mSv). The results were obtained from personal monitoring data for all categories except aviation, which utilized information related to airline crews from U.S. Department of Labor and DOT.

For all occupational groups reviewed, the average annual effective dose received is but a fraction (<10%) of the annual occupational limit of 50 mSv recommended by NCRP (1993a). For most occupational workers, the annual dose is less than the value of 1 mSv recommended by NCRP (1993a) for members of the public. For 2006, the total occupational collective effective dose is 1,400 person-Sv. As stated in Section 7.1.2, the occupational collective effective doses derived from personal monitoring data are

TABLE 7.6—*Summary of annual occupational doses for government.*

Government Workers	2003	2004	2005	2006
Monitored workers	93,079	117,523	133,162	122,367
Workers with recordable dose	16,433	17,307	15,128	15,055
Collective effective dose (person-Sv)	7.2	14.0	5.7	7.8
Average effective dose (mSv)	0.44	0.81	0.38	0.52

TABLE 7.7—*Summary of annual occupational doses for DOE workers.*

DOE Workers	2003	2004	2005	2006
Monitored workers	102,509	100,011	98,040	91,280
Workers with recordable dose	17,484	15,739	16,136	12,953
Collective effective dose (person-Sv)	14.4	10.9	9.9	8.1
Average effective dose (mSv)	0.83	0.70	0.61	0.63

TABLE 7.8—Summary of annual occupational doses for the military.

Subcategory	Data	2003	2004	2005	2006
Air Force	Monitored workers	6,745	6,992	6,679	6,598
	Workers with recordable dose	917	2,079	896	961
	Collective effective dose (person-Sv)	0.8	1.1	0.5	0.6
	Average effective dose (mSv)	0.9	0.5	0.6	0.8
Army	Monitored workers	13,392	13,707	12,680	12,018
	Workers with recordable dose	1,725	1,663	1,774	1,622
	Collective effective dose (person-Sv)	1.2	1.1	1.1	1.0
	Average effective dose (mSv)	0.70	0.66	0.62	0.62
Navy Nuclear Propulsion[a,b]	Monitored workers	43,656	45,405	44,983	45,964
	Collective effective dose (person-Sv)	19.3	20.5	19.6	20.0
USN/Marines[a]	Monitored workers	6,489	6,341	5,954	5,965
	Collective effective dose (person-Sv)	1.3	1.4	1.3	1.3
Total	Collective effective dose (person-Sv)	22.6	24.1	22.5	22.9

[a]For Naval nuclear propulsion and the U.S. Navy/Marines, the number of monitored individuals with recordable doses (*i.e.*, above the minimum detectable level) was not discernible from the monitored population. The average effective dose is not presented.

[b]Data from 2004 were used for 2005 and 2006 for the two small components of the Navy Nuclear Propulsion subcategory [Nuclear reactors (DOE laboratory) and Nuclear reactors (prototype exposures); not shown] as it was the latest available.

likely underestimated, in part because some individuals who are monitored, but do not have a recordable dose above the minimum detectable level, may have received several tenths of a millisievert annually. For example, if the average annual effective dose in 2006 for all workers with doses below the minimum detectable level (nearly 2.6 million) were assumed to be 0.1 mSv, 260 person-Sv would be added to the occupational collective effective dose making it 1,660 person-Sv.

It is worth noting that for the categories in which doses were monitored (except commercial nuclear power and the DOE component of government and DOE) a small fraction of workers received an annual dose exceeding 50 mSv.[29] In 2006 the percentage of workers in each category exceeding 50 mSv was 0.07 % in medical, 0.1 % in industrial and commerce, 0.08 % in education and research, and 0.03 % in government and DOE (but no workers from DOE).

---

[29]NCRP (1993a) has an additional cumulative limit with age [*i.e.*, 10 mSv × age (years)] that would apply to these workers.

8. Summary and Conclusions

Radiation exposure of the U.S. population results from a variety of sources. For the purpose of this Report, the following five categories (noting the individuals exposed) were used:

- ubiquitous background radiation (members of the public)
- medical exposure (patients)
- consumer products and activities (members of the public)
- industrial, security, medical, educational and research activities (members of the public)
- occupational exposure (workers)

These categories are very similar in organization to those used in NCRP (1987a) for exposure to the U.S. population in the early 1980s. However, they do differ in their detailed components. For ubiquitous background radiation, more is known about radon levels in the United States and their related doses than before. For medical exposure, computed tomography (CT) and interventional procedures were just beginning to be utilized in the early 1980s, and now they are common. For consumer products and activities, an effort to include cigarette smoking and commercial air travel has been made. The industrial, security, medical, educational and research activities included in this Report and NCRP (1987a) are not identical, and for occupational exposure, considerable information from personal monitoring services is now available, but the contributions from both these categories are very small.

8.1 Population Doses for 2006

Table 8.1 summarizes the results for collective effective dose (S) (person-sievert and percent of total); effective dose per individual in the U.S. population (E_{US}) (millisievert and percent of total); and, when possible, average effective dose for the exposed group (E_{Exp}) (millisievert) for 2006. The estimates are annual values for the five categories (and major subcategories). Some additional data are provided on number of medical procedures and number of persons exposed.

TABLE 8.1—Collective effective dose (S), effective dose per individual in the U.S. population (E_{US}), and average effective dose for the exposed group (E_{Exp}) for 2006 (annual values for percent are rounded to the nearest 1 %).

Exposure Category	S (person-Sv)	E_{US} (mSv)	Percent of Total S or E_{US}	E_{Exp} (mSv)	Number of Procedures (millions)	Number of People Exposed
Ubiquitous background	933,000	3.11	50	3.11		300 million
Internal, inhalation (radon and thoron)	684,000	2.28	37 (73)[a]	2.28		
External, space	99,000	0.33	5 (11)[a]	0.33		
Internal, ingestion	87,000	0.29	5 (9)[a]	0.29		
External, terrestrial	63,000	0.21	3 (7)[a]	0.21		
Medical[b]	899,000	3.00	48	—	395	
Computed tomography	440,000	1.47	24 (49)[c]	—	67[d] (17 %)	
Nuclear medicine	231,000	0.77	12 (26)[c]	—	18 (5 %)	
Interventional fluoroscopy	128,000	0.43	7 (14)[c]	—	17 (4 %)	
Conventional radiography and fluoroscopy	100,000	0.33	5 (11)[c]	—	293 (74 %)	
Consumer[e]	39,000	0.13	2	0.001 – 0.3		Table 5.8
Industrial, security, medical, educational and research[f]	1,000	0.003	0.05	0.001 – 0.01		Table 6.3

TABLE 8.1—(continued).

Exposure Category	S (person-Sv)	E_{US} (mSv)	Percent of Total S or E_{US}	E_{Exp} (mSv)	Number of Procedures (millions)	Number of People Exposed
Occupational	*1,400*	*0.005*	*0.08*	*1.1*		*1,216,000*
Medical	550			0.8		735,000
Aviation	530			3.1		173,000
Commercial nuclear power	110			1.9		59,000
Industry and commerce	110			0.8		134,000
Education and research	60			0.7		84,000
Government, DOE, military	40			0.6		31,000
Total	*1,873,400* *(1,870,000)*	*6.248* *(6.2)*				

[a]Numbers in parentheses are percent for ubiquitous background category only.
[b]A separate analysis for external-beam radiotherapy is presented in Section 4.6, but is excluded from the totals presented here, as explained in Section 4.6.
[c]Numbers in parentheses are percent for medical category only.
[d]Number of CT scans (Section 4.2).
[e]Includes exposure to members of the public due to: building materials, commercial air travel, cigarette smoking, mining and agriculture, combustion of fossil fuels, highway and road construction materials, and glass and ceramics.
[f]Includes exposure to members of the public due to: nuclear-power generation; DOE installations; decommissioning and radioactive waste; industrial, medical, educational and research activities; contact with nuclear-medicine patients; and security inspection systems.

The total from all sources for 2006 is 1,870,000 person-Sv for S and 6.2 mSv for E_{US}, using a U.S. population of 300 million for 2006. These are significant increases over NCRP (1987a) estimates. Nearly all the S or E_{US} (98 %) results from ubiquitous background (50 %) and medical exposure of patients (48 %). Consumer products and activities account for 2 % and the other two categories contribute very little (on the order of 0.1 %). This distribution is presented in Figure 8.1.

The major sources are radon and thoron (37 %) (primarily radon), CT (24 %), nuclear medicine (12 %); other ubiquitous background sources (external plus internal) (13 %), and other medical exposure (interventional fluoroscopy plus conventional radiography and fluoroscopy) (12 %). This distribution is presented in Figure 8.2.

Of particular note in Table 8.1 is the observation that while the number of CT scans is only 17 % of the total procedures for the medical category,[30]   CT contributes nearly one-half (49 %) of

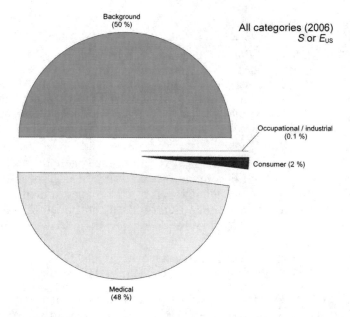

Fig. 8.1. Distribution of S or E_{US} for the categories of exposure for 2006. The percent values have been rounded to the nearest 1 %, except those <1 %. The total for S is 1,870,000 person-Sv and the total for E_{US} is 6.2 mSv, using a U.S. population of 300 million for 2006 [see Table 8.1 for the values of S (person-sievert) and E_{US} (millisievert)].

[30]Excludes dental bitewing and full-mouth procedures.

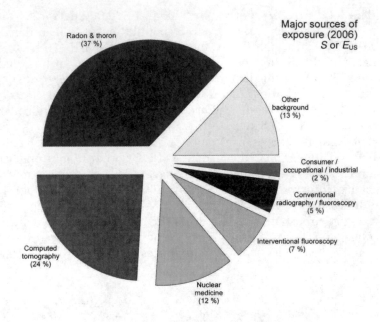

Fig. 8.2. Distribution of S or E_{US} for the major sources of exposure for 2006. The percent values have been rounded to the nearest 1 %. The total for S is 1,870,000 person-Sv and the total for E_{US} is 6.2 mSv, using a U.S. population of 300 million for 2006. The other background category consists of the external (space and terrestrial) and internal subcategories [see Table 8.1 for the values of S (person-sievert) and E_{US} (millisievert)].

the S or E_{US} for medical exposure, and nearly one-quarter (24 %) of the S or E_{US} for all sources of exposure. In a similar manner, while nuclear medicine consists of only 5 % of these medical procedures it contributes over one-quarter (26 %) of the S or E_{US} for medical exposure, and 12 % of the S or E_{US} for all sources of exposure.

8.2 Comparison of Population Doses for 2006 and the Early 1980s

Figures 8.3 and 8.4 present the distributions for the categories and major sources from the early 1980s, respectively.

Table 8.2 compares the results for S or E_{US} as reported by NCRP (1987a) for the early 1980s and in this Report for 2006. The estimates are annual values for the five categories (and major subcategories). Table 8.3 gives the magnitude of the changes in S or E_{US} for the five categories between NCRP (1987a) and this Report as ratios of the 2006 values to the values for the early 1980s. Of particular note are the following comparisons:

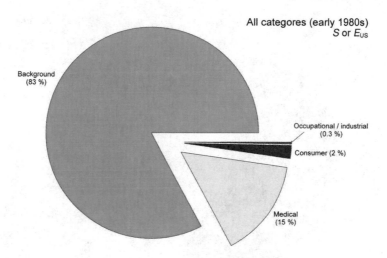

Fig. 8.3. Distribution of S or E_{US} for the categories of exposure for the early 1980s (NCRP, 1987a). The percent values have been rounded to the nearest 1 %, except those <1 %. The total for S is 835,000 person-Sv and the total for E_{US} is 3.6 mSv, using a U.S. population of 230 million for the early 1980s [see Table 8.2 for the values of S (person-sievert) and E_{US} (millisievert)].

- Total S (all sources) is 1,870,000 and 835,000 person-Sv for 2006 and the early 1980s, respectively. The increase for 2006 is a factor of ~2.2 (124 %). This includes an increase due only to the number of individuals in the U.S. population, which increased a factor of 1.3 (30 %) from 230 million in 1980 to 300 million in 2006.
- Total E_{US} (all sources) is 6.2 and 3.6 mSv for 2006 and the early 1980s, respectively. The increase for 2006 is a factor of ~1.7 (72 %). This differs from the ratio for S because of the normalization to an individual in the U.S. population, thus removing the effect of the population increase. The remaining increase is due solely to additional exposure that was not experienced in the early 1980s.
- S for ubiquitous background alone is 933,000 and 690,000 person-Sv for 2006 and the early 1980s, respectively, which is a factor of 1.35 (35 %). This corresponds approximately to the population increase. Therefore, E_{US} for ubiquitous background is 3.1 and 3 mSv for 2006 and the early 1980s, respectively, and nearly the same.
- S for medical exposure alone is 899,000 person-Sv for 2006 and 123,000 person-Sv for the early 1980s. The increase for

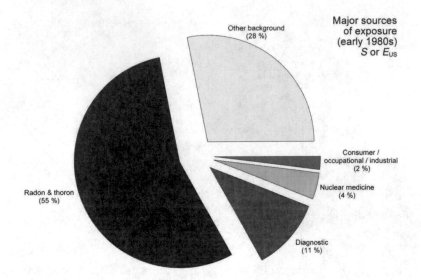

Fig. 8.4. Distribution of S or E_{US} for the major sources of exposure for the early 1980s (NCRP, 1987a). The percent values have been rounded to the nearest 1 %. The total for S is 835,000 person-Sv and the total for E_{US} is 3.6 mSv, using a U.S. population of 230 million for 1980 [see Table 8.2 for the values of S (person-sievert) and E_{US} (millisievert)].

2006 is a factor of 7.3 (630 %). This also includes an increase due only to population growth. The increase in medical exposure accounts for the large majority (776,000 person-Sv) of the overall increase (1,035,000 person-Sv) in S from the early 1980s.

- E_{US} for medical exposure is 3 and 0.53 mSv for 2006 and the early 1980s, respectively. The increase for 2006 is a factor of 5.7 (470 %). With the increase due to population growth removed, this represents the much increased utilization of the medical modalities of CT, nuclear-medicine, and inter-ventional-fluoroscopic procedures compared with the early 1980s.

The occupational category suggests a reduction in the values of S and E_{US} compared to the early 1980s, but that category and the remaining two categories (*i.e.*, consumer; and industrial, security, medical, educational and research) consist of relatively small contributions from disparate aggregated sources and further conclusions cannot be drawn.

TABLE 8.2—*Comparison of collective effective dose (S) and effective dose per individual in the U.S. population (E_{US}) as reported in NCRP (1987a) and in this Report (annual values for percent are rounded to the nearest 1 %)*

Exposure Category	This Report [for 2006]			NCRP (1987a)[a] [for the early 1980s]		
	S (person-Sv)	E_{US} (mSv)	Percent of Total S or E_{US}	S (person-Sv)[a]	E_{US} (mSv)[a]	Percent of Total S or E_{US}
Ubiquitous background	933,000	3.11	50	690,000	3.0	83
Radon and thoron[b]	684,000	2.28	37	460,000	2.0	55
Other	249,000	0.83	13	230,000	1.0	28
Medical	899,000	3.00	48	123,000	0.53	15
CT (2006)	440,000	1.47	24			
Conventional radiography and fluoroscopy (2006)	100,000	0.33	5			
All diagnostic (1980)				91,000[c,d]	0.39	11
Nuclear medicine	231,000	0.77	12	32,000[d]	0.14	4
Interventional fluoroscopy (2006)	129,000	0.43	7			
Consumer	39,000	0.13	2	12,000 – 29,000	0.05 – 0.13	<2
Industrial, security, medical, educational and research	1,000	0.003	0.05	200[e]	0.001	0.03

TABLE 8.2—(continued).

Exposure Category	This Report [for 2006]			NCRP (1987a)[a] [for the early 1980s]		
	S (person-Sv)	E_{US} (mSv)	Percent of Total S or E_{US}	S (person-Sv)[a]	E_{US} (mSv)[a]	Percent of Total S or E_{US}
Occupational	1,400	0.005[f]	0.08	2,000	0.009[f]	0.3
Total	1,870,000[g]	6.2[g]		835,000	3.6	

[a]The quantities used in NCRP (1987a) were expressed in H_E.
[b]Radon plus thoron for 2006; radon only for the early 1980s.
[c]Included 3,700 person-Sv from CT and 4,200 person-Sv from interventional fluoroscopy [listed as "other" in NCRP (1987a)].
[d]Values differ slightly from those reported in NCRP (1989a) and Table 4.19.
[e]Consisted of the nuclear fuel cycle and miscellaneous environmental sources.
[f]The values of E_{Exp} are 1.1 mSv for 2006 and 2.3 mSv for the early 1980s.
[g]Rounded values.

TABLE 8.3—*Magnitude of changes in collective effective dose (S) and effective dose per individual in the U.S. population (E_{US}) between the early1980s (NCRP, 1987a) and 2006 (this Report).*

Exposure Category	S (person-Sv)[a]			E_{US} (mSv)[a]		
	(1) 2006	(2) Early 1980s	Ratio (1)/(2)	(1) 2006	(2) Early 1980s	Ratio (1)/(2)
Ubiquitous background	933,000	690,000	1.35	3.11	3.00	1.04
Medical	899,000	123,000	7.3	3.00	0.53	5.7
Consumer	39,000	12,000 – 29,000	—[b]	0.13	0.05 – 0.13	—[b]
Industrial, security, medical, educational and research	1,000	200	—[b]	0.003	0.001	—[b]
Occupational	1,400	2,000	—[b]	0.005	0.009	—[b]
Total	1,870,000[c]	835,000	2.2	6.2[c]	3.6	1.7

[a]The quantities used in NCRP (1987a) were expressed in H_E.
[b]Not listed; disparate aggregated sources.
[c]Rounded values.

8.3 Uncertainties in Estimating the Dose Quantities

Uncertainty in the dose quantities presented in this Report are due to uncertainty in the underlying measurements from which these quantities are estimated, in the dosimetric models and their parameters, in the number of individuals exposed, and in the assumptions made in the absence of information.

With regard to exposure from the ubiquitous background radiation category, the greatest uncertainty is with estimating effective dose from exposure to radon, thoron, and their short-lived decay products. There also are uncertainties associated with the estimated effective dose from internally-deposited uranium and thorium due to a scarcity of human tissue data. Because of the complexity of intake routes, and differing uptakes of the various radioactive elements in the natural series decay chains, different approaches have yet to be reconciled. There are uncertainties for estimating effective dose for external irradiation associated with shielding by buildings, irradiation by building materials, and portions of time spent out- and indoors.

In the assessment of effective dose and collective effective dose for the medical exposure of patients category, the largest sources of uncertainty are in the number of procedures and the effective dose for each type of examination. For 2006, no information was readily available for the actual number of patients, only for the number of procedures. Additional uncertainty arises because effective doses are based on various types of measurements using standard phantoms and representative clinical technique factors. The effective doses to patients may differ significantly from those determined in that manner. In nuclear medicine, uncertainties in effective dose arise because of assumptions made regarding the transfer of the radionuclide between different metabolic or physiologic compartments in the human body, especially in diseased patients, as well as in radiation transport calculations, the quantity of impurities in the radiopharmaceutical and the amount of administered activity.

For the consumer products and activities category, and the industrial, security, medical, educational and research activities category, large uncertainties arise because of the lack of measurements and records for assessing exposure to members of the public. For the occupational exposure category uncertainties and a general bias toward underestimation of effective dose are introduced because of a number of reasons, including:

- not every supplier of personal monitoring systems was included;

- workers may not wear their personal monitors at all times;
- monitoring programs do not exist for some occupationally-exposed work groups; and
- dosimetry may or may not be issued or audited.

Additional reasons are listed in Section 7.1.2.

A detailed uncertainty analysis was possible for only the ubiquitous background radiation category (Table 3.14). The uncertainty for other exposure categories cannot be inferred from that analysis. At the present time, uncertainty analysis for all the other categories is limited primarily to identification of the contributing factors.

Appendix A

Conversions from International System of Quantities and Units to Previous System

Absorbed dose, kerma
  1 Gy = 100 rad
  1 mGy = 100 mrad
Effective dose, equivalent dose
  1 Sv = 100 rem
  1 mSv = 100 mrem
  1 μSv = 0.1 mrem
Exposure
  1 C kg^{-1} = 3,876 R
  1 C kg^{-1} min^{-1} = 3,876 R min^{-1}
Activity
  1 Bq = 27 pCi
  1 Bq m^{-3} = 0.027 pCi L^{-1}
  1 MBq (1 × 10^6 Bq) = 0.027 mCi
  1 Bq kg^{-1} = 0.027 pCi g^{-1}
Relationship (free-in-air) between air kerma and exposure
  1 Gy (air kerma) results from 114 R (exposure)
  1 mGy results from 0.114 R
Working level and working level month
  1 WL = 2.08 × 10^{-5} J m^{-3} = 1.3 × 10^5 MeV L^{-1} (potential alpha-energy concentration)
  1 WLM = 3.54 × 10^{-3} J h m^{-3} = 2.21 × 10^7 MeV L^{-1} (potential alpha-energy exposure)

Appendix B

Radionuclides in Domestic Water Supplies

Radium, uranium and radon may be present in public and domestic (private) water supplies throughout the United States. Between July 1, 1984 and October 31, 1986, EPA sampled 990 public water supplies as part of the National Inorganic and Radionuclide Survey (NIRS) (Longtin, 1988).

NIRS data are presented as population-weighted average concentrations for each state and for the United States. Population-weighted means that for each water system sampled, the concentration was multiplied by the population served by that system. The result was summed for all systems and divided by the sum of the population over all sites sampled for that state. Longtin (1988) reported that 30 to 90 % of the systems in a given state showed concentrations below the minimum reporting level, but he assumed that those results were equal to the minimum reporting level. This assumption overestimates the level of occurrence, introducing a bias on the high side. However, for systems with multiple sources, the distribution sampling method used by Longtin (1988) may bias the results low for some consumers who are near the start of the distribution system and receive water from a point-of-entry with elevated radionuclide concentrations. Although the sampling was done in 1986, NIRS data are still the most complete and current empirical data available on radionuclides in public drinking water supplies.

B.1 Radium and Uranium in Drinking Water

The range of doses using NIRS data is presented in Table B.1. The range was selected by using the states with the lowest and

TABLE B.1—*Annual effective doses (E) and collective effective doses (S) (by age) in the U.S. population from radium and uranium in public water supplies.*

Age (y)	Number of People Exposed (thousands)[a]	E (minimum – maximum) (μSv)[b]	S^c (person-Sv) (using average concentrations)
0 – 1	3,526	154 – 768	822
>1 – 2	3,502	26 – 134	140
>2 – 7	17,272	21 – 109	558
>7 – 12	16,757	25 – 132	651
>12 – 17	18,020	50 – 278	1,438
>17	196,485	11 – 67	3,590

[a]Values are 85 % of the estimated 2006 population based on the 2000 U.S. Census (USCB, 2006c). The total 2006 population is 300 million.

[b]Represents the range of concentrations of radium and uranium for U.S. community water systems.

[c]Based on population-weighted U.S. averages of 33 Bq m^{-3} for ^{226}Ra, 52 Bq m^{-3} for ^{228}Ra, 52 Bq m^{-3} for ^{224}Ra, and 41 Bq m^{-3} for total uranium.

highest population-weighted averages for each radionuclide. Consumption rates for each age range were taken from Table A2 of *Estimated Per Capita Water Ingestion in the United States* (EPA, 2000b). The dose conversion coefficients were taken from ICRP Publication 72 (ICRP, 1996), to convert to effective dose (E). Based on the reconnaissance survey conducted by USGS in 1998, it was assumed that ^{224}Ra concentrations were equal to ^{228}Ra concentrations (Barringer *et al.*, 2001). Since uranium concentrations were reported as a mass concentration (μg L^{-1}), they were converted to an activity concentration (Bq L^{-1}) of ^{238}U by multiplying by 0.025 Bq μg^{-1} (Longtin, 1988). Uranium-234 concentrations were assumed to be equal to that of ^{238}U based on the assumption of natural abundance (Longtin, 1988). Hess *et al.* (1985) reported ^{234}U to ^{238}U activity ratios of <1 to >20, which suggests a large variability depending on the chemistry of the local aquifer. The contribution to E from ^{235}U was negligible and was not included in these estimates. Eighty-five percent of the U.S. population uses public water supplies (Hutson *et al.*, 2005). Therefore, the population values used for the age distribution are 85 % of the estimated 2006 values in each age range based on the 2000 U.S. Census (USCB,

2006c). The total 2006 population is 300 million. Note that E for an infant (age 0 to 1 y) is over 10 times that for an adult, even accounting for the lower consumption rate of infants. However, S is much smaller for infants than adults due to the smaller population size.

USGS reports that 15 % of the total population of the United States consumes drinking water from private wells (Hutson *et al.*, 2005). USGS analyzed data for ^{222}Rn and uranium from domestic wells that were sampled from 1986 to 2004 as part of the National Water-Quality Assessment Program, the USGS Cooperative Water Program, National Research Program, and the Toxic Substances Hydrology Program (Focazio *et al.*, 2006). Radium-226, radium-228, and radium-224 concentrations in domestic wells were obtained directly from the same USGS National Water-Quality Assessment Program.[31] Not all water samples were analyzed for radon, uranium and radium. Uranium was analyzed in samples from 2,390 wells, while radon was analyzed in samples from 4,820 wells. Radium-226, radium-228, and radium-224 were analyzed in samples from 558, 391, and 553 wells, respectively. The concentrations of uranium and radon are higher in these private wells than in the community water supplies analyzed by Longtin (1988). The concentration distribution of radium in the national survey was higher in community water supplies than the domestic wells sampled. This difference may be due to a bias in domestic well selection focused towards volatile organic compound detection where aquifers were shallow and unconfined, which may have corresponded to a few radium-affected areas, as well as substantial sampling of domestic wells from confined aquifers with chemistry not conducive to radium mobility.[31]

The concentrations for private wells are not population weighted. The range of doses was determined based on the minimum and maximum reported values. In the case of radon, the minimum value used was determined by assessing the lowest positive value (407 Bq m^{-3}), which was comparable with EPA assessment of the method's minimum detectable concentration (444 Bq m^{-3}). The lowest minimum detectable concentration was used as the minimum for uranium and the radium family. The values of E resulting from this occurrence data are presented in Tables B.2 and B.3 for uranium and radium, respectively, and for radon in Section B.2.

Although the uranium and radon data in Focazio *et al.* (2006) were not originally designed to be a statistical representation of national occurrence of domestic water supplies, the data encompass

[31]Szabo, Z. (2007). Personal communication (New Jersey Water Science Center, U.S. Geological Survey, Trenton, New Jersey).

TABLE B.2—*Annual effective doses (E) and collective effective doses (S) in the U.S. population from uranium in private wells.*

Age (y)	Number of People Exposed (thousands)[a]	E (minimum – maximum) (μSv)[b]	S^c (person-Sv) (using average concentration)
0 – 1	622	0.02 – 1,122	7
>1 – 2	618	0.007 – 349	2
>2 – 7	3,048	0.006 – 318	10
>7 – 12	2,957	0.005 – 288	9
>12 – 17	3,180	0.008 – 426	14
>17	34,674	0.008 – 424	154

[a]Values are 15 % of the estimated 2006 population based on the 2000 U.S. Census (USCB, 2006c). The total 2006 population is 300 million.

[b]Represents the range of concentrations of total uranium for U.S. private wells of between 0.5 Bq m^{-3} (0.01 μg L^{-1}) and 25,782 Bq m^{-3} (520 μg L^{-1}).

[c]Based on average U.S. total uranium concentration of 270 Bq m^{-3} (5.44 μg L^{-1}).

TABLE B.3—*Annual effective doses (E) from radium in private wells.[a]*

Age (y)	E (minimum – maximum) (μSv)[b]
0 – 1	0.35 – 2,900
>1 – 2	0.60 – 480
>2 – 7	0.48 – 390
>7 – 12	0.58 – 480
>12 – 17	1.2 – 1,000
>17	0.27 – 210

[a]S for the U.S. population was not determined because the data were not representative of the U.S. average concentration of radium.

[b]Represents the range of concentrations for U.S. private wells of 0.67 to 407 Bq m^{-3} for ^{226}Ra, 0.74 to 688 Bq m^{-3} for ^{228}Ra, and 0.92 to 159 Bq m^{-3} for ^{224}Ra.

large parts of the United States including at least some wells in every state and Puerto Rico. Therefore, the average value from the data was used to determine S for the U.S. population from private wells for uranium (Table B.2) and radon (Tables B.5 and B.7) (Section B.2).

B.2 Radon in Water

Radon is a naturally-occurring radioactive gas, and may be found in drinking water and indoor air. Radon is a decay product of natural uranium present in some rocks and soil. If groundwater travels through uranium-bearing rock, the radon will dissolve in the groundwater. Whenever water is used in a home such as for showering, washing clothes, and flushing toilets, some of the radon is released from the water and mixes with the indoor air where it is inhaled by the consumer. Drinking water containing dissolved radon is also a source of exposure to internal organs after ingestion.

Most of the radon in indoor air comes directly from soil that is in contact with or beneath the basement or foundation. Radon enters homes through openings that are in contact with the ground, such as cracks in the foundation, small openings around pipes, and sump pits. This is discussed in Section 3 as part of the exposure from ubiquitous background radiation.

To determine the dose from radon in water, the concentration of radon in air that results from a given concentration of radon in water, termed the transfer coefficient, must be determined. NAS/NRC (1999a), *Risk Assessment of Radon in Drinking Water,* concluded that the transfer coefficient is between 0.8×10^{-4} and 1.2×10^{-4} and is dependent on many factors including room volume, water usage, and ventilation rate. NAS/NRC (1999a) recommended that EPA continue to use 1×10^{-4} as the best central estimate of the transfer coefficient. This means that typical use of water containing radon at 10,000 Bq m^{-3} will, on average, increase the air radon concentration by 1 Bq m^{-3}.

Effective dose[32] from radon decay products in air for adults is determined in this Report using a conversion coefficient of 10 mSv WLM^{-1} (Section 3.3.4.10). WLM is defined as the exposure to 1 WL for a working month (170 h). WL is a measure of the energy from a specified amount of alpha-particle emitting short-lived radon progeny in 1 L of air. For a more detailed discussion of WLM, WL and E from inhaled radon, see Sections 3.3.4.1 and 3.3.4.10. In order to determine the WLM from a given concentration of radon

[32]The committed effective dose component from internal exposure.

in water, the transfer coefficient of 10,000 to 1 (as discussed above), and an equilibrium factor of 40 % is assumed (Section 3.3.4.4). The occupancy factor for a year was determined by using EPA *Exposure Factors Handbook* value of 16.4 h indoors at home per day (EPA, 1997). It was assumed that a person spends 350 d y^{-1} at home (EPA, 1997).

Using NIRS data for population-weighted averages, the minimum and maximum *E* from radon in public water supplies was calculated for the United States for inhalation (Table B.4) and ingestion (Table B.5). The estimated annual *S* (inhalation plus ingestion) for adults using the average concentration is 8,700 person-Sv. For average U.S. concentration of radon in private wells, the estimated annual *S* (inhalation plus ingestion) for adults is ~14,000 person-Sv. The separate annual contributions from inhalation and ingestion to *E* for adults from radon in private water supplies are given in Tables B.6 and B.7, respectively.

B.3 Summary

NIRS data and dose conversion coefficients from ICRP [1996 (for radium and uranium)] and NAS/NRC [1999a (for radon)] were used to estimate *S* due to radium, uranium and radon in community water for the 2006 estimated U.S. population (USCB, 2006c).

Since public drinking water is regulated with respect to radium and uranium by EPA, the dose from radium and uranium should be an insignificant contributor to the total radiation exposure of the U.S. population, provided that these public water supplies are in compliance with EPA maximum contaminant levels. All systems are required to be in compliance by 2008. However, private well water is unregulated, as well as radon in water from public or private wells. Although private wells serve a small portion of the population, individuals who consume water from these private wells could receive significant doses. Some private well water contains much greater amounts of radon than public water supplies (*e.g.*, radon levels over 37×10^6 Bq m^{-3} have been observed in water in the Appalachian Highlands). The resultant annual *E* to an individual from such a concentration can be as high as 135 mSv.

Higher doses to some individuals could also result from consumption of public water supplies that draw from groundwater with elevated radon concentrations. Longtin (1988) found that radon concentrations in water from large public water supplies (serving >1,000 people) are less than concentrations in small public water supplies (those serving <1,000 people). However, the resulting contributions to collective effective doses would be higher for

TABLE B.4—*Annual inhalation contribution to effective dose (E) and collective effective dose (S) for adults from radon in water from public water supplies.*

Concentration in Water (Bq m^{-3})	Concentration in Air (Bq m^{-3})	Working Level	Working Level Month	E (mSv)	S (person-Sv)
Minimum: 3,704	0.37	4 × 10^{-5}	1.3 × 10^{-3}	0.01	
Maximum: 99,018	10	1.1 × 10^{-3}	0.036	0.36	
Average: 9,222	0.92	9.9 × 10^{-5}	3.3 × 10^{-3}	0.03[a]	6,484[a]

[a]The values 0.03 and 6,484 are E_{Exp} and S, respectively, for this population. The value for S is based on the adult population (age >17 y) given in Table B.1.

TABLE B.5—*Annual ingestion contribution to effective dose (E) and collective effective dose (S) from radon in water from public water supplies.*

Age (y)	Number of People Exposed (thousands)	E (minimum – maximum) (μSv)[a]	S (person-Sv)[b] (using average concentration)
0 – 1	3,526	18 – 485	160
>1 – 2	3,502	9 – 247	81
>2 – 7	17,272	5 – 145	234
>7 – 12	16,757	3 – 92	143
>12 – 17	18,020	4 – 97	163
>17	196,485	4 – 121	2,217

[a]Represents the minimum and maximum concentrations of radon in water for public water supplies of 3,700 and 98,919 Bq m^{-3}, respectively. Dose conversion coefficients obtained from NAS/NRC (1999a).
[b]Based on average U.S. radon concentration of 9,213 Bq m^{-3}.

TABLE B.6—*Annual inhalation contribution to effective dose (E) and collective effective dose (S) for adults from radon in water from private water supplies.*

Concentration in Water (Bq m^{-3})	Concentration in Air (Bq m^{-3})	Working Level	Working Level Month	E (mSv)	S (person-Sv)
Minimum: 407	0.04	4.4×10^{-6}	1.5×10^{-4}	1.5×10^{-3}	
Maximum: 33,703,703	3,370	0.36	12	120	
Average: 78,740	7.87	8.5×10^{-4}	0.03	0.3[a]	10,402[a]

[a]The values 0.3 and 10,402 are E_{Exp} and S, respectively, for this population.

TABLE B.7—*Annual ingestion contribution to effective dose (E) and collective effective dose (S) from radon in water from private water supplies.*

Age (y)	Number of People Exposed (thousands)	E (minimum – maximum) (μSv)[a]	S (person-Sv)[b] (using average concentration)
0 – 1	622	2 – 165,096	240
>1 – 2	618	1 – 84,092	121
>2 – 7	3,048	59 – 49,476	352
>7 – 12	2,957	38 – 31,302	216
>12 – 17	3,180	40 – 33,167	246
>17	34,674	50 – 41,230	3,340

[a]Represents the minimum and maximum concentrations of radon in water for U.S. private water supplies.
[b]Based on average U.S. radon concentration of 78,740 Bq m^{-3}.

the large public water supplies because of the much larger number of individuals served.

The estimated annual S from average concentrations of uranium, radium and radon in the United States for consuming community water is 33,700 person-Sv [16,700 person-Sv for public water supplies (sum of entries in Tables B.1, B.4, and B.5) plus 17,000 person-Sv for private water supplies (sum of entries in Tables B.2, B.3, B.6, and B.7)].[33]

[33]The sum of 15,100 person-Sv from Tables B.2, B.6, and B.7 was adjusted arbitrarily to 17,000 person-Sv to include a small contribution from radium that could not be directly calculated (Table B.3).

Appendix C

Computed Tomography Dose Indices and Dose Length Product

The computed tomography dose index ($CTDI$) (Shope *et al.*, 1981) is the primary dose metric in computed tomography (CT). $CTDI$ represents the average absorbed dose at the midpoint of a range along the longitudinal axis spanned in a sequence of contiguous exposures, each exposure made in an axial-scanning mode (*i.e.*, where there is no table movement during irradiation). As $CTDI$ is equivalent to the longitudinal integral of dose contributions (per total beam width) associated with a single rotation of the x-ray tube around the system isocenter, $CTDI$ is typically measured with a fixed-length (usually 100 mm) ionization chamber centrally positioned at the fan-beam plane during a single rotation. $CTDI_{100}$ is the name for this index of dose based on a convention of a 100 mm range of integration along the longitudinal axis (Bongartz *et al.*, 2004; IEC, 2002; Jessen *et al.*, 2000). Specifically, $CTDI_{100}$ has units of absorbed dose (milligray in air) within a standard cylindrical dosimetry phantom made of polymethyl methacrylate [*i.e.*, acrylic, Plexiglas® (Evonik Industries, Darmstadt, Germany), Perspex® or Lucite® (Lucite International, Southampton, United Kingdom)]. Phantom diameters of 16 cm and 32 cm, respectively, correspond to dimensions associated with an adult head and body. The value of $CTDI_{100}$ varies across the field-of-view. For the body phantom, $CTDI_{100}$ is typically a factor of two higher near the phantom surface than along the central axis. With the phantom central axis aligned with the axis of rotation, and with the phantom positioned centrally at the fan-beam plane, measurements are made along the phantom central (c) axis and along peripheral (p) axes located 10 mm below the phantom surface. The average $CTDI_{100}$ across the field-of-view of the phantom is given by the weighted $CTDI_{100}$ (*i.e.*, $CTDI_w$) (Bongartz *et al.*, 2004; IEC, 2002; Jessen *et al.*, 2000), which is approximated as follows:

$$CTDI_w = \frac{1}{3} CTDI_{100,c} + \frac{2}{3} CTDI_{100,p}. \qquad (C.1)$$

$CTDI_w$ has been a useful indicator of radiation output of a scanner operating at a peak kilovoltage and milliampere-second.

In order to represent dose for a specific scan protocol, which almost always involves a series of rotations, it is essential to take into account any gaps or overlaps between the radiation dose profiles from consecutive rotations of the x-ray source. This is accomplished with use of a dose descriptor known as the volume $CTDI_w$ (*i.e.*, $CTDI_{vol}$) (IEC, 2002), which, for axial-mode CT scanning is given as follows:

$$CTDI_{vol} = \left(N\frac{T}{I} \right)(CTDI_w), \qquad (C.2)$$

where:

N = number of slices imaged simultaneously during a rotation

T = nominal width of each slice

I = table travel between each successive gantry rotation

In helical-mode CT scanning, the table moves during x-ray rotation and data acquisition; the ratio of table travel per rotation to the nominal total beam width (NT) is referred to as pitch (p). For helical-mode scanning:

$$CTDI_{vol} = \frac{CTDI_w}{p}. \qquad (C.3)$$

$CTDI_w$ represents the index $CTDI_{100}$ of absorbed dose as an average over the field-of-view of the phantom within the x-y plane. By accounting for variation in dose along the central axis (z-axis) as well as over the x-y plane, $CTDI_{vol}$ represents an index of absorbed dose as an average over the volume of the phantom central section.

To better represent the overall energy delivered by a given scan protocol, the $CTDI_{vol}$ (milligray) can be integrated over the scan length (L) (centimeters) to compute DLP (mGy cm), where:

$$DLP = CTDI_{\text{vol}} \, L \qquad\qquad\qquad (C.4)$$

DLP is an index of total energy absorbtion associated with a specific scan acquisition. Thus, while an abdominal CT scan might have the same $CTDI_{\text{vol}}$ as an abdominal-and-pelvic CT scan, the latter examination would have a higher *DLP*, proportional to the longer longitudinal range of anatomy covered during scanning.

A more detailed discussion on the measurement and reporting of radiation dose in CT is found in *The Measurement, Reporting, and Management of Radiation Dose in CT* (McCollough *et al.*, 2008).

Appendix D

Supporting Data for Section 4 (Medical Exposure of Patients)

TABLE D.1—*Projections included in specific conventional radiographic and fluoroscopic examinations.*

CPT[a]	Description[b]	Examination[b]	Projections[b]
74000	Radiologic examination, abdomen; single AP view	Abdomen	AP abdomen, oblique, cone
74022	Radiologic examination, abdomen; complete acute abdomen series, including supine, erect, and/or decubitus views, single view chest	Abdomen	PA chest, 2 AP abdomen
74020	Radiologic examination, abdomen; complete, including decubitus and/or erect views	Abdomen	2 AP abdomen
74010	Radiologic examination, abdomen; AP and additional oblique and cone views	Abdomen	AP abdomen, oblique, cone
71010	Radiologic examination, chest; single view, frontal	Chest	PA

TABLE D.1—(continued).

CPT[a]	Description[b]	Examination[b]	Projections[b]
71020	Radiologic examination, chest; two views, frontal and lateral;	Chest	PA, lateral
74230	Swallowing function, with cineradiography/videoradiography	UGI	2 min, PA, oblique
74220	Radiologic examination, esophagus	UGI	1 min, 3 films, PA, oblique
74250	Radiologic examination, small intestine; includes multiple serial films	UGI	2 min, 6 abdomen, 1 cone
74246	Radiological examination, GI tract; upper, air contrast, with specific high density barium, effervescent agent, with or without glucagon; with or without delayed films, without KUB	UGI	3 min, 12 10 × 12 coned films
74240	Radiologic examination, GI tract, upper; with or without delayed films, without KUB	UGI	2 min, 8 coned films
74247	Radiological examination, GI tract, upper; air contrast, with specific high density barium, effervescent agent, with or without glucagon; with or without delayed films, with KUB	UGI	3 min, 12 films
74249	Radiological examination, GI tract, upper; air contrast, with specific high density barium, effervescent agent, with or without glucagon; with small intestine follow-through	UGI	2 min, 12 films
74245	Radiologic examination, GI tract, upper; with small intestine, includes multiple serial films	UGI	4 min, 8 coned, 4 14 × 17

Code	Description		
74241	Radiologic examination, GI tract, upper; with or without delayed films, with KUB	UGI	2 min, 8 coned 10 × 12
74290	Cholecystography, oral contrast	Biliary	1 min, 4 coned films
74270	Radiologic examination, colon; barium enema, with or without KUB	Barium enema	3 min, 4 abdomen 14 × 17, 8 coned 10 × 12
74280	Radiologic examination, colon; air contrast with specific high density barium, with or without glucagon	Barium enema	3 min, 4 abdomen 14 × 17, 8 coned 10 × 12
70220	Radiologic examination, sinuses, paranasal, complete, minimum of three views	Other HNF	2 PA, 1 lateral
70210	Radiologic examination, sinuses, paranasal, less than three views	Other HNF	PA, lateral
70360	Radiologic examination, neck; soft tissue	Other HNF	Lateral
70160	Radiologic examination, nasal bones; complete, minimum of three views	Other HNF	PA, lateral
70150	Radiologic examination, facial bones; complete, minimum of three views	Other HNF	2 PA, lateral
70371	Complex dynamic pharyngeal and speech evaluation by cinefluorography or video recording	Other HNF	3 min, PA, oblique
70030	Radiologic examination, eye; for detection of foreign body	Other HNF	PA
70200	Radiologic examination, orbits; complete, minimum of four views	Other HNF	2 PA, 2 oblique

TABLE D.1—(continued).

CPT[a]	Description[b]	Examination[b]	Projections[b]
70110	Radiologic examination, mandible; complete, minimum of four views	Other HNF	2 PA, 2 lateral, 10 × 12
70140	Radiologic examination, facial bones; less than three views	Other HNF	PA, lateral
70100	Radiologic examination, mandible; partial, less than four views	Other HNF	PA, 2 lateral
70330	Radiologic examination, temporomandibular joint; open and closed mouth, bilateral	Other HNF	PA, 4 lateral
70370	Radiologic examination, pharynx or larynx; including fluoroscopy and/or magnification technique	Other HNF	2 min, PA, 2 lateral
70320	Radiologic examination, teeth; complete, full mouth	Dental	
70355	Orthopantogram	Dental	
70300	Radiologic examination, teeth; single view	Dental	
70350	Cephalogram, orthodontic	Dental	
70310	Radiologic examination, teeth; partial examination, less than full mouth	Dental	
73560	Radiologic examination, knee; one or two views	Knee	AP lateral
73562	Radiologic examination, knee; three views	Knee	AP, lateral sunrise

73564	Radiologic examination, knee; complete, four or more views	Knee	2 AP, 1 lateral sunrise patella
73550	Radiologic examination, femur; two views	Knee	AP, lateral
73565	Radiologic examination, knee; both knees, standing, AP	Knee	2 AP
73030	Radiologic examination, shoulder; complete, minimum of two views	Shoulder	AP axillary
73060	Radiologic examination, humerus; minimum of two views	Shoulder	AP lateral
73020	Radiologic examination, shoulder; one view	Shoulder	AP
73000	Radiologic examination, clavicle; complete	Shoulder	AP
73010	Radiologic examination, scapula; complete	Shoulder	1 AP, 1 oblique coned
73050	Radiologic examination, acromioclavicular joints; bilateral, with or without weighted distraction	Shoulder	2 AP, upper 1/3 chest only
73510	Radiologic examination, hip; unilateral, complete, minimum of two views	Hip	AP, oblique
73500	Radiologic examination, hip; unilateral, one view	Hip	AP
73530	Radiologic examination, hip; during operative procedure	Hip	AP
73520	Radiologic examination, hips; bilateral, minimum of two views of each hip, including AP view of pelvis	Hip	1 pelvis, 2 hip AP, 2 oblique hip
72170	Radiologic examination, pelvis; one or two views	Pelvis	AP pelvis

TABLE D.1—(continued).

CPT[a]	Description[b]	Examination[b]	Projections[b]
72220	Radiologic examination, sacrum and coccyx; minimum of two views	Pelvis	AP pelvis coned 10 × 12, lateral coned sacrum 10 × 12
72190	Radiologic examination, pelvis; complete, minimum of three views	Pelvis	AP, 2 oblique
72202	Radiologic examination, sacroiliac joints; three or more views	Pelvis	AP coned 10 × 12 and 2 oblique 10 × 12
72200	Radiologic examination, sacroiliac joints; less than three views	Pelvis	2 oblique coned 10 × 12
73540	Radiologic examination, pelvis and hips, infant or child, minimum of two views	Pelvis	2 AP pelvis
72040	Radiologic examination, spine, cervical; two or three views	CS	AP, lateral
72050	Radiologic examination, spine, cervical; minimum of four views	CS	AP, lateral, 2 oblique
72020	Radiologic examination, spine; single view, specify level	CS	Lateral
72052	Radiologic examination, spine, cervical; complete, including oblique and flexion and/or extension studies	CS	AP, 3 lateral, 2 oblique
72100	Radiologic examination, spine, lumbosacral; two or three views	LS	AP, 1 lateral, 1 coned lateral 10 × 12

72110	Radiologic examination, spine, lumbosacral; minimum of four views	LS	AP, 2 oblique, 1 spot lateral
72114	Radiolcgic examination, spine, lumbosacral; complete, including bending views	LS	AP, 3 lateral
72120	Radiologic examination, spine, lumbosacral; bending views only, minimum of four views	LS	AP, 3 lateral
70250	Radiologic examination, skull; less than four views	Skull	PA, lateral
70260	Radiologic examination, skull; complete, minimum of four views	Skull	3 AP, lateral
72070	Radiolcgic examination, spine; thoracic, two views	TS	AP, lateral
72072	Radiologic examination, spine; thoracic, three views	TS	AP, 2 lateral
72080	Radiologic examination, spine; thoracolumbar, two views	TS	AP, lateral
72074	Radiologic examination, spine; thoracic, minimum of four views	TS	AP, lateral, 2 obliques
72069	Radiologic examination, spine; thoracolumbar, standing (scoliosis)	TS	AP
76075	DEXA, bone density study, one or more sites; axial skeleton (*e.g.*, hips, pelvis, spine)	DEXA	
74420	Urography, retrograde; with or without KUB	IVP	3 AP abdomen
74400	Urography (pyelography); intravenous, with or without KUB, with or without tomography	IVP	4 AP abdomen, 5 coned 10 × 12

TABLE D.1—(continued).

CPT[a]	Description[b]	Examination[b]	Projections[b]
74415	Urography, infusion; drip technique and/or bolus technique; with nephrotomography	IVP	4 AP abdomen, 5 coned 10 × 12
74410	Urography, infusion; drip technique and/or bolus technique	IVP	6 AP

[a]CPT = Common Procedural Terminology (AMA, 2004).

[b]
AP	=	anterior-posterior view	IVP =	intravenous pyelogram
CS	=	cervical spine	KUB =	kidney, ureter and bladder
DEXA	=	dual-energy x-ray absorptiometry	LS =	lumbosacral spine
GI	=	gastrointestinal	PA =	posterior-anterior view
HNF	=	head and neck films	TS =	thoracic spine
			UGI =	upper gastrointestinal

TABLE D.2—*Data used to obtain effective dose estimates for fluoroscopically-guided diagnostic and interventional procedures.*

Groups/Subgrcups	Examinations	Kerma-Area Product (KAP) (Gy cm^2)	Dose Conversion Coefficient (DCC$_E$) [mSv (Gy cm^2)$^{-1}$]	Effective Dose (E) (mSv)
Nonvascular procedures				
Urinary studies	Cystometrography	7	0.18	1.3[a]
	Cystography	10	0.18	1.8[a]
	Excretion urography, micturating cysto-urethrogram	6.4	0.18	1.2[a]
	Urethrography	6	0.18	1.1[a]
	Urinary tract			2.5 – 7[b]
Myelography	Myelography	12.3	0.2	2.5[a]
				4[c]
	Discography			1.3[a]
	Lumbar radiculography			3.7[a]
	Endoscopic retrograde cholangiopancreatography	15	0.26	3.9[a]
		14.5	0.26	3.8[d]
	Arthrograms	1.7	0.1	0.17[a]

TABLE D.2—(continued).

Groups/Subgroups	Examinations	Kerma-Area Product (KAP) (Gy cm²)	Dose Conversion Coefficient (DCC_E) [mSv (Gy cm²)⁻¹]	Effective Dose (E) (mSv)
Orthopedic and joints		0.06 – 0.15	0.01	<0.025[a]
Obstetrics and gynecology	Pelvimetry	1.4	0.29	0.41[a]
	Hysterosalpingogram	4	0.29	1.2[a]
Biopsy	Pathological specimen			1.6[a]
	Biopsy	6	0.26	1.6[a]
	Small bowel biopsy	1	0.26	0.26[a]
	Venous sampling			0.4[a]
Vertebroplasty		78 (mean) 6.6 – 335 (range)	0.2	15.6[e] (mean) 1.3 – 67 (range)
Noncardiac diagnostic procedures				
Peripheral vascular	Arteriography (all types)	27.2 26.3	0.26	7.1[a] 4.0[f]
	Runoffs			3.5[g]
	Phlebography/venography of a limb	3.7	0.1	0.37[a]

Neurologic (including carotid)	Phlebography (leg-pelvis)			0.5 – 2[b]
	Carotid, cerebral angiography	48.5	0.087	4[a]
		28	0.028	0.78[a]
	Carotid angiogram	34.6	0.087	3.0[a]
	Cerebral angiogram	91.8	0.087	8.0[a]
Renal	Antegrade pyelography	3.5	0.18	0.6[a]
	Nephrostogram	9	0.18	1.6[a]
	Retrograde pyelogram	13	0.18	2.3[a]
	Renal angiogram	48.5	0.26	12.6[a]
Carotid and aortic arch	Thoracic aortography, arch angiogram	34.5	0.12	4.1[a]
	Abdominal aortography	98	0.26	25.5[a] 14[h]
Other peripheral				0.37 – 7.1[a]
Neurologic (excluding carotid)	Cervical spine	0.49	0.13	0.064[a]
	Thoracic spine	4.2	0.19	0.80[a]
	Lumbar spine	5.7	0.21	1.2[a]
Pulmonary	Pulmonary arteriography	47	0.12	5.6[a]
	Pulmonary angiogram	73	0.12	8.8[e]

TABLE D.2—(continued).

Groups/Subgroups	Examinations	Kerma-Area Product (KAP) (Gy cm^2)	Dose Conversion Coefficient (DCC_E) [mSv (Gy cm^2)$^{-1}$]	Effective Dose (E) (mSv)
Arterial pressures				7[a]
	Venacavogram	21	0.12	2.5[a]
Noncardiac interventional vascular procedures				
Vascular access				4.5[g]
				7.4[i]
Percutaneous transluminal angioplasty (PTA)		17.8	0.26	4.6[a]
		19.5	0.26	5.1[d]
Stents	Renal/visceral PTA (all) with stent	241 (mean) 75 – 464 (range)	0.26	63[e] (mean) 19.5 – 121 (range)
	Iliac PTA (all) with stent	245 (mean) 42 – 657 (range)	0.26	64[e] (mean) 11 – 171 (range)
	Carotid stent	161 (mean) 32 – 515 (range)	0.087	14[e] (mean) 2.8 – 45 (range)
	Bile duct, dilation and stenting	54	0.26	14[a]
	Stenting	47.9	0.26	12.5[d]

Inferior vena cava filters			
Filter placement only	54 (mean) 6.1 – 203 (range)	0.26	14[e] (mean) 5.2 – 160 (range)
Pulmonary angiography with filter	103 (mean) 71 – 119 (range)	0.12	12[e] (mean) 8.5 – 14 (range)
Embolization			
Bronchial artery embolization	138 (mean) 72 – 315 (range)	0.12	17[e] (mean) 8.6 – 38 (range)
Hepatic chemoembolization	270 (mean) 20 – 616 (range)	0.26	70[e] (mean) 5.2 – 160 (range)
Pelvic arterial embolization	299 (mean) 38 – 624 (range)	0.26	78[e] (mean) 9.9 – 162 (range)
Pelvic vein embolization: ovarian vein	169 (mean)	0.26	44[e] (mean)
Other tumor embolization	327 (mean) 87 – 972 (range)	0.26	84[e] (mean) 23 – 252 (range)
Embolization	91.5 / 114	0.26 / 0.26	23.8[a] / 29.6[d]
Thrombolytic therapy	13.5	0.26	3.5[a]
Cardiac procedures			
Diagnostic arteriography	14 – 63	0.12	3.1 – 10.6[a] / 5 – 9[j]

TABLE D.2—(continued).

Groups/Subgroups	Examinations	Kerma-Area Product (KAP) (Gy cm²)	Dose Conversion Coefficient (DCC_E) [mSv (Gy cm²)$^{-1}$]	Effective Dose (E) (mSv)
Intervention	Angioplasty	26	0.26 0.20[k]	6.8[a]
	Percutaneous transluminal coronary angioplasty	58	0.26	15.1[a] 6 – 15[j]
			0.18[l] 0.20[m] 0.28[n]	10[o] 22[p]
		63.4	0.26	16.5[d]
	Embolization	75	0.26	19.5[a]
	Cardiac radiofrequency ablation	30	0.1 0.14[r]	3[q]
			0.18 – 0.2[k] 0.21 – 0.23[m]	21[s] 17.3[a]
		33.1	0.19	6.3[a]
		48.7 (mean) 6.4 – 230 (range)		15.2 (mean)[t] 2.1 – 59.6 (range)[t]

Procedure			
Transjugular intrahepatic portosystemic shunt	206	0.26	53.6[a]
	431 (mean)	0.26	112[e] (mean)
	89 – 1,013 (range)		23 – 263 (range)
	182[u]		19[v]
	161		84[i]
	524		
Diagnostic procedures	12.5 (mean)		3.2 (mean)[t]
	4.5 – 117 (range)		1.3 – 23.9 (range)[t]
Pacemaker insertion	7	0.1	0.7[a]
			0.7[u]

Footnotes apply to all data listed on a given row.

[a]Hart and Wall (2002).
[b]Regulla and Eder (2005).
[c]RSNA (2008).
[d]Marshall et al. (2000).
[e]Miller et al. (2003).
[f]Thwaites et al. (1996).
[g]Bor et al. (2004).
[h]Chu et al. (1998).
[i]McParland (1998).
[j]Bogaert et al. (2008).
[k]Broadhead et al. (1997).
[l]Betsou et al. (1998).
[m]Neofotistou et al. (1998).
[n]Delichas et al. (2003).
[o]Pukkila and Karila (1990).
[p]Lindsay et al. (1992).
[q]Schultz and Zoetelief (2005).
[r]McFadden et al. (2002).
[s]Rosenthal et al. (1998).
[t]Efstathopoulos et al. (2006).
[u]Williams (1997).
[v]Zweers et al. (1998).

TABLE D.3—*Distribution of nuclear-medicine procedures by CPT code and category in 2004 Medicare data.*

Nuclear-Medicine Procedures			Medicare 2004		
Organ, System or Condition	CPT Code	Description[a]	Total Procedures	Percent of Total Procedures	Procedures per 100,000 Medicare Population
Bone	78102	Bone marrow	10,383	0.206	3
	78103	Bone marrow	353	0.007	1
	78104	Bone marrow	448	0.009	1
	78300	Bone limited	40,057	0.793	118
	78305	Bone multiple	20,258	0.401	60
	78306	Bone: whole body	722,175	14.3	2,124
	78315	Bone 3-phase	139,592	2.77	411
	78320	Bone SPECT	22,739	0.450	73
		Total bone	*956,005*	*18.9*	
	78350	DEXA	2,614	0.052	8
	78351	DEXA	0	0	0
Cardiac	78428	Shunt	878	0.017	3
	78460	Perfusion	6,933	0.137	20
	78461	Perfusion	25,590	0.507	75

78464	Perfusion SPECT	89,287	1.77	263
78465	Perfusion SPECT	2,930,450	58.0	8,618
78472	Blood pool	88,911	1.76	261
78473	Blood pool	5,953	0.118	18
78478	Profusion in addition to primary code	0	0	0
78480	Profusion in addition to primary code	0	0	0
78481	Blood pool	25,655	0.508	75
78483	Blood pool	7,526	0.149	22
78494	Blood pool	5,432	0.107	16
78459	PET metabolism	539	0.010	2
78491	PET perfusion	0	0	
78492	PET Perfusion	0	0	
78496	Blood pool in addition to primary code[b]	0	0	
	Total cardiac	3,187,154	63.1	
78580	Perfusion blood pool	0	0	

Lung

TABLE D.3—(continued).

Organ, System or Condition	Nuclear-Medicine Procedures		Medicare 2004		
	CPT Code	Description[a]	Total Procedures	Percent of Total Procedures	Procedures per 100,000 Medicare Population
	78584	VQ xenon perfusion in addition to primary code[b]	23,388	0.463	69
	78585	VQ xenon	114,186	2.26	336
	78586	Ventilation aerosol	820	0.016	2
	78587	Ventilation aerosol	7321	0.145	22
	78588	VQ aerosol	85,957	1.70	253
	78591	Ventilation single	882	0.017	3
	78593	VQ aerosol	16,409	0.325	43
	78594	Ventilation xenon	7,601	0.151	22
	78596	VQ quantitative	11,150	0.221	33
		Total lung	*267,714*	*5.30*	
Thyroid	78000	Uptake	4,076	0.081	12
	78001	Multiple uptake	2,555	0.051	8

Code	Description			
78003	Uptake	558	0.011	2
78006	Image + single uptake	31,400	0.622	92
78007	Image + multiple uptake	38,428	0.761	113
78010	Image	12,994	0.257	38
78011	Image + flow	483	0.010	1
78015	Image mets limited	214	0.004	1
78018	Image mets	7,971	0.158	23
78020	Image mets	778	0.015	2
	Total thyroid	*99,457*	*1.97*	
Renal				
78700	Kidney static	1,868	0.037	5
78701	Kidney + flow	3,023	0.060	9
78704	Renogram	4,430	0.088	13
78707	Renogram	41,127	0.815	121
78708	Renogram	22,032	0.436	65
78709	Renogram	8,694	0.172	26
78715	Kidney flow	912	0.018	3
78710	SPECT kidney	200	0.004	1
78760	Testicular	155	0.003	0

TABLE D.3—(*continued*).

Organ, System or Condition	CPT Code	Description[a]	Total Procedures	Percent of Total Procedures	Procedures per 100,000 Medicare Population
				Medicare 2004	
	78761	Testicular	245	0.005	1
		Total renal	*82,686*	*1.64*	
GI	78201	Liver static	669	0.013	2
	78202	Liver + flow	546	0.011	2
	78205	Liver SPECT	2,913	0.058	9
	78206	Liver SPECT	781	0.015	2
	78215	Liver and spleen	14,922	0.296	44
	78216	Liver and spleen	2,211	0.044	7
	78220	Hepatobiliary	180,600	3.58	531
	78260	Esophagus motility	263	0.005	1
	78261	Gastric mucosa	134	0.003	0
	78262	GE reflux	578	0.011	2
	78624	Gastric emptying	46,849	0.928	138

Nuclear-Medicine Procedures

78278	Blood loss	50,049	0.991	147
78290	Intestine	2,138	0.042	6
78291	LaVeen shunt	319	0.006	1
78299	Unlisted	185	0.004	1
	Total GI	*303,157*	*6.05*	
Brain				
78600	Static limited	107	0.002	0
78601	Static + flow limited	304	0.006	1
78605	Static complete	265	0.005	1
78606	Static + flow complete	918	0.018	3
78607	SPECT	8,586	0.170	25
78610	Flow only	296	0.006	1
78615	Flow only	598	0.012	2
78608	PET FDG	15	0.000	0
78609	PET perfusion	0	0	0
78630	CSF	5,156	0.102	15
74635	CSF	488	0.010	1
78645	CSF	1,119	0.022	3
78650	CSF leak	281	0.006	1

TABLE D.3—(*continued*).

Organ, System or Condition	CPT Code	Description[a]	Total Procedures	Percent of Total Procedures	Procedures per 100,000 Medicare Population
				Medicare 2004	
Infection		*Total brain*	*18,133*	*0.359*	*47*
	78805	Inflammation limited	16,133	0.320	87
	78806	Inflammation whole body	29,470	0.583	6
	78807	SPECT	1,928	0.038	
		Total infection	*47,531*	*0.942*	
Tumor					
Non-FDG tumor	78075	Adrenal	205	0.004	1
	78070	Parathyroid	27,662	0.548	81
	78800	Tumor limited	3,640	0.072	11
	78801	Tumor multiple	1,835	0.036	4
	78802	Tumor: whole body	10,890	0.216	32
	78803	Tumor SPECT	8,845	0.175	26
	78804	Tumor multiple days	2,202	0.044	6
	78195	Lymphatics	28,466	0.564	87

	Code	Description			
PET	78810	FDG	35	0.0007	0
		Total tumor	83,780	*1.66*	
		Total Medicare diagnostic nuclear medicine	*5,048,231*		
Therapy	79000	Hyperthyroid	11,158		33
	79001	Hyperthyroid	250		1
	79020	Hyperthyroid	189		1
	79030	Thyroid cancer gland ablation	3,455		10
	79035	Thyroid cancer	1,117		3
	79100	Polycythemia vera	164		0
	79200	Intracavitary	27		0
	79400	Nonthyroid, nonhematological	1,257		4
	79999	Unlisted	43		0
		Total Medicare nuclear-medicine unsealed-radionuclide therapy	*17,660*		

aCSF   =   cerebrospinal fluid   GI   =   gastrointestinal
DEXA   =   dual-energy x-ray absorptiometry   PET   =   positron emission tomography
FDG   =   fluoroceoxyglucose   SPECT   =   single-photon emission computed tomography
GE   =   gastroesophageal   VQ   =   ventilation-perfusion scan
bThese are "add on" codes for purposes of billing and do not represent additional administrations of radiopharmaceuticals.

TABLE D.4—*Number of paid exams, procedures or visits and percent for general groups by different data set.*

Nuclear-Medicine Description	Medicare 2004		IMV 2005 (IMV, 2006c)		VA 2006	
	Total Paid Exams	Percent of Total	Visits	Percent of Total	Procedures	Percent of Total
Bone	956,005	17.66	3,450,000	20.0	46,572	11.8
Dual-energy x-ray absorptiometry	2,614	0.05			1,706	0.43
Cardiac	3,194,508	58.6	9,800,000	56.9	325,716	82.2
Lung	267,714	4.92	740,000	4.30	3,263	0.82
Thyroid	99,457	1.83			6,383	1.61
Renal	82,686	1.52	470,000	2.73	5,618	1.42
Gastrointestinal	303,157	5.57	1,210,000	7.03	3,623	0.92
Brain	18,133	0.33			1,378	0.35
Infection	47,531	0.87	380,000	2.21	1,518	0.38
Tumor	360,542	6.62	340,000	1.97	204	0.05
Other			830,000	4.82		
Therapy	17,600	<0.01			51.0	0.01
Total nuclear medicine	5,447,302	100	17,220,000	100	396,032	100

TABLE D.5—Radionuclides, administered activity, dose conversion coefficient and effective dose per procedure in nuclear medicine.[a,b]

CPT Code	Nuclear-Medicine Procedure Description[c]	Radiopharmaceutical[d]	Administered Activity (MBq)	Dose Conversion Coefficient (mSv MBq^{-1})	Effective Dose per Procedure (mSv)
Bone					
78102	Bone marrow	^{99m}Tc SC	370	0.0094	3.5
78103	Bone marrow	^{99m}Tc SC	370	0.0094	3.5
78104	Bone marrow	^{99m}Tc SC	370	0.0094	3.5
78300	Bone limited	^{99m}Tc MDP	1,110	0.0057	6.3
78305	Bone multiple	^{99m}Tc MDP	1,110	0.0057	6.3
78306	Bone: whole body	^{99m}Tc MDP	1,110	0.0057	6.3
78315	Bone 3-phase	^{99m}Tc MDP	1,110	0.0057	6.3
78320	Bone SPECT	^{99m}Tc MDP	1,110	0.0057	6.3
78350	DEXA	None			
78351	DEXA	None			
Cardiac					
78428	Shunt	^{99m}Tc RBC	1,110	0.007	7.8
78460	Perfusion	^{99m}Tc MIBI/^{201}Tl 75/25	1,480/150	0.0085/0.22	17.7

TABLE D.5—(continued).

Nuclear-Medicine Procedure		Radiopharmaceutical[d]	Administered Activity (MBq)	Dose Conversion Coefficient (mSv MBq^{-1})	Effective Dose per Procedure (mSv)
CPT Code	Description[c]				
78461	Perfusion	^{99m}Tc MIBI/^{201}Tl 75/25	1,480/150	0.0085/0.22	17.7
78464	Perfusion: SPECT	^{99m}Tc MIBI/^{201}Tl 75/25	1,480/150	0.0085/0.22	17.7
78465	Perfusion: SPECT	^{99m}Tc MIBI/^{201}Tl 75/25	1,480/150	0.0085/0.22	17.7
78472	Blood pool	^{99m}Tc RBC	1,110	0.007	7.8
78473	Blood pool	^{99m}Tc RBC	1,110	0.007	7.8
78478	Perfusion in addition to primary code		0		0
78480	Perfusion in addition to primary code		0		0
78481	Blood pool	^{99m}Tc RBC	1,110	0.007	7.8
78483	Blood pool	^{99m}Tc RBC	1,110	0.007	7.8
78494	Blood pool	^{99m}Tc RBC	1,110	0.007	7.8
78459	PET metabolism	^{18}F FDG	740	0.019	14.1
78496	Blood pool in addition to primary code				0

Lung

Code	Study	Radiopharmaceutical			
78580	Perfusion blood pool	99mTc MAA	185	0.011	2.0
78584	VQ xenon	99mTc MAA	185	0.011	2.0
		133Xe	740	0.00074	0.5
78585	VQ xenon	99mTc MAA	185	0.011	2.0
		133Xe	740	0.00074	0.5
78586	Ventilation aerosol	99mTc DTPA	1,300	0.007	9.1
78587	Ventilation aerosol	99mTc DTPA	1,300	0.007	9.1
78588	VQ aerosol	99mTc MAA	185	0.011	2.0
		99mTc MAA	1,300	0.007	9.1
78591	Ventilation single	133Xe	740	0.00074	0.5
78593	VQ aerosol	99mTc MAA	185	0.011	2.0
		99mTc DTPA	1,300	0.007	9.1
78594	Ventilation xenon	133Xe	740	0.0008	0.6
78596	VQ quantitative	99mTc MAA	185	0.011	2.0

Thyroid

Code	Study	Radiopharmaceutical			
78000	Uptake	123I	7.4	0.0075	0.06

TABLE D.5—(continued).

CPT Code	Nuclear-Medicine Procedure Description[c]	Radiopharmaceutical[d]	Administered Activity (MBq)	Dose Conversion Coefficient (mSv MBq^{-1})	Effective Dose per Procedure (mSv)
78001	Multiple uptake	^{123}I	7.4	0.0075	0.06
78003	Uptake	^{123}I	7.4	0.0075	0.06
78006	Image + single uptake	^{123}I	25	0.0075	0.2
78007	Image + multiple uptake	^{123}I	25	0.0075	0.2
78010	Image	^{99m}Tc O$_4$/^{123}I 50/50	370/25	0.013/0.075	6.7
78011	Image + flow	^{99m}Tc O$_4$/^{123}I 50/50	370/25	0.013/0.075	6.7
78015	Image mets ltd	^{131}I	185	0.062	11.5
78018	Image mets	^{131}I	185	0.062	11.5
78020	Image mets	^{131}I	185	0.062	11.5
Renal					
78700	Kidney static	^{99m}Tc DTPA/^{99m}Tc MAG3 50/50	370	0.0049/0.007	2.2

7870	Kidney + flow	^{99m}Tc DTPA/^{99m}Tc MAG3 50/50	370	0.0049/0.007	2.2
78704	Renogram	^{99m}Tc DTPA/^{99m}Tc MAG3 50/50	370	0.0049/0.007	2.2
78707	Renogram	^{99m}Tc DTPA/^{99m}Tc MAG3 50/50	370	0.0049/0.007	2.2
78708	Renogram	^{99m}Tc DTPA/^{99m}Tc MAG3 50/50	370	0.0049/0.007	2.2
78709	Renogram	^{99m}Tc DTPA/^{99m}Tc MAG3 50/50	370	0.0049/0.007	2.2
78715	Kidney flow	^{99m}Tc DTPA/^{99m}Tc MAG3 50/50	370	0.0049/0.007	2.2
78710	SPECT kidney	^{99m}Tc Glucohep/DMSA 50/50	370	0.0054/0.0088	2.6
78760	Testicular	^{99m}Tc O$_4$	1,110	0.013	14.4
78761	Testicular	^{99m}Tc O$_4$	1,110	0.013	14.4
GI					
78201	Liver static	^{99m}Tc SC	222	0.0094	2.1
78202	Liver + flow	^{99m}Tc SC	222	0.0094	2.1
78205	Liver SPECT	^{99m}Tc SC	222	0.0094	2.1

TABLE D.5—(*continued*).

	Nuclear-Medicine Procedure		Administered Activity (MBq)	Dose Conversion Coefficient (mSv MBq^{-1})	Effective Dose per Procedure (mSv)
CPT Code	Description[c]	Radiopharmaceutical[d]			
78206	Liver SPECT	^{99m}Tc SC	222	0.0094	2.1
78215	Liver SPECT	^{99m}Tc SC	222	0.0094	2.1
78216	Liver spleen	^{99m}Tc SC	222	0.0094	2.1
78220	Hepatobiliary	^{99m}Tc DISIDA	185	0.017	3.1
78260	Esophagus motility	^{99m}Tc SC	11.1	0.024	0.3
78261	Gastric mucosa	^{99m}Tc O$_4$	370	0.13	48.1
78262	GE reflux	^{99m}Tc SC	11.1	0.0094	0.1
78624	Gastric emptying	^{99m}Tc SC eggs	14.8	0.024	0.4
78278	Blood loss	^{99m}Tc RBC	1,110	0.007	7.8
78290	Intestine	^{99m}Tc O$_4$	370	0.013	4.8
78291	LaVeen shunt	^{99m}Tc MAA	74	0.011	0.8
78299	Unlisted				0
Brain					
78600	Static limited	^{99m}Tc HMPAO	740	0.0093	6.9

Code	Description	Agent	Dose		Value
78601	Static + flow limited	^{99m}Tc HMPAO	740	0.0093	6.9
78605	Static complete	^{99m}Tc HMPAO	740	0.0093	6.9
78606	Static + flow complete	^{99m}Tc HMPAO	740	0.0093	6.9
78607	SPECT	^{99m}Tc HMPAO	740	0.0093	6.9
78610	Flow cnly	^{99m}Tc DTPA	740	0.0049	3.6
78615	Flow cnly	^{99m}Tc DTPA	740	0.0049	3.6
78608	PET FDG	^{18}F FDG	740	0.019	14.1
78630	CSF	^{111}In DTPA	18.5	0.021	0.4
74635	CSF	^{111}In DTPA	18.5	0.021	0.4
78645	CSF	^{111}In DTPA	18.5	0.021	0.4
78650	CSF leak	^{111}In DTPA	18.5	0.021	0.4
Infection					
78805	Inflammation limited	^{99m}Tc WBC/^{111}In WBC/^{67}Ga 33/33/33	740/18.5/220	0.017/0.36/0.1	8.5
78806	Inflammation whole body	^{99m}Tc WBC/^{111}In WBC/^{67}Ga 33/33/33	740/18.5/220	0.017/0.36/0.1	8.5
78807	SPECT	^{99m}Tc WBC/^{111}In WBC/^{67}Ga 33/33/33	740/18.5/220	0.017/0.36/0.1	8.5

TABLE D.5—(*continued*).

Nuclear-Medicine Procedure		Administered Activity (MBq)	Dose Conversion Coefficient (mSv MBq^{-1})	Effective Dose per Procedure (mSv)
CPT Code	Description[c]			
Radiopharmaceutical[d]				
Non-FDG tumor				
78075	Adrenal			
	^{131}I MIBG	60	0.14	8.4
	^{123}I MIBG	400	0.013	5.2
78070	Parathyroid			
	^{99m}Tc sestamibi	740	0.0085	6.3
78800	Tumor limited			
	^{67}Ga citrate/^{111}In octreotide 50/50	220/222	0.1/0.12	25
78801	Tumor multiple			
	^{67}Ga citrate/^{111}In octreotide 50/50	220/222	0.1/0.12	25
78802	Tumor whole body			
	^{67}Ga citrate/^{111}In octreotide 50/50	220/222	0.1/0.12	25
78803	Tumor SPECT			
	^{67}Ga citrate/^{111}In octreotide 50/50	220/222	0.1/0.12	25
78804	Tumor multiple days			
	^{67}Ga citrate/^{111}In octreotide 50/50	220/222	0.1/0.12	25
78195	Lymphatics			
	^{99m}Tc SC	370	0.0094	3.5

PET					
78810	FDG	^{18}F FDG	740	0.019	14.1

[a]Collected data for this Report is presented as specific types of procedures (CPT code). Unfortunately for a number of procedures there are several different radionuclides that could have been used. In these circumstances, since national data are not available, it was necessary to apply judgment derived from nuclear-medicine practices in a few large hospitals regarding the ratio for the different radionuclides. The percentage ratio assumed is shown after the radiopharmaceuticals. The dose conversion coefficients can then be used and then weighted to arrive at an estimate of absorbed and effective dose for the specific procedure. For the cardiac studies using ^{99m}Tc the dose conversion coefficient for sestamibi were assumed rather than tetrofosmin.

[b]In addition to the dose conversion coefficients it is also necessary to know the amount of administered activity. Suggested ranges of administered activity are available both in textbooks and the SNM (2008) website. Most nuclear-medicine departments have standing physician directed orders for the amount to be administered for different studies. There are no surveys available regarding the actual administered activity in the United States. Typically, however, many departments use activities near or at the high end of suggested activity ranges in order to optimize patient throughput and image quality.

[c]CSF = cerebrospinal fluid
DEXA = dual-energy x-ray absorptiometry
FDG = fluorodeoxyglucose
GE = gastroesophageal
GI = gastrointestinal
MAA = macro aggregated albumin
PET = positron emission tomography
SPECT = single-photon emission computed tomography
VQ = ventilation-perfusion scan

[d]DISIDA = diisopropyl iminodiacetic acid
DMSA = dimercaptosuccinic acid
DTPA = diethylenetriamine pentaacetic acid
FDG = fluorodeoxyglucose
HMPAO = exametazine (hexamethylenepropylene-amineoxime)
MAG3 = mertiatide (mercaptoacetylglycyl-glycyl-glycine)
MDP = methylene diphosphonate
MIBG = metaiodobenzylguanidine
MIBI = methoxyisobutyl isonitrile
RBC = red blood cells
SC = sulphur colloid
WBC = white blood cells

TABLE D.6—Change in numbers of procedures (in thousands) and percentage since 1972 for in vivo diagnostic nuclear-medicine examinations.

Procedure	1973[a]		1982[a]		2005[b]	
	Number	Percent of Total Exams	Number	Percent of Total Exams	Number	Percent of Total Exams
Bone	125	3.6	1,811	24.5	3,450	20
Cardiac	33	1.0	950	12.8	9,800	57
Lung	417	11.9	1,191	16.1	740	4
Thyroid	460	13.1	677	9.1	—	<2
Renal	122	3.5	236	3.2	470	3
GI	535	15.2	1,603	21.7	1,210	7
Brain	1,510	43.0	812	11.0	—	<2
Infection					380	2
Tumor	14	0.4	121	1.6	340	2
Other	294	8.4			—	<2
Total	3,510	100	7,400	100	17,200	100

[a]NCRP (1989a).
[b]IMV (2006c).

Appendix E

Descriptions of Diagnostic and Therapeutic Nuclear-Medicine Procedures

E.1 Diagnostic Procedures

E.1.1 Cerebrovascular

The most common nuclear-medicine imaging procedures of the brain can be divided into three different categories:

- Planar brain imaging employs radiopharmaceuticals that are perfusion agents and usually is only done for brain death studies. There are several radiopharmaceuticals that can be used for this purpose.
- SPECT brain perfusion imaging uses lipophilic radiopharmaceuticals that cross the blood-brain barrier to localize in normal brain tissue and pathologic processes in proportion to cerebral blood flow. The two most common radiopharmaceuticals used are ^{99m}Tc exametazine (HMPAO) and ^{99m}Tc bicisate (ECD).
- PET metabolic brain imaging uses functional positron-emitting radiopharmaceuticals, such as ^{18}F fluorodeoxyglucose (FDG; a glucose analogue) and neuroreceptor agents.

E.1.2 Thyroid and Parathyroid

Thyroid imaging and iodine uptake studies are primarily designed to assess the ability of the thyroid or a thyroid nodule to trap or organify compounds. Currently either ^{123}I or ^{99m}Tc pertechnetate is used for diagnostic purposes.

Parathyroid imaging is done almost exclusively for localization of parathyroid adenomas that are causing hypercalcemia. The most commonly used radiopharmaceutical is ^{99m}Tc sestamibi.

E.1.3 *Cardiac*

The most common use of nuclear medicine in cardiac imaging is to assess blood perfusion of the myocardium. The most common radiopharmaceuticals used are ^{99m}Tc sestamibi, ^{99m}Tc tetrofosmin, and less commonly ^{201}Tl chloride. The different analyses can be done with a single administration of radiopharmaceutical and billed as a single examination, but often appears in billing data with add-on codes, which can lead to confusion in determining the actual number of procedures and radiopharmaceutical injections. Less commonly, dual-injection stress-rest studies are performed.

The positron-emitting radiopharmaceuticals including ^{13}N ammonia and ^{82}Rb chloride can be used to assess myocardial perfusion. Fluorine-18 FDG can be used for evaluation of myocardial metabolism. Most of these techniques also are used to simultaneously evaluate left ventricular wall motion.

Another common cardiac nuclear-medicine examination is done by tagging red blood cells (RBC) with ^{99m}Tc to assess left ventricular function and ejection fraction.

E.1.4 *Pulmonary*

Evaluation of pulmonary function is performed by inhalation of a radiopharmaceutical for ventilation [usually ^{99m}Tc diethylenetriamine pentaacetic acid (DTPA) aerosol or ^{133}Xe gas] and intravenous injection of a different radiopharmaceutical for evaluation of lung perfusion [^{99m}Tc macro aggregated albumin (MAA)]. In the last 5 y CT has replaced the vast majority of nuclear-medicine lung scans.

E.1.5 *Gastrointestinal*

Several very different types of diagnostic nuclear-medicine examinations may be performed, depending upon the suspected GI problem. Liver/spleen scans employ ^{99m}Tc sulfur colloid to image and evaluate the reticuloendothelial system. With the advent and growth of CT scanning this examination has also experienced a rapid decrease in frequency.

Hepatobiliary scans using ^{99m}Tc diisopropyl iminodiacetic acid (DISIDA) are commonly used to diagnose cholecystitis, biliary obstruction, and biliary leaks. GI studies performed with technetium tagged red cells can localize intestinal bleeding sites and evaluate hepatic hemagiomas. There are also studies that employ various radiopharmaceuticals to evaluate gastroesophageal reflux and esophageal and stomach motility.

E.1.6 *Musculoskeletal*

Essentially all bone scans use ^{99m}Tc diphosphonates [usually methylene diphosphonate (MDP)]. The most common indication is to evaluate for the presence and or progression of metastases from tumors, and occasionally to evaluate for primary bone tumors, bone infections, or suspected fractures that cannot be found by x-ray procedures.

E.1.7 *Genitourinary System and Adrenal Glands*

Genitourinary applications of nuclear medicine are most commonly for evaluation of the function of the kidneys, to distinguish obstruction of the ureter from a dilated but nonobstructed collecting system, and to evaluate renal artery stenosis in hypertensive patients. Less common applications include evaluation of renal transplants and ureteral reflux. The radiopharmaceuticals in common use include ^{99m}Tc DTPA and ^{99m}Tc MAG3 (mertiatide). Imaging of the kidneys is usually performed by CT but there arc occasional circumstances when nuclear medicine can be helpful. Occasionally, adrenal cortical or adrenal medullary imaging is used for evaluation of adrenal hyperplasia or functional neoplasms.

E.1.8 *Inflammation and Infection Imaging*

Evaluation of suspected abscesses is usually begun with CT scanning. When this is unsuccessful there are nuclear-medicine techniques that can be helpful. Historically, ^{67}Ga citrate was used but it has been largely replaced by the use of ^{99m}Tc or ^{111}In-labeled white blood cells (WBC). A small quantity of the cells arc harvested from the patient, labeled and reinjected.

E.1.9 *Tumor Imaging*

Often nuclear-medicine examination data simply refer to the number of examinations done for tumor imaging. While there are a number of positron-emitting radionuclides available today, the short half-life (^{11}C, 20.3 min; ^{13}N, 10 min; ^{15}O, 124 s) or need for expensive generator systems (^{82}Rb) has resulted in ^{18}F FDG (half-life of 110 min) being used for the overwhelming majority of PET scans. This indicator of glucose metabolism is used primarily for staging and therapy evaluation in a wide variety of tumors, including breast cancer, lung cancer, colorectal cancer, lymphoma, and melanoma.

Fluorine-18 FDG has largely supplanted the use of ^{67}Ga citrate for evaluation of lymphoma, hepatoma, and some other cancers. However, ^{111}In pentetreotide is used for some specific types of tumors such as carcinoid. Iodine-123 or iodine-131 metaiodobenzylguanidine (MIBG) is useful for rare tumors including pheochromocytoma and neuroblastoma. Technetium-99m sestamibi is used for localization of parathyroid adenomas and occasionally is still used for breast tumors. Thallium-201 chloride is usually used for Kaposi's sarcoma and brain tumors. Iodine-123 and iodine-131 sodium iodide remain the standard for imaging thyroid cancer metastases. Use of monoclonal antibodies for various tumors has been in and out of vogue with their current use being primarily for lymphoma evaluation and therapy.

Estimation of the radiation dose from this category of procedures is the most difficult because there are many different radiopharmaceuticals that can be used based upon the suspected tumor type. Fortunately, the overall contribution of this category is small compared with the total frequency and radiation dose for all nuclear-medicine examinations.

E.2 Therapeutic Procedures

E.2.1 *Thyroid*

Hyperfunction of the thyroid gland (hyperthyroidism) can be treated with antithyroid drugs, surgery, or with radioiodine. In the United States radioiodine treatment of hyperthyroidism is the most common form of nuclear-medicine therapy.

Thyroid cancer often spreads to local lymph nodes, lungs, and bone. Many thyroid cancers will accumulate iodine (although to a lesser extent than normal thyroid tissue). Following complete surgical excision of the cancer and the thyroid gland, radioiodine may be given to destroy any residual iodine-accumulating thyroid and cancer cells. This is the second most common form of therapy with unsealed radionuclides.

The 2004 Medicare data indicate that 2 % of nuclear-medicine procedures were ^{131}I therapy but this is likely an underestimate of the true situation as the majority of patients receiving iodine therapy for hyperthyroidism are young or middle age females and, thus, not included in the Medicare data.

E.2.2 *Bone Metastases Therapy*

Several cancers (such as prostate and breast) have a predilection for diffuse spread throughout the skeleton. There are a number of radiopharmaceuticals that will localize in the metastatic lesions to provide palliation (but not cure). The usual radiopharmaceuticals used are ^{153}Sm ethylene diamine tetramethylene phosphonate (EDTMP), ^{89}Sr chloride, ^{186}Re hydroxyethylene-diphosphonate (HEDP), and ^{117m}Sn DTPA.

E.2.3 *Intracavitary Therapy*

Intracavitary therapy is usually used to treat diffusely spread tumors in confined anatomical spaces or to treat arthritis and synovitis. For tumor therapy there may be direct injection of ^{198}Au colloids or even ^{131}I- or ^{90}Y-labeled antibodies into confined anatomical spaces (such as the pleural space or the peritoneal cavity). For treatment of arthritis or synovitis there is direct instillation of ^{90}Y ferric hydroxide macroaggregate (FHMA), ^{165}Dy FHMA, or ^{169}Er colloid into the joint space.

E.2.4 *Polycythemia Vera*

This is a relatively rare disease that is characterized by overproduction of red and white blood cells by the bone marrow. Phosphate-32 is given intravenously and localizes in the bone and the beta emissions result in mild bone marrow suppression and reduction in production of many blood elements.

E.2.5 *Intra-arterial Therapy*

Some tumors (such as hepatomas) are highly vascularized and may not be amenable to surgery or chemotherapy. In these circumstances it is possible to place a catheter in the arterial supply and inject insoluble radiolabeled particles that lodge in the arterioles and capillaries of the tumor and provide a local radiation dose. The radionuclides most commonly used are ^{131}I-labeled oil contrast and ^{90}Y glass or resin microspheres.

E.2.6 *Radioimmunotherapy*

This type of therapy uses radiolabeled antibodies directed against tumor specific antigens. These agents are gaining in popularity and are currently being used for treatment of chemotherapy resistant lymphomas. The antibodies are labeled with ^{131}I or ^{90}Y and injected intravenously in relatively large activities, but can also be labeled with other beta-particle, Auger-electron, or alpha-particle emitting radionuclides.

Appendix F

Supporting Data for Section 6.3 (U.S. Department of Energy Installations)

TABLE F.1—*Estimated annual effective dose equivalent (H_E) (individual and collective) to persons within 80 km for operating DOE sites.*

DOE Site	Years for Which Data Applies	H_E, MEI[a] (range) (µSv)	H_E, MEI[a] (average) (µSv)	Average H_E, Individual (µSv)	Average Collective H_E (all years) (person-Sv)	Most Recent Collective H_E (person-Sv)	Year of Most Recent Collective H_E
Ames Laboratory	1990 – 2004	<0.1	<0.01	NA	<0.00001	<0.00001	2004
Argonne National Laboratory	1990 – 2004	0.3 – 34	5.6	0.009	0.074	0.038	2004
Ashtabula Environmental Management Project	1998 – 2001	<0.1 – 0.6	0.20	NA	NA	NA	NA

Site							
Battelle Columbus Laboratories	1990 – 2001	<0.1 – 0.6	0.12	<0.001	0.00032	0.00001	2001
Bettis Atomic Power Laboratory	1990 – 2001	24 – 28	26	0.009	0.029	0.012	2001
Brookhaven National Laboratory	1990 – 2004	0.4 – 10	4.3	0.006	0.029	0.0016	2004
Colonie Interim Storage Site	1990 – 1992	2.3 – 15	7.1	0.017	0.013	0.040	1992
Energy Technology Engineering Center	1990 – 2001	<0.1	0.01	<0.001	0.00024	0.00001	2001
Fermi National Accelerator Laboratory	1990 – 1994	0.1 – 160	48	0.004	0.032	0.00026	1994
Fernald Environmental Management Project	1990 – 2001	7 – 120	58	0.005	0.012	0.021	1994
Grand Junction Project Office	1990 – 2001	<0.1 – 1.9	0.83	0.029	0.00243	0.00006	2001
Hanford Site	1990 – 2003	0.1 – 0.6	0.23	0.014	0.0052	0.0050	2003
Hazelwood Interim Storage Site	1990 – 1992	1 – 9	3.8	0.050	0.012	0.011	1992

TABLE F.1—(continued).

DOE Site	Years for Which Data Applies	H_E, MEI[a] (range) (μSv)	H_E, MEI (average) (μSv)	Average H_E, Individual (μSv)	Average Collective H_E (all years) (person-Sv)	Most Recent Collective H_E (person-Sv)	Year of Most Recent Collective H_E
Idaho National Engineering Laboratory	1990 – 2001	<0.1 – 0.7	0.17	0.015	0.0031	0.0059	2001
Inhalation Toxicology Research Institute	1990 – 1994	<0.1	<0.01	NA	NA	NA	NA
Knolls Atomic Power Laboratory: Kesselring	1990 – 2001	1	1	0.002	0.001	0.001	2001
Knolls Atomic Power Laboratory: Schenectady	1990 – 2001	1	1	0.001	0.0018	0.001	2001
Knolls Atomic Power Laboratory: Windsor	1990 – 2001	1	1	<0.001	0.001	0.001	1999
Laboratory for Energy Related Health Research	1990 – 2001	<0.1 – 0.9	0.19	<0.001	0.0021	<0.00001	2001
Lawrence Berkeley Laboratory	1990 – 2004	0.1 – 3	11	0.012	0.021	0.0002	2004

Lawrence Livermore National Laboratory	1990 – 2001	0.2 – 2.8	0.95	0.003	0.0077	0.0016	2001
Lawrence Livermore National Laboratory: Site 300	1990 – 2001	0.1 – 0.8	0.37	0.028	0.072	0.094	2001
Los Alamos National Laboratory	1990 – 2001	31 – 190	80	0.08	0.018	0.016	2001
Maywood Interim Storage Site	1990 – 1992	6.3 – 13	10.4	0.003	0.029	0.045	1992
Miamisburg Environmental Management Project	1998 – 2001	1.1 – 12	4.3	0.007	0.022	0.028	2001
Middlesex Sampling Plants	1990 – 1993	2.3 – 26	13.60	<0.001	0.0028	0.0028	1990
MIT Bates Linear Accelerator	1991 – 1992	<0.1 – 3	1.5	NA	NA	NA	NA
Monticello Mill Tailings Site	1990 – 1999	120 – 370	248	NA	0.62	0.48	1999
Mound Laboratory	1990 – 1994	0.3 – 2.8	2.08	0.031	0.031	0.019	1994
Naval Reactor Facility	1990 – 2001	<0.1	<0.01	<0.001	<0.00001	<0.00001	2001
Nevada Test Site	1990 – 2002	<0.1 – 6.3	1.6	0.07	0.0024	0.0044	2001

TABLE F.1—(continued).

DOE Site	Years for Which Data Applies	H_E, MEI[a] (range) (μSv)	H_E, MEI (average) (μSv)	Average H_E, Individual (μSv)	Average Collective H_E (all years) (person-Sv)	Most Recent Collective H_E (person-Sv)	Year of Most Recent Collective H_E
New Brunswick Site	1991	1	1.0	<0.001	0.0004	0.0004	1991
Niagara Falls Storage Site	1990 – 1992	<0.1 – 4.4	2.5	0.005	0.0013	0.00077	1992
Oak Ridge Reservation	1990 – 2004	13.5 – 110	41	0.47	0.171	0.104	2004
Paducah Gaseous Diffusion Plant	1990 – 2002	6.9 – 62	34	<0.001	0.00002	0.00003	1998
Pantex Plant	1991 – 2004	<0.1 – 1.6	0.17	0.001	0.00023	<0.00001	2004
Pinellas Plant	1990 – 1994	<0.1 – 1	0.24	0.009	0.0079	0.00097	1994
Portsmouth Gaseous Diffusion Plant	1990 – 2001	0.2 – 29	8.5	0.033	0.020	0.002	2001
Princeton Plasma Physics Laboratory	1990 – 2003	0.1 – 6.8	2.7	0.001	0.019	0.053	2001
RMI Company Extrusion Plant	1990 – 1994	<0.1 – 1	0.23	<0.001	0.00002	<0.00001	1994

Site							
Rockwell International: Desoto Site	1990 – 1994	<0.1 – 5.2	1.57	<0.001	<0.00001	<0.00001	1994
Rockwell International: Santa Susana	1990 – 1994	<0.1 – 0.7	0.26	<0.001	0.00001	0.00001	1994
Rocky Flats Plant	1990 – 1994	1 – 5.2	3.76	0.019	0.043	0.0026	1994
Sandia: Albuquerque	1998 – 2001	<0.1	0.02	0.003	0.0018	0.00068	2001
Sandia: Livermore	1990 – 1994	0.1 – 2.5	1.3	0.002	0.01	0.007	1994
Sandia: Tonopah	1990 – 2001	<0.1 – 29	5.2	0.007	0.00001	0.00005	1994
Savannah River Site	1990 – 2004	1.8 – 4.6	2.51	0.10	0.064	0.060	2004
Stanford Linear Accelerator Center	1990 – 2004	20 – 400	74	0.6	0.20	0.229	2004
Thomas Jefferson National Accelerator Facility	1998 – 2004	1 – 70	35.6	0.001	0.00013	0.00025	2001
Waste Isolation Pilot Plant	1998 – 2001	<0.1	<0.01	NA	NA	NA	NA
Wayne Interim Storage Site	1990 – 1992	6 – 8.4	7.2	<0.001	0.00051	0.00022	1991
Weldon Spring Site	1990 – 2001	0.3 – 76	24.3	0.029	0.0024	0.001	2001

TABLE F.1—(continued).

DOE Site	Years for Which Data Applies	H_E, MEI[a] (range) (μSv)	H_E, MEI (average) (μSv)	Average H_E, Individual (μSv)	Average Collective H_E (all years) (person-Sv)	Most Recent Collective H_E (person-Sv)	Year of Most Recent Collective H_E
West Valley Demonstration Project	1990 – 2004	0.2 – 2.3	0.63	0.001	0.0016	0.002	2004
Total collective H_E for all sites					1.59	1.29	

[a]MEI = maximally-exposed individual.

Glossary

absorbed dose: The energy imparted to matter by ionizing radiation per unit mass of irradiated material at the point of interest. In the SI system the unit is $J\ kg^{-1}$ with the special name gray (Gy). The special unit previously used was rad. 1 Gy = 100 rad.

absorbed fraction: The fraction of the photon energy emitted within a specified volume of material that is absorbed by the volume. The absorbed fraction depends on the source distribution, the photon energy, and the size, shape, and composition of the volume.

accelerator: A device that accelerates charged particles (*e.g.*, protons, electrons) to high speed in order to produce ionization or nuclear reactions in a target; often used for the production of certain radionuclides or directly for radiation therapy. The cyclotron and the linear accelerator are types of accelerators.

activation: Production of radionuclides by absorption of radiations (*e.g.*, photons, neutrons or alpha particles) by atomic nuclei.

activity: The number of spontaneous nuclear transformations occurring in an amount of radionuclide in a particular energy state in a given time interval. The unit for activity in the SI system is reciprocal second (s^{-1}) (*i.e.*, one nuclear transformation per second), with the special name becquerel (Bq). The special unit previously used was curie (Ci); 1 Ci = 3.7 × 10^{10} Bq.

administered activity: The amount, in terms of activity, of a radionuclide given to a patient during a diagnostic or therapeutic procedure.

Agreement State: Any state with which the U.S. Nuclear Regulatory Commission (NRC) has entered into an effective licensing agreement under Section 274(b) of the Atomic Energy Act of 1954, as amended, to enable the state to regulate source, special nuclear, and byproduct materials.

air kerma: (see *kerma*).

alpha particle: A positively charged particle ejected spontaneously from the nuclei of some radioactive elements. It is identical to a helium nucleus with a mass number of 4 and an electric charge of +2. Alpha particles from radioactive decay (<10 MeV) have low penetrating power and a short range (*e.g.*, a few centimeters in air).

angiography: The radiographic visualization of blood vessels following introduction of contrast material.

as low as reasonably achievable: A principle of radiation protection philosophy that requires that exposures to ionizing radiation be kept as low as reasonably achievable, economic and societal factors being taken into account. The protection from radiation exposure is as low as reasonably achievable when the expenditure of further resources

306

would be unwarranted by the reduction in exposure that would be achieved.

atomic number: The number of positively charged protons in the nucleus of an atom.

attenuation: The reduction of radiation intensity upon passage of radiation through matter.

background radiation: (see *ubiquitous background radiation*).

becquerel (Bq): The special name for the unit of activity in the SI system [*i.e.*, one nuclear transformation per second (s^{-1})]. The special unit previously used was curie (Ci); 3.7×10^{10} Bq = 1 Ci; 37 MBq (megabecquerels) = 1 mCi (millicurie)

beta particle: An energetic electron emitted spontaneously from nuclei in the decay of many radionuclides.

bioassay: A technique used to identify, quantify and/or specify the location of radionuclides in the body by direct (*in vivo*) or indirect (*in vitro*) analysis of tissues or excretions from the body.

brachytherapy: Method of radiation therapy in which an encapsulated source is utilized to deliver gamma or beta radiation at a distance up to a few centimeters either by surface, intracavitary or interstitial application.

bronchial epithelium: The surface layer of cells lining the conducting airways of the lung. The thickness decreases with bronchial generation from 80 μm in the trachea to 15 μm in the finest airways.

cancer: A general term for over 100 diseases characterized by abnormal cells and altered control of proliferation of malignant cells.

carcinogenesis: Induction of cancer (*e.g.*, by radiation or other agent).

cardiac catheterization: Passage of a small catheter through a vessel in an arm, leg or neck and into the heart, permitting the securing of blood samples, determination of intracardiac pressure, detection of cardiac anomalies, and injection of contrast media for imaging of vessels.

cephalometric: Referring to images of the head, primarily the dentofacial structures, usually obtained in lateral and posteroanterior orientation. The images are used to measure and study maxillofacial growth and maxilla-mandible relationships.

charged particle: An atomic or subatomic quantity of matter (*e.g.*, electron, proton, alpha particle, ionized atom) having a net positive or negative electrical charge of one or more elementary units of charge.

cinefluorography: The production of motion picture photographic records of the image formed on the output phosphor of an image intensifier by the action of x rays transmitted through the patient.

cleanup: Decontamination and removal of radioactive or other hazardous materials from a contaminated site. Sometimes used to refer to the more general concept of remediation (see *decommissioning*).

coefficient of variation: The ratio of the standard deviation to the mean.

collective effective dose (*S*) **(person-Sv):** Most frequently the product of the mean effective dose for a population and the number of persons in the population, but, more precisely, and preferably, the sum of all individual effective doses in the population of concern.

colloid: Small, insoluble and nondiffusible particle (as a single large molecule or mass of smaller molecules) in solid, liquid or gaseous form that remains in suspension in a surrounding solid, liquid or gaseous medium of different matter.

commercial waste (radioactive): Radioactive waste generated in any activity by a nongovernmental entity. Often refers to waste containing source, special nuclear, or byproduct material regulated by the U.S. Nuclear Regulatory Commission or an Agreement State, but also may refer to waste containing naturally-occurring and accelerator-produced radioactive material that is currently regulated only by the states.

committed effective dose: Effective dose due to absorbed doses in the specified organs or tissues over a specified period of time following an intake of a radionuclide by ingestion, inhalation, or dermal absorption. The time period over which the committed effective dose is calculated normally is 50 y for intakes by adults or from age-at-intake to age 70 y for intakes by other age groups.

computed radiography: An imaging technique in which photo-stimulable phosphor plates are used as the image receptor for an x-ray image. The plate is then placed in a separate device and interrogated with a laser focused to a small area. The resultant stimulated light emission, proportional to the x-ray dose at that point, is detected and the signal digitized to form an array of pixels representing the x-ray image.

computed tomography (CT): An imaging procedure that uses multiple x-ray transmission measurements and a computer program to generate tomographic images of the patient.

computed tomography dose index (*CTDI*): A dose index quantity obtained by integrating over the dose profile resulting from a single computed tomography axial rotation. When obtained using a 10 cm (100 mm) long ionization chamber, it is designated $CTDI_{100}$. When normalized per milliampere-second (mAs), it is designated $_{n}CTDI_{100}$.

confidence interval (CI): A measure of the extent to which an estimate of dose or other parameter is expected to lie within a specified interval (*e.g.*, a 90 % confidence interval of a dose estimate means that, based on available information, the probability is 0.9 that the true but unknown dose lies within the specified interval).

contamination (radioactive): Radioactive material that is present in undesired locations such as on the surface of or inside structures, areas, objects or individuals.

conventional fluoroscopy: An imaging technique using x rays to visualize the dynamics of bodily functioning. For example, a material with high x-ray absorption is injected or ingested and fluoroscopy is used to monitor the progress of the material through the blood vessels or gastrointestinal tract. The image receptor can be either an image intensifier and video camera tube, or a large-area solid-state detector.

conventional radiography: An imaging technique where the image receptor consists of a combination of (usually two) intensifying(s) screens in intimate contact with a photographic film (usually a dual-emulsion film). After exposure to the x-ray image, the photographic film is then processed in chemical solutions. Photographic film is relatively insensitive to x rays; the light from the intensifying screens produces most of the film optical density (also referred to as screen-film radiography).

conversion coefficient: The quotient of a dose quantity under specied conditions and an associated field quantity (*e.g.*, air kerma or fluence).

critical group: Subgroup of an exposed or potentially exposed population that receives or is expected to receive the highest dose due to exposure.

curie (Ci): The special unit previously used for activity (see *activity* and *becquerel*).

decommissioning: The process of closing down a facility followed by reducing the residual quantities of radioactive material to a level that permits the release of the property for either limited (restricted) or unrestricted use.

deep dose equivalent: Dose equivalent at a tissue depth of 1 cm. Also called personal dose equivalent at a depth of 1 cm. The unit for deep dose equivalent in the SI system is $J\ kg^{-1}$, with the special name sievert (Sv).

dental bitewing: An intraoral radiograph that demonstrates the crowns, necks and coronal thirds of the roots of both upper and lower teeth, so named because the patient bites upon a tab or "wing" projecting from the center of the image-receptor packet.

depleted uranium: Uranium with an isotopic content of <0.7 % ^{235}U; typically depleted uranium contains ~0.2 % ^{235}U.

deterministic effects: Effects that occur in all individuals who receive greater than a threshold dose; the severity of the effect varies with the dose above the threshold. Examples are radiation-induced cataracts (lens of the eye) and radiation-induced erythema (skin).

detriment: (see *radiation detriment*).

digital radiography: An imaging technique using an x-ray sensitive plate integrated into the x-ray imaging system. The plate converts the absorbed x-ray image into an electrical charge map which is then digitized to form an array of pixels representing the x-ray image. The image information is presented in a digital array rather than on film.

direct exposure x-ray (film) images: A dual-emulsion photographic film is exposed directly to x rays, without the use of intensifying screens. The radiation dose required for direct exposure imaging is 10 to 20 times higher than is required with screen-film imaging since the photographic film is relatively insensitive to x-ray exposure.

disposal: Placement of waste in a facility designed to isolate waste from the accessible environment without an intention to retrieve the waste, irrespective of whether such isolation permits recovery of waste.

dose (radiation dose): A general term used when the context is not specific to a particular dose quantity. When the context is specific, the name or symbol for the quantity is used (*e.g.*, mean absorbed dose, effective dose).

dose equivalent (H): The product of the absorbed dose (D) at a point and the quality factor (Q) at that point for the radiation type (*i.e.*, $H = DQ$). The unit of dose equivalent is J kg^{-1} with the special name sievert (Sv).

dose-length product (DLP): A dose index quantity obtained using the following formula:

$$DLP = \frac{L}{p}\left(\frac{1}{3}CTDI_{100,c} + \frac{2}{3}CTDI_{100,p}\right), \qquad (G.1)$$

where L is the length of patient scanned, p is the pitch, and $CTDI_{100,c}$ and $CTDI_{100,p}$ are $CTDI_{100}$ values determined at the center and periphery of a standardized phantom (see *pitch* and *computed tomography dose index*).

dose limit: A limit on dose that is applied for exposure to individuals in order to prevent the occurrence of radiation-induced deterministic effects or to limit the probability of radiation-related stochastic effects.

dose rate (radiation dose rate): Dose delivered per unit time. Can refer to any dose quantity (*e.g.*, absorbed dose, dose equivalent).

dosimeter: Dose measuring device (see *personal monitoring*).

dosimetric model: (1) For intakes of radionuclides into the body, model that estimates the dose in various organs and tissues per disintegration of a radionuclide in a specified source organ (site of deposition or transit in the body). (2) For external exposure, model that estimates the dose rate in organs and tissues per unit activity concentration of a radionuclide in an environmental medium.

dosimetry: The science or technique of determining radiation dose.

effective dose (E): The sum over specified organs and tissues of the products of the equivalent dose in a tissue (H_T) and the tissue weighting factor for that tissue or organ (w_T):

$$E = \sum_T w_T H_T . \qquad (G.2)$$

The tissue weighting factors have been developed from a reference population of equal numbers of both males and females and a wide range of ages (ICRP, 1991). Effective dose (E) applies only to stochastic effects. The unit is the joule per kilogram (J kg^{-1}) with the special name sievert (Sv). ICRP (2007a) revised the w_T values and the w_R values (see *equivalent dose*) used in effective dose; when the ICRP (2007a) formulation is cited in this Report, it is denoted as E^*.

effective dose equivalent (H_E): The sum over specified organs and tissues of the products of the mean dose equivalent in a tissue (H_T) and the weighting factor for that tissue or organ (w_T):

$$H_E = \sum_T w_T H_T . \qquad (G.3)$$

The formulation differs from ICRP (1991) and is defined in ICRP (1977). Now superseded in ICRP and NCRP recommendations by *effective dose*, but the formulation is still in use by most federal and state agencies.

electron: Subatomic charged particle. Negatively charged electrons are parts of stable atoms. Both negatively and positively charged electrons (positrons) may be expelled from the radioactive atom when it disintegrates (see *beta particle*).

element: Any substance that cannot be separated into different substances by ordinary chemical methods. Elements are distinguished by the number of protons in the nucleus of atoms.

entrance air kerma (or **entrance skin exposure**)**:** Air kerma (or exposure) measured free-in-air at the location of the entry surface of an irradiated person or phantom in the absence of the person or phantom.

equilibrium factor: The ratio of the actual potential alpha-energy concentration to the potential alpha-energy concentration that would prevail if all the decay products in each of the radon progeny decay series were in equilibrium with the parent radon.

equivalent dose (H_T)**:** Mean absorbed dose in a tissue or organ $(D_{T,R})$ weighted by the radiation weighting factor (w_R) for the type and energy of radiation incident on the body:

$$H_T = \sum_R w_R D_{T,R} \ ,\qquad\qquad (G.4)$$

The SI unit of equivalent dose is the joule per kilogram ($J \ kg^{-1}$) with the special name sievert (Sv). $1 \ Sv = 1 \ J \ kg^{-1}$.

exempt: Excluded from regulation as hazardous or radioactive material.

exposure: A general term used to express the act of being exposed to ionizing radiation. In this Report, exposure also refers to inhalation intake (*e.g.*, for radon) expressed in working level months (see *working level month*). Exposure is also a defined ionizing radiation quantity. It is a measure of the ionization produced in air by x or gamma rays. The unit of exposure is coulomb per kilogram ($C \ kg^{-1}$). The special name for exposure is roentgen (R), where $1 \ R = 2.58 \times 10^{-4} \ C \ kg^{-1}$.

exposure assessment: A specification of the population potentially exposed to ionizing radiation and the pathways and routes by which exposure can occur, and quantification of the magnitude, duration and timing of the exposures and resulting doses.

external dose: Dose to organs or tissues of an organism due to radiation sources outside the body.

fallout: In the context of this Report, the radioactive material falling from the atmosphere to Earth's surface after a nuclear event, such as a weapons test or accident.

field size: The geometrical projection of the x-ray beam on a plane perpendicular to the central ray of the distal end of the limiting diaphragm, as seen from the center of the front surface of the source.

film: A thin, transparent sheet of polyester or similar material coated on one or both sides with an emulsion sensitive to radiation and light.

fission (nuclear): A nuclear transformation characterized by the splitting of a nucleus into at least two other nuclei and the release of a relatively large amount of energy.

fluence: The number of particles or photons per unit of a cross-sectional area (units of m^{-2}).

fluoroscopy: A medical x-ray procedure used for observation of the internal features of the body by means of the fluorescence produced on a screen by a continuous field of x rays transmitted through the body.

food chain: The hierarchical order of groups of organisms based on what each group eats.

galactic cosmic radiation: The charged-particle radiation outside the magnetosphere comprised of 2 % electrons and positrons, and 98 % nuclei, the latter component consisting (by fluence) of 87 % protons, 12 % helium ions, and 1 % high atomic number, high-energy particles.

gamma rays: Electromagnetic radiation emitted by the atomic nucleus. Gamma rays have high penetrating ability compared with alpha and beta particles.

genetic effects: Changes in reproductive cells that may result in detriment to offspring.

geometric mean (GM): The geometric mean of a set of n values is the nth root of the product of the n values [$e.g.$, the geometric mean of (a,b) is the square root (second root) of a times b, which is written $(a \times b)^{1/2}$].

geometric standard deviation (GSD): In a lognormal distribution, the exponential of the standard deviation of the associated normal distribution (always ≥ 1).

gray (Gy): The special name for the SI unit J kg^{-1} ($i.e.$, energy imparted per unit mass of a material). 1 Gy = 1 J kg^{-1}.

groundwater: Water below the land surface in a zone of saturation that is under a pressure equal to or greater than atmospheric pressure.

half-life: The time in which one-half of the atoms (on average) of a particular radioactive substance disintegrate into another nuclear form (also called physical or radiological half-life).

hereditary effects: Effects expressed in offspring due to alteration of reproductive cells in the parent(s).

image intensifier: An x-ray image receptor which increases the brightness of a fluoroscopic image by electronic amplification and image minification.

image quality: The overall clarity of a radiographic image. Image sharpness, image contrast, and image noise are three common measures of image quality.

image receptor: A system for deriving a diagnostically usable image from the x rays transmitted through the patient. Examples: screen-film system, photostimulable storage phosphor, solid-state detector.

internal dose: Dose to organs or tissues of an organism due to intakes of radionuclides ($e.g.$, by ingestion, inhalation, or dermal absorption).

internal exposure: Exposure to radiation originating from a source within the body (*e.g.*, as a result of intakes of radionuclides into the body by inhalation or ingestion).

International System of Quantities and Units [Systeme Internationale (SI)]: The International System of Quantities and Units as defined by the General Conference of Weights and Measures in 1960 and periodically revised since. These units are generally based on the meter/kilogram/second units, with special quantities for radiation including the becquerel, gray and sievert.

intraoral radiography: Radiography with an image receptor placed intraorally and lingually or palatally to the teeth.

in vivo: From Latin "in life"; refers to a procedure carried out in the living body, as opposed to a procedure done outside the body (*in vitro*) (*e.g.*, in a test tube).

ionization chamber: A device for detection of ionizing radiation or for measurement of exposure, air kerma, or absorbed dose (or their corresponding rates).

ionizing radiation: Particulate or electromagnetic radiation that is capable of removing electrons from a neutral atom or molecule either directly or indirectly, resulting in an excess charge.

irradiation: The process of exposure to radiation.

isotope: One of several nuclides having the same number of protons in their nuclei, but different nuclear mass numbers due to different numbers of neutrons in the nucleus.

kerma (kinetic energy released per unit mass) (K): The sum of the initial kinetic energies of all the charged particles liberated by uncharged particles in a mass of material. The unit for kerma is J kg^{-1}, with the special name gray (Gy). Kerma can be quoted for any specified material at a point in free space or in an absorbing medium (*e.g.*, air kerma).

kerma-area product (KAP): The incident air kerma (in gray or milligray) times the cross-sectional area of the x-ray beam (in cm^2).

landfill: A disposal facility or part of a facility where waste is placed in or on land and which is not a pile, a land treatment facility, a surface impoundment, an underground injection well, a salt dome formation, a salt bed formation, an underground mine, a cave, or a corrective action management unit.

leachate: The water that has been in contact with sediment or soil and whose chemical characteristics have been affected by properties of the sediment or soil, as well as the duration of contact.

license: Permission issued by the U.S. Nuclear Regulatory Commission (NRC) or an Agreement State in accordance with applicable laws or regulations.

linear accelerator (electron): A device that accelerates electrons along a linear path into an electron target or converter where the energy is converted into bremsstrahlung or x-ray photons.

lognormal distribution: A set of values whose logarithms are normally distributed is said to be lognormally distributed. The lognormal distribution is asymmetric. It is bounded at the lower end by zero because the logarithm is defined only for positive numbers.

low-level radioactive waste: A general term for a wide range of radioactive waste that contain low concentrations of radionuclides, where the low concentrations are defined by U.S. regulations.

magnification (in medical x-ray imaging): An imaging procedure carried out with magnification usually produced by purposeful introduction of distance between the subject and the image receptor.

mammography: An x-ray examination of the breast.

maximally-exposed individual (MEI): Individual assumed to receive the highest dose from exposure to radiation.

mean: Sum of the measured values divided by the number of measurements. The mean value is also often called the (arithmetic) average value. The mean of a distribution is the weighted average of the possible values of the random variable.

mean absorbed dose: The mean absorbed dose in an organ or tissue, obtained by integrating or averaging absorbed doses at points in the organ or tissue.

mean glandular dose: The energy deposited per unit mass of glandular tissue (the radiosensitive tissue in the breast) averaged over all the glandular tissue in the breast (*i.e.*, the mean absorbed dose to glandular tissue).

median: Of a set of n values, the median is the value that is as frequently exceeded (by other values in the set) as not. The median value of a distribution is the 50th percentile.

medical facility: A hospital, clinic or other facility that provides medical services.

member of the public: An individual who is not already considered occupationally exposed by a radiation source or practice under consideration. When being irradiated as a result of medical care, patients are a separate category.

migration: The movement of substances in the environment, usually by means of air, surface water, or groundwater.

mill tailings: Residues from chemical processing of uranium or thorium ores for their source material content. Mill tailings are a form of byproduct material, as defined in the Atomic Energy Act.

minimum detectable level: A general term for the lowest value of a quantity that a measurement device is capable of detecting.

model: Mathematical or physical representation of an environmental or biological system, sometimes including specific numerical values for parameters of the system.

monitor: To determine the level of ionizing radiation or radioactive contamination. Also, a device used for this purpose.

monitoring: Periodic or continuous determination of exposure rate or dose rate in an area (area monitoring), or of the exposure received by a person (personal monitoring), or the measurement of contamination levels.

Monte-Carlo simulation: Computation of a probability distribution of an output of a model on the basis of repeated calculations using random sampling of input variables from specified probability distributions.

naturally-occurring radioactive material (NORM): Materials found in the natural environment containing inherent concentrations of radionuclides. Examples include materials containing long-lived radioactive isotopes of the elements uranium, thorium and potassium, and of their decay products (*e.g.*, the elements radium and radon) that have always been present in Earth's crust.

negligible individual dose: A level of effective dose to an individual per source or practice that may be ignored. This term was defined in NCRP Report No. 116 (NCRP, 1993a) and its recommended value is 0.01 mSv.

neutron: An uncharged elementary particle having a mass slightly greater than a proton that is usually stable when within the nucleus but is unstable otherwise.

normal distribution: The normal distribution is an unbounded symmetric distribution, characterized by its mean and standard deviation. In a normal distribution, the median is equal to the mean.

nuclear fuel cycle: Activities associated with production, utilization and disposition of fuel for nuclear reactors, including power reactors, research reactors, and defense and isotope production reactors, and byproducts related to such activities.

nuclide: A species of atom having specied numbers of neutrons and protons in its nucleus.

occupational exposures: Radiation exposures to individuals that are incurred in the workplace as a result of situations that can reasonably be regarded as being the responsibility of management (radiation exposures associated with medical diagnosis of or treatment for the individual are excluded).

optically-stimulated luminescent dosimeter: A dosimeter containing a crystalline solid for measuring radiation dose. When used for personal dosimetry, filters (absorbers) are included to help characterize the types of radiation encountered. When irradiated with intense light, optically-stimulated luminescent crystals that have been exposed to ionizing radiation give off light proportional to the energy they received from the radiation.

panoramic examination: A method of radiography by which continuous curved tomograms of the maxillary and mandibular dental arches and their associated structures may be obtained.

pathway: Route or mechanism of transport of contaminants in the environment, the means of release of contaminants from a facility, or the means of exposure of humans or other organisms.

personal dose equivalent: (see *deep dose equivalent*).

personal monitoring: The use of a small radiation detector that is worn by an individual. Common personal dosimeters contain film, thermoluminescent, or optically-stimulated luminescent materials as the radiation detection device.

person-sievert (person-Sv): The unit of collective effective dose.

phantom: A volume of tissue- or water-equivalent material used to simulate the absorption and scattering characteristics of the patient's body or portion thereof.

photon: Quantum of electromagnetic radiation, having no charge or mass, that exhibits both particle and wave behavior, such as a gamma or x ray.

pitch (p): In computed tomography (CT), the ratio of the patient translation per gantry rotation to the nominal beam width for the CT scan.

positron: An antiparticle equal in mass to an electron and having an equal but positive charge.

positron emission tomography (PET): An imaging technique using radionuclides that emit positrons (positively charged electrons), whose annihilation photons are imaged in coincidence to form tomographic views of the body.

precision: Acceptable degree of uncertainty of an estimate with respect to an actual event or outcome (result).

probability distribution: Estimate of the likelihood of occurrence of different possible values of a measured value, a model parameter, or model output.

projection: The direction of the central ray (*e.g.*, mediolateral, craniocaudal) in an x-ray exam.

protective devices (medical exposure): Devices such as gloves, aprons and gowns made of radiation absorbing materials, used to reduce occupational radiation exposure in medical procedures.

proton: An elementary nuclear particle with a positive charge equal to the charge of an electron and a mass equal to the nucleus of the ^{1}H atom.

quality assurance: Process of ensuring proper documentation of data, interpretations of data, which are embodied in assumptions, and computer codes.

quality control: The routine performance of tests and tasks and the interpretation of data from the tests of equipment function and the corrective actions taken.

rad: The special unit previously used for absorbed dose; 100 rad = 1 Gy (see *gray*).

radiation (ionizing): Electromagnetic radiation (x or gamma rays) or particulate radiation (alpha particles, beta particles, electrons, positrons, protons, neutrons, and heavy charged particles) capable of producing ions by direct or secondary processes in passage through matter.

radiation detriment: Measure of stochastic effects from exposure to ionizing radiation that takes into account the probability of fatal cancers, probability of severe hereditary effects in future generations, probability of nonfatal cancers weighted by the lethality fraction, and relative years of life lost per fatal health effect.

radiation weighting factor (w_R): A factor used to allow for differences in the biological effectiveness between different radiations when calculating equivalent dose (H_T) (see *equivalent dose*). These factors are independent of the tissue or organ irradiated.

radioactive decay: The spontaneous transformation of one nuclide into a different nuclide or into a different energy state of the same nuclide. The process results in a decrease, with time, of the number of original radioactive atoms in a sample. Decay generally involves the emission from the nucleus of alpha particles, beta particles, or gamma rays.

radioactive series: A succession of nuclides, each of which transforms by radioactive decay into the next until a stable nuclide results. The first member is called the parent and the subsequent members of the series are called progeny, daughters or decay products.

radioactive waste: Solid, liquid or gaseous materials of no value that contain radionuclides, either anthropogenic or naturally-occurring, and are regulated as hazardous material due to the presence of radionuclides.

radiograph: A film or other record produced by the action of x rays on a sensitized surface.

radiography: The production of images on film or other media by the action of x rays transmitted through a patient.

radiology: That branch of healing arts and sciences that deals with the use of images in the diagnosis and treatment of disease.

radionuclide: An unstable (radioactive) nuclide. A nuclide is a species of atom characterized by the constitution of its nucleus (*i.e.*, the number of protons and neutrons, and the energy content).

radiopharmaceutical: A radioactive substance administered to a patient for diagnostic or therapeutic nuclear-medicine procedures. A radiopharmaceutical contains two parts, the radionuclide and the pharmaceutical (*e.g.*, ^{99m}Tc DTPA). In some cases the two are one (*e.g.*, ^{133}Xe gas).

radon (and **radon progeny**): Radon is a colorless, odorless, naturally-occurring, and gaseous element resulting from radioactive decay of isotopes of radium. Radon is also the common name for the specific radionuclide ^{222}Rn and is used throughout this Report in that context. Radon progeny are short-lived decay products of ^{222}Rn (*i.e.*, ^{218}Po, ^{214}Pb, ^{214}Bi, and ^{214}Po).

relative biological effectiveness: A factor used to compare the biological effectiveness of absorbed doses from different types of ionizing radiation, determined experimentally. Relative biological effectiveness is the ratio of the absorbed dose of a reference radiation (usually taken as 250 kVp x rays) to the absorbed dose of the radiation in question required to produce the same level of an identical biological effect in a particular experimental organism or tissue.

rem: The special unit previously used for the quantities equivalent dose and effective dose (or effective dose equivalent); 100 rem = 1 Sv (see *sievert*).

remediation: Actions taken to reduce risks to human health or the environment posed by the presence of radioactive or hazardous chemical contaminants at a site including, but not restricted to, excavation of contaminated soil, removal of contaminants from building surfaces or equipment, stabilization of buried waste, and installation of engineered barriers (*e.g.*, caps on waste trenches) to reduce the potential for migration of contaminants.

residual (contamination or dose): Radioactive material in structures, materials, soils, groundwater, and other media at a site resulting from activities under the site operator's control, especially radioactive material remaining at a site after decommissioning and remediation. Residual radioactive material does not include naturally-occurring radioactive material in its undisturbed state.

roentgen (R): The special name for the unit of exposure. Exposure is a specific quantity of ionization (charge) produced by the absorption of x- or gamma-radiation energy in a specified mass of air under standard conditions. 1 R = 2.58×10^{-4} coulomb per kilogram (C kg^{-1}).

screen-film radiography: (see *conventional radiography*).

sealed source: Radioactive material encased in a capsule designed to prevent leakage or escape of the material.

sestamibi: Sestamibi [Cardiolite® (E.I. du Pont de Nemours and Company, Wilmington, Delaware)] labeled with ^{99m}Tc. Used to visualize some types of breast cancer utilizing a gamma camera.

sievert (Sv): The special name (in the SI system) for the unit of equivalent dose and effective dose (or effective dose equivalent); 1 Sv = 1 J kg^{-1}. 1 Sv = 100 rem (see *rem*).

single-photon emission computed tomography (SPECT): An imaging technique in which one or more gamma cameras sample a region of the body from several angles, producing tomographic images ("slices") of the region.

solar cycle: The solar-activity cyclic behavior, usually represented by the number of sunspots visible on the solar photosphere. The average length of solar cycles since 1900 is 11.4 y.

solar particles: Penetrating particulate ionizing radiation that originates from the sun.

source (or radiation source): Radiation-producing equipment or an aggregate of radioactive nuclei.

source term: Rate of release of radionuclides from a waste-disposal facility, usually over time.

space radiation: Penetrating ionizing radiation, both particulate and electromagnetic, that originates in outer space.

specific activity: Activity of a radionuclide per unit mass of the radionuclide; also may refer to activity of a radionuclide per unit mass of material in which the radionuclide is dispersed.

standard deviation (SD): Square root of the variance. In a set of n measurements, the variance (s^2) is the sum of the squared deviations from the mean divided by $(n - 1)$ (see *mean*).

standard deviation (error) of the mean: The square root of the variance divided by the number of observations: $(s^2/n)^{1/2}$. An equivalent definition is that the standard deviation of the mean is the standard deviation divided by the square root of the number of observations $(s/n^{1/2})$.

standard error: The standard deviation of an estimate considered as a random variable. The standard deviation of the mean is often known as the standard error.

stochastic: Of, pertaining to, or arising from chance; involving probability; random.

stochastic effects: Effects, the probability of which, rather than their severity, is assumed to be a function of dose without a threshold. For example, cancer and hereditary effects of radiation are regarded as being stochastic.

surface water: Water on or above the land surface (*e.g.*, rivers, streams, lakes, ponds, oceans).

tailings: Waste or refuse left in various processes of milling or mining. Tailings often contain a significant portion of the radioactive material present in the undisturbed ore.

technologically-enhanced naturally-occurring radioactive material (TENORM): Naturally-occurring radioactive material whose concentrations of radionuclides are increased by or as a result of past or present human practices. TENORM does not include background radiation or the naturally-occurring radionuclides in rocks or soils. TENORM also does not include uranium or thorium in source material as defined in the Atomic Energy Act of 1954 and NRC regulations.

terrestrial: Of or relating to Earth or its inhabitants; of or relating to land as distinct from air or water; living on or in or growing from land.

thermoluminescent dosimeter (TLD): A dosimeter containing a phosphor for measuring dose. When used for personal dosimetry, filters (absorbers) are included to help characterize the types of radiation. When heated, TLDs that have been exposed to ionizing radiation give off light proportional to the energy absorbed.

thorium: A naturally radioactive element. Thorium-232 is the parent of one radioactive series, and specific thorium nuclides are members of the three naturally-occurring radionuclide series.

thoron (and thoron progeny): Thoron is the common name for the specific radionuclide ^{220}Rn and is used throughout this Report. Thoron progeny are short-lived decay products of ^{220}Rn (*i.e.*, ^{216}Po, ^{212}Pb, ^{212}Bi, and ^{212}Po).

threshold dose: (see *deterministic effects*).

tissue weighting factor (w_T)**:** A factor that indicates the ratio of the risk of stochastic effects attributable to irradiation of a given organ or tissue (T) to the total risk when the whole body is uniformly irradiated. When calculating effective dose equivalent, tissue weighting factor represents the risk of fatal cancers or severe hereditary effects. When calculating effective dose, tissue weighting factor represents total detriment.

tomography: A special technique to show in detail images of structures lying in a predetermined plane of tissue, while blurring or eliminating detail in images of structures in other planes.

total effective dose equivalent (TEDE): The sum of the deep dose equivalent (for external exposures) and the committed effective dose equivalent (from intakes of radionuclides) (NRC, 2007a). TEDE accumulates over a period of time that includes external irradiation as well as committed doses due to radionuclide intakes during that period of time.

ubiquitous background radiation: As used in this Report, includes external exposure from space radiation (solar particles and cosmic rays), external exposure from terrestrial radiation (primarily ^{40}K and the ^{238}U and ^{232}Th decay series), internal exposure from inhalation of radon and thoron and their progeny, and internal exposure from radionuclides in the body.

uncertainty: Lack of sureness or confidence in predictions of models or results of measurements. Uncertainties may be categorized as Type A, which are those due to stochastic variation, or Type B, which are those due to lack of knowledge founded on an incomplete characterization, understanding or measurement of a system.

uranium: A naturally radioactive element. In natural ores, it consists of 0.7 % ^{235}U, 99.3 % ^{238}U, and a small amount of ^{234}U.

variability: A heterogeneity, diversity or range that characterizes a measured value or parameter (*e.g.*, differences in body weight in a population). Further study cannot reduce variability but may provide greater confidence in quantitative characterizations of variability (see *uncertainty*).

veterinary medicine: The branch of medicine that deals with the diagnosis and treatment of diseases and injuries of animals by a licensed veterinarian.

view (radiographic): The image on film resulting from projection of the x-ray beam through a patient, usually named according to the direction of the x-ray beam relative to the body (*e.g.*, antero-posterior).

working level (WL): Any combination of short-lived radon (^{222}Rn) daughter products in 1 L of air that will result in the emission of exactly 1.30×10^5 MeV (million electron volts) of potential alpha energy (ICRP, 1993). 1 WL will result in the emission of 2.08×10^{-5} J m^{-3}.

working level month (WLM): A cumulative exposure, equivalent to exposure to 1 WL for a working month (170 h) (*i.e.*, 2.08×10^{-5} J h m^{-3} $\times$ 170 h = 3.54×10^{-3} J h m^{-3}).

x rays: Penetrating electromagnetic radiation having a range of wavelengths (energies) that are similar to those of gamma photons. X rays are usually produced by interaction of the electron field around certain nuclei or by the slowing down of energetic electrons. Once formed, there is no physical difference between x- and gamma-ray photons; however, there is a difference in their origin.

Abbreviations, Acronyms and Symbols

ε_p	potential alpha-energy exposure (time integral)
AEA	Atomic Energy Act of 1954
AP	antero-posterior view
bb	bronchiolar region of the respiratory tract
BB	bronchial region of the respiratory tract
BMI	body mass index
BWR	boiling water reactor
C	observed concentration of radon gas
CAARS	Cargo Advanced Automated Radiography System
CCP	coal combustion product
c_{eq}	equilibrium equivalent concentration of radon gas
C_i	radon-gas concentration in each location i
C_K	potassium concentration (grams of potassium per kilogram of body mass)
c_p	potential alpha-energy concentration
CPT	Common Procedural Terminology
CS	cervical spine
CSF	cerebrospinal fluid
CT	computed tomography
$CTDI$	computed tomography dose index
$CTDI_{100}$	computed tomography dose index using a 10 cm (100 mm) long ionization chamber
$CTDI_{vol}$	computed tomography dose index based on volume (*i.e.*, volume $CTDI_w$)
$CTDI_w$	weighted $CTDI_{100}$
DCC_E	dose conversion coefficient from kerma-air product to effective dose
DEXA	dual-energy x-ray absorptiometry
DISIDA	diisopropyl iminodiacetic acid
DLP	dose-length product
DMSA	dimercaptosuccinic acid
DTPA	diethylenetriamine pentaacetic acid
E	effective dose [ICRP (1991) formulation]
E^*	effective dose [ICRP (2007a) formulation)]
ECD	bicisate (L,L-ethyl cysteinate dimer)
EDTMP	ethylene diamine tetramethylene phosphonate

E_{Exp}	average effective dose to an individual in a group exposed to a specific source
E_{p}	unit potential alpha-energy exposure
E_{US}	effective dose per individual in the U.S. population
FDG	fluorodeoxyglucose
FHMA	ferric hydroxide macroaggregate
GE	gastroesophageal
GI	gastrointestinal
GM	geometric mean
GSD	geometric standard deviation
H_{E}	effective dose equivalent
HMPAO	exametazine (hexamethylenepropylene-amineoxime)
HNF	head and neck films
H_{T}	equivalent dose
IMRT	intensity modulated radiotherapy
IMV	IMV Medical Information Division
ISCORS	Interagency Steering Committee on Radiation Standards
i.v.	intravenous
IVP	intravenous pyelogram
KAP	kerma-area product
KUB	kidney, ureter and bladder
L	length of patient scanned (scan length)
LAT	lateral view
l_{II}	building attenuation factor
LINAC	linear electron accelerator
LNEP	large national employer plan
LS	lumbosacral spine
MAA	macro aggregated albumin
MAG3	mertiatide (mercaptoacetylglycyl-glycyl-glycine)
MDCT	multidetector computed tomography
MDP	methylene diphosphonate
MEI	maximally-exposed individual
MIBG	metaiodobenzylguanidine
MIBI	methoxyisobutyl isonitrile
MSW	municipal solid waste
NEXT	Nationwide Evaluation of X-Ray Trends
NII	nonintrusive inspection
NIRS	National Inorganic and Radionuclide Survey
NJDEP	New Jersey Department of Environmental Protection
NORM	naturally-occurring radioactive material
NRRS	National Residential Radon Survey
NURE	National Uranium Resource Evaluation
p	pitch
PA	postero-anterior view
PET	positron emission tomography

PFNA	pulsed fast-neutron analysis
POTW	publicly-owned treatment works
PTA	percutaneous transluminal angioplasty
PWR	pressurized water reactor
RBC	red blood cells
S	collective effective dose
SC	sulphur colloid
SD	standard deviation
SI	Systeme Internationale (International System of Quantities and Units)
SNM	Society of Nuclear Medicine
SPECT	single-photon emission computed tomography
TEDE	total effective dose equivalent
TENORM	technologically-enhanced naturally-occurring radioactive material
TLD	thermoluminescent dosimeter
TS	thoracic spine
VACIS®	Vehicle and Cargo Inspection System
VQ	ventilation-perfusion scan
UGI	upper gastrointestinal
WBC	white blood cells
WL	working level
WLM	working level month
w_R	radiation weighting factor
w_T	tissue weighting factor

References

ABD EL-AZIZ, N., KHATER, A.E.M. and AL-SEWAIDAN, H.A. (2005). "Natural radioactivity contents in tobacco," pages 407 to 408 in *High Levels of Natural Radiation and Radon Areas: Radiation Dose and Health Effects*, International Congress Series Vol. 1276 (Elsevier, New York).

ABU-JARAD, F. and FAZAL-UR-REHMAN (2003). "Detection of ^{210}Po on filter papers 16 years after use for collection of short-lived radon progeny in a room," J. Environ. Radioact. **67**(1), 27–33.

ACAA (2002). American Coal Ash Association. *ACAA Releases 2002 Coal Combustion Products Production and Use Figures*, http://acaa.affiniscape.com/associations/8003/files/acaa_2002_ccp_svy(11-25-03).pdf (accessed February 4, 2009) (American Coal Ash Association, Aurora, Colorado).

ACE (2008). U.S. Army Corps of Engineers. *About FUSRAP*, http://www.lrb.usace.army.mil/fusrap (accessed February 4, 2009) (U.S. Army Corps of Engineers, Buffalo, New York).

ACHEY, B., MILLER, K., ERDMAN, M. and KING, S. (2004). "Potential dose to nuclear medicine technologists from ^{99m}Tc-DTPA aerosol lung studies," Health Phys. **86**(Suppl. 2), S85–S87.

AEA (1954). U.S. Atomic Energy Act. Public Law 83-703 (August 30), 68 Stat. 919, as amended (U.S. Government Printing Office, Washington).

AHQR (2007). Agency for Healthcare Quality and Research. *Medical Expenditure Panel Surveys, 2001–2004*, http://www.meps.ahrq.gov/mepsweb/index.jsp (accessed December 28, 2007) (U.S. Department of Health and Human Services, Rockville, Maryland).

ALTSHULER, B., NELSON, N. and KUSCHNER, M. (1964). "Estimation of lung tissue dose from the inhalation of radon and daughters," Health Phys. **10**(12), 1137-1161.

AMA (2004). American Medical Association. *CPT 2004: Current Procedural Terminology, Standard Edition*, 4th ed. (American Medical Association, Chicago, Illinois).

ANDERSEN, B., STREET, L. and WILHELMSEN, R. (1998). *1997 LMITCO Environmental Monitoring Program Report for the Idaho National Engineering and Environmental Laboratory*, INEEL/EXT-98-00305, http://www.energystorm.us/1997_Lmitco_Environmental_Monitoring_Program_Report_For_The_Idaho_National_Engineering_And_Environmental_Laboratory-r19234.html?searchTerms=1997~lmitco (accessed February 3, 2009) (U.S. Department of Energy, Washington).

ANSI (2002). American National Standards Institute. *Radiation Safety for Personnel Security Screening Systems ("People Scanners")*, ANSI/HPS N43.17-2002 (Health Physics Society, McLean, Virginia).

ARVELA, H., HYVONEN, H., LEMMELA, H. and CASTREN, O. (1995). "Indoor and outdoor gamma radiation in Finland," Radiat. Prot. Dosim. **59**(1), 25–32.

BALTER, S., OETGEN, M., HILL, A., DALTON, J., SACHER, A., LIPSZTEIN, R., COLLINS, M. and MOSES, J. (2000). "Personnel exposure during gamma endovascular brachytherapy," Health Phys. **79**(2), 136–146.

BALTER, S., SCHUELER, B.A., MILLER, D.L., COLE, P.E., LU, H.T., BERENSTEIN, A., ALBERT, R., GEORGIA, J.D., NOONAN, P.T., RUSSELL, E.J., MALISCH, T.W., VOGELZANG, R.L., GEISINGER, M., CARDELLA, J.F., ST. GEORGE, J., MILLER, G.L., III and ANDERSON, J. (2004). "Radiation doses in interventional radiology procedures: The RAD-IR Study: Part III: Dosimetric performance of the interventional fluoroscopy units," J. Vasc. Interv. Radiol. **15**(9), 919–926.

BARRINGER, T.H., DEPAUL, V.T., FOCAZIO, M.J., KRAEMER, T.F., MULLIN, A.H. and SZABO, Z. (2001). *Occurrence of Selected Radionuclides in Ground Water Used for Drinking Water in the United States: A Reconnaissance Survey, 1998,* Water-Resources Investigations Report 00-4273 (U.S. Geological Survey, Denver).

BEHLING, U.H. and HILDEBRAND, J.E. (1986). *Radiation and Health Effects: A Report on the TMI-2 Accident and Related Health Studies* (GPU Nuclear Corporation, Middletown, Pennsylvania).

BERG, J., LAMB, C.R. and O'CALLAGHAN, M.W. (1990). "Bone scintigraphy in the initial evaluation of dogs with primary bone tumors," J. Am. Vet. Med. Assoc. **196**(6), 917–920.

BETSOU, S. EFSTATHOPOULOS, E.P., KATRITISIS, D., FAULKNER, K. and PANAYIOTAKIS, G. (1998). "Patient radiation doses during cardiac catheterization procedures," Br. J. Radiol. **71**(846), 634–639.

BLACK, S.C. and BRETTHAUER, E.W. (1968). "Polonium-210 in tobacco," Radiol. Health Data Rep. **9**(3), 145–152.

BLANCHARD, R.L., HANS, J.M., KAUFMAN, R.F., EADIE, G.G., FOWLER, T.W., HORTON, T.R., SMITH, J.M. and MAGNO, P.J. (1983). *Potential Health and Environmental Hazards of Uranium Mine Wastes*, EPA Report 520/1-83-007 (National Technical Information Service, Springfield, Virginia).

BOGAERT, E., BACHER, K. and THIERENS, H. (2008). "Interventional cardiovascular procedures in Belgium: Effective dose and conversion factors," Radiat. Protect. Dosim. **129**(1–3), 77–82.

BOHAN, M., YUE, N. and NATH, R. (2001). "On the need for massive additional shielding of a catheterization laboratory for the implementation of high dose rate ^{192}Ir intravascular brachytherapy," Cardiovas. Radiat. Med. **2**(1), 39–41.

BOICE, J.D., JR., BLETTNER, M. and AUVINEN, A. (2000). "Epidemiologic studies of pilots and aircrew," Health Phys. **79**(5), 576–584.

BOLTNEVA, L.I., NZZAROV, I.M. and FRIDMAN, SH.D. (1974). "The cosmic radiation dose at the earth's surface." Izvestiya (English edition) 4, 250–255.

BONGARTZ, G., GOLDING, S.J., JURIK, A.G., LEONARDI, M., VAN PERSIJN VAN MEERTEN, E., RODRIGUEZ, R., SCHNEIDER, K., CALZADO, A., GELEIJNS, J., JESSEN, K.A., PANZER, W., SHRIMPTON, P.C. and TOSI, G. (2004). *European Guidelines for Multislice Computed Tomography*, http://www.msct.eu/CT_Quality_ Criteria.htm (accessed February 4, 2009) (European Commission, Luxembourg).

BOR, D., SANCAK T., OLGAR, ELCIMl, Y., ADANALI, A., SANLIDILEK, U. and AKYAR, S. (2004). "Comparison of effective doses obtained from dose-area product and air kerma measurements in interventional radiology," Br. J. Radiol. **77**(916), 315–322.

BOU SERHAL, C., VAN STEENBERGHE, D., BOSMANS, H., SANDERINK, G.C.H., QUIRYNEN, M. and JACOBS, R. (2001). "Organ radiation dose assessment for conventional spiral tomography: A human cadaver study," Clin. Oral Implants Res. **12**(1), 85–90.

BRENNER, D.J., MILLER, R.C., HUANG, Y. and HALL, E.J. (1995). "The biological effectiveness of radon-progeny alpha particles. III. Quality factors," Radiat. Res. **142**(1), 61–69.

BRIX, G., NAGEL, H.D., STAMM, G., VEIT, R., LECHEL, U., GRIEBEL, J. and GALANSKI, M. (2003). "Radiation exposure in multi-slice versus single-slice spiral CT: Results of a nationwide survey," Eur. Radiol. **13**(8), 1979–1991.

BROADHEAD, D.A., CHAPPLE, C.L., FAULKNER, K., DAVIES, M.L. and MCCALLUM, H. (1997). "The impact of cardiology on the collective effective dose in the North of England," Br. J. Radiol. **70**(833), 492–497.

BRUGMANS, M.J.P., BUIJIS, W.C.A.M., GELEIJNS, J. and LEMBRECHTS, J. (2002). "Population exposure to diagnostic use of ionizing radiation in The Netherlands," Health Phys. **82**(4), 500–509.

BTS (2008). Bureau of Transportation Statistics. *Data Library: Aviation,* http://www.transtats.bts.gov (accessed February 4, 2009) (U.S. Department of Transportation, Washington).

BUCKLEY, J. (2005). *Status of the Decommissioning Program, 2004 Annual Report. Final Report*, NUREG-1814 (National Technical Information Service, Springfield, Virginia).

BUCKLEY, J. (2007). *Status of the Decommissioning Program, 2006 Annual Report*, NUREG-1814, rev. 1 (U.S. Nuclear Regulatory Commission, Washington).

BUCKLEY, D.W., BELANGER, R., MARTIN, P.E., NICHOLAW, K.M. and SWENSON, J.B. (1980). *Environmental Assessment of Consumer Products Containing Radioactive Material*, NUREG/CR-1775 (U.S. Nuclear Regulatory Commission, Washington).

BUNGE, R.E. and HERMAN, C.L. (1985). *Radiation Experience Data (RED): Documentation and Results of the 1980 Survey of U.S. Hospitals*, DHEW Pub FDA 86-8253 (National Technical Information Service, Springfield Virginia).

BURLING, D., HALLIGAN, S., TAYLOR, S.A., USISKIN, S. and BAR-TRAM, C.I. (2004). "CT colonography practice in the UK: A national survey," Clin Radiol. **59**(1), 39–43.

CAGNON, C.H., BENEDICT, S.H., MANKOVICH, N.J., BUSHBERG, J.T., SEIBERT, J.A. and WHITING, J.S. (1991). "Exposure rates in high-level-control fluoroscopy for image enhancement," Radiology **178**, 643–646.

CBO (2005). Congressional Budget Office. *The Potential Cost of Meeting Demand for Veterans' Health Care*, http://www.cbo.gov/ftpdocs/61xx/doc6171/03-23-Veterans.pdf (accessed February 4, 2009) (Congressional Budget Office, Washington).

CBP (2004). U.S. Customs and Borders Protection. *Programmatic Environmental Assessment for Gamma Imaging Inspection Systems. Final Report*, http://www.cbp.gov/xp/cgov/border_security/port_activities/cargo_exam/vacis (accessed February 3, 2009) (U.S. Department of Homeland Security, Washington).

CDC (2006). Centers for Disease Control and Prevention. *National Oral Health Surveillance System, Dental Visit*, http://apps.nccd.cdc.gov/nohss/ListV.asp?qkey=5&DataSet=2 (accessed February 4, 2009) (Centers for Disease Control and Prevention, Atlanta, Georgia).

CERCLA (1980). Comprehensive Environmental Response, Compensation and Liability Act. Public Law 96-510 (December 11), 94 Stat. 2909, as amended (U.S. Government Printing Office, Washington).

CHAPPLE, C.L., FAULKNER, K., LEE, R.E., and HUNTER, E.W. (1992). "Results of a survey of doses to paediatric patients undergoing common radiological examinations," Br. J. Radiol. **65**(771), 225–231.

CHEN, J., TOKONAMI, S., SORIMACHI, A., TAKAHASHI, H. and FAL-COMER, R. (2008). "Preliminary results of simultaneous radon and thoron tests in Ottawa," Radiat. Prot. Dosim. **130**(2), 253–256.

CHIESA, C., DE SANTIS, V., CRIPPA, F., SCHIAVINI, M., FRAIGOLA, C.E., BOGNI, A., PASCALI, C., DECISE, D., MARCHESINI, R. and BOMBARDIERI, E. (1997). "Radiation dose to technicians per nuclear medicine procedure: Comparison between technetium-99m, gallium-67, and iodine-131 radiotracers and fluorine-18 fluorodeoxyglucose," Eur. J. Nucl. Med. **24**(11), 1380–1389.

CHU, R.Y.L., PARRY, C., THOMPSON, W., III and LOEFFLER, C. (1998). "Patient doses in abdominal aortogram and aorta femoral runoff examinations," Health Phys. **75**(5), 487–491.

CMS (2006). Centers for Medicare and Medicaid Services. *Physician / Supplier Procedure Summary Master File*, http://www.cms.hhs.gov/NonIdentifiableDataFiles/06_PhysicianSupplierProcedureSummaryMasterFile.asp (accessed February 4, 2009) (U.S. Department of Health and Human Services, Baltimore, Maryland).

CNS (2003). Chem-Nuclear Systems. *Environmental Radiological Performance Verification of the Barnwell Waste Disposal Facility Summary*, BEDL-03-003 (Chem-Nuclear Systems, Columbia, South Carolina).

COHEN, B.L. (1992). "Compilation and integration of studies of radon levels in U.S. homes by states and counties," Crit. Rev. Environ. Control **22**, 243–364.

COHEN, B.L. (1996). *Index*, ftp://ftp.pitt.edu/users/b/l/blc (accessed February 4, 2009) (University of Pittsburgh, Pennsylvania).

COHEN, B.S., EISENBUD, M. and HARLEY, N.H. (1980). "Measurement of the alpha-radioactivity on the mucosal surface of the human bronchial tree," Health Phys. **39**(4), 619–632.

COHNEN, M., POLL, L., PUTTMANN, C., EWEN, K. and MODDER, U. (2001). "Radiation exposure in multi-slice CT of the heart," Rofo **173**(4), 295–299.

COHNEN, M., POLL, L.J., PUTTMANN, C., EWEN, K., SALEH, A. and MODDER, U. (2003). "Effective doses in standard protocols for multi-slice CT scanning," Eur. Radiol. **13**(5), 1148–1153.

CONWAY, B.J., MCCROHAN, J.L., ANTONSEN, R.G., RUETER, F.G., SLAYTON, R.J. and SULEIMAN, O.H. (1992). "Average radiation dose in standard CT examinations of the head: Results of the 1990 NEXT survey," Radiology **184**, 135–140.

CRAWLEY, M.T. and ROGERS, A.T. (1994). "A comparison of computed tomography practice in 1989 and 1991," Br. J. Radiol. **67**(801), 872–876.

CRCPD (2008). Conference of Radiation Control Program Directors, Inc. *Nationwide Evaluation of X-Ray Trends (NEXT)*, http://crcpd.org/NEXT.asp (accessed February 3, 2009) (Conference of Radiation Control Program Directors, Inc., Frankfort, Kentucky).

CRISTY, M. and ECKERMAN, K.F. (1987). *Specific Absorbed Fractions of Energy at Various Ages from Internal Photon Sources*, ORNL/TM-8381, Vol. 1–7 (Oak Ridge National Laboratory, Oak Ridge, Tennessee).

CS (2007). CensusScope. *Age Distribution, 2000*, http://www.censusscope.org/us/s1/chart_age.html (accessed February 4, 2009) (Social Science Data Analysis Network, Ann Arbor, Michigan)

CUSMA, J.T., BELL, M.R., WONDROW, M.A., TAUBEL, J.P. and HOLMES, D.R. JR. (1999). "Real-time measurement of radiation exposure to patients during diagnostic coronary angiography and percutaneous interventional procedures," J. Am. Coll. Cardiol. **33**, 427–435.

DARBY, S., HILL, D., DEO, H., AUVINEN, A., BARROS-DIOS, J.M., BAYSSON, H., BOCHICCHIO, F., FALK, R., FARCHI, S., FIGUEIRAS, A., HAKAMA, M., HEID, I., HUNTER, N., KREIENBROCK, L., KREUZER, M., LAGARDE, F., MAKELAINEN, I., MUIRHEAD, C., OBERAIGNER, W., PERSHAGEN, G., RUOSTEENOJA, E., SCHAFFRATH ROSARIO, A., TIRMARCHE, M., TOMASEK, L., WHITLEY, E., WICHMANN, H.E. and DOLL, R. (2006). "Residential radon and lung cancer—detailed results of a collaborative analysis of individual data on 7148 persons with lung cancer and 14,208 persons without lung cancer from 13 epidemiologic studies in Europe," Scand. J. Work. Environ. Health **32**(Suppl. 1), 1–84.

DARNLEY, A.G., DUVAL, J.S. and CARSON, J.M. (2003). *The Surface Distribution of Natural Radioelements Across the USA and Parts of Canada: A Contribution to Global Geochemical Baselines*, http://cgc.rncan.gc.ca/gamma/dist/index_e.php (accessed February 4, 2009) (Natural Resources Canada, Ottawa, Ontario).

DELICHAS, M.G., PSARRAKOS, K., MOLYVDA-ATHANASSOPOULOU, E., GIANNOGLOU, G., HATZIIOANNOU, K. and PAPANASTASSIOU, E. (2003). "Radiation doses to patients undergoing coronary angiography and percutaneous tranluminal coronary angioplasty," Radiat. Prot. Dosim. **103**(2), 149–154.

DESIDERI, D., MELI, M.A., FEDUZI, L. and ROSELLI, C. (2007). "^{210}Po and ^{210}Pb inhalation by cigarette smoking in Italy," Health Phys. **92**(1), 58–63.

DICKSON, E.D., LEWIS, D.E. and HAGEMEYER, D.A. (2007). *Occupational Radiation Exposure at Commercial Nuclear Power Reactors and Other Facilities 2006. Thirty-Ninth Annual Report*, NUREG-0713, Vol. 28, http://www.nrc.gov/reading-rm/doc-collections/nuregs/staff/sr0713/v28/sr0713.pdf (accessed February 4, 2009) (National Technical Information Service, Springfield, Virginia).

DIGNUM, P.H. and VAN LINGEN, A. (1997). "PET and radiation protection," Tijdsch. Nucl. Geneesdk. **20**, 172–173.

DOE (1991). U.S. Department of Energy. *Waste Isolation Pilot Plant Site Environmental Report for Calendar Year 1990*, DOE/WIPP 91-008 (U.S. Department of Energy, Washington).

DOE (1994). U.S. Department of Energy. *Environmental Management: Pinellas Plant Annual Site Environmental Report for Calendar Year 1993*, MMSC-EM-94146, http://www.osti.gov/energycitations/servlets/purl/10161399-zpqy16/native (accessed February 3, 2009) (U.S. Department of Energy, Washington).

DOE (1995). U.S. Department of Energy. *Waste Isolation Pilot Plant: Site Environmental Report for Calendar Year 1994*, DOE/WIPP 95-2094, http://www.osti.gov/energycitations/servlets/purl/171302-Wk8tBG/webviewable (accessed February 3, 2009) (U.S. Department of Energy, Washington).

DOE (1996). U.S. Department of Energy. *Waste Isolation Pilot Plant Site Environmental Report for Calendar Year 1995*, DOE/WIPP 96-2182, http://www.osti.gov/energycitations/servlets/purl/366467-UiKfyc/webviewable (accessed February 3, 2009) (U.S. Department of Energy, Washington).

DOE (1997a). U.S. Department of Energy. *Site Environmental Report for Calendar Year 1996*, GJO-97-11-FOS, FJO-GJ-44, http://www.osti.gov/energycitations/servlets/purl/501529-1p843H/webviewable (accessed February 3, 2009) (U.S. Department of Energy, Washington).

DOE (1997b). U.S. Department of Energy. *West Valley Demonstration Project: Site Environmental Report for Calendar Year 1996*, DOE/NE/44139-T4, http://www.osti.gov/energycitations/servlets/purl/569063-Xj7Yu1/webviewable (accessed February 3, 2009) (U.S. Department of Energy, Washington).

DOE (2000). U.S. Department of Energy. *Site Environmental Report for Calendar Year 1999 DOE Operations at the Boeing Company Rocketdyne*, RD00-159, http://www.etec.energy.gov/Health-and-Safety/Documents/ASERS/ASER_1999.PDF (accessed February 3, 2009) (U.S. Department of Energy, Washington).

DOE (2001a). U.S. Department of Energy. *Summary Site Environmental Report, Radiological Doses and Releases, 1990–1994*, DOE/EH-0644, http://www.hss.energy.gov/nuclearsafety/env/reports/aser/aser1994.pdf (accessed February 3, 2009) (U.S. Department of Energy, Washington).

DOE (2001b). U.S. Department of Energy. *Waste isolation Pilot Plant CY 2000 Site Environmental Report*, DOE/WIPP 01-2225, http://www.osti.gov/energycitations/servlets/purl/814883-NIoizo/native (accessed February 3, 2009) (U.S. Department of Energy, Washington).

DOE (2002). U.S. Department of Energy. *Waste Isolation Pilot Plant 2001 Site Environmental Report*, DOE/WIPP 02-2225, http://www.osti.gov/energycitations/servlets/purl/813477-FKcYPc/native (accessed February 3, 2009) (U.S. Department of Energy, Washington).

DOE (2003). U.S. Department of Energy. *Waste Isolation Pilot Plant Site Environmental Report Calendar Year 2002*, DOE/WIPP 03-2225, http://www.wipp.energy.gov/library/ser/2002ASER.pdf (accessed February 3, 2009) (U.S. Department of Energy, Washington).

DOE (2004). U.S. Department of Energy. *Summary Annual Site Environmental Report, Radiological Doses and Releases, 1998–2001*, DOE/EH-0692, http://www.hss.energy.gov/nuclearsafety/env/reports/aser/aser2001.pdf (accessed February 3, 2009) (U.S. Department of Energy, Washington).

DOE (2005). U.S. Department of Energy. *2004 Site Environmental Report for Pantex Plant*, DOE/AL/66620-2004, http://www.pantex.com/ucm/groups/exweb/@exweb/@regcomp/documents/web_content/ex_aser_2004.pdf (accessed February 3, 2009) (BWXT Pantex, Amarillo, Texas).

DOE (2006a). U.S. Department of Energy. *DOE Occupational Radiation Exposure, 2006 Report*, http://www.hss.energy.gov/CSA/Analysis/rems/annual/2006_Occupational_Radiation_Exposure_Report.pdf (accessed February 3, 2009) (U.S. Department of Energy, Washington).

DOE (2006b). U.S. Department of Energy. *About the Department of Energy, Major DOE Laboratories and Field Facilities*, http://www.cfo.doe.gov/strategicplan/doelabs.htm (accessed February 3, 2000) (U.S. Department of Energy, Washington).

DOE (2007). U.S. Department of Energy *DOE Laboratory Accreditation Program, Library*, http://www.hss.energy.gov/CSA/CSP/doelap/library/library.html (accessed February 3, 2009) (U.S. Department of Energy, Washington).

DOL (2005). U.S. Department of Labor. *Occupational Employment Statistics*, http://data.bls.gov/OES (accessed February 4, 2009) (U.S. Department of Labor, Washington).

DOL (2008). U.S. Department of Labor. *Occupational Employment Statistics*, http://www.bls.gov/oes/home.htm (accessed February 3, 2009) (U.S. Department of Labor, Washington).

DOYLE, J.F. (1972). "The aerial radiological measuring system program," page 589 to 606 in *The Natural Radiation Environment, II*, Adams, J.A.S., Lowder, W.M. and Gesell, T.F., Eds., CONF-720805 (National Technical Information Service, Springfield, Virginia).

DUVAL, J .S. and RIGGLE, F.E. (1999). *Profiles of Gamma-Ray and Magnetic Data from Aerial Surveys Over the Conterminous United States*, DDS-31 (U.S. Geological Survey, Denver).

DUVAL, J.S., CARSON, J.M., HOLMAN, P.B. and DARNLEY, A.G. (2005). *Terrestrial Radioactivity and Gamma-Ray Exposure in the United States and Canada.*, U.S. Geological Open-File Report 2005-1413, http://pubs.usgs.gov/of/2005/1413/namrad.htm#Introduction.htm (accessed February 3, 2009) (U.S. Geological Survey, Reston, Denver).

ECKERMAN, K.F. and RYMAN, J.C. (1993). *Federal Guidance Report No. 12, External Exposure to Radionuclides in Air, Water, and Soil: Exposure-to-Dose Coefficients for General Application, Based on the 1987 Federal Radiation Protection Guidance*, EPA 402-R-93-081, http://ordose.ornl.gov/documents/fgr12.pdf (accessed February 3, 2009) (U.S. Environmental Protection Agency, Washington).

ECKERMAN, K.F. and SJOREEN, A.L. (2004). *Radiological Toolbox User's Manual*, ORNL/TM-2004/27, http://ordose.ornl.gov/documents/tboxman.pdf (accessed February 3, 2009) (National Technical Information Service, Springfield, Virginia).

ECKERMAN, K.F. and SJOREEN, A.L. (2006). *Radiological Toolbox User's Manual*, ORNL/TM-2004/27R1, http://www.nrc.gov/about-nrc/regulatory/research/manual.pdf (accessed February 3, 2009) (National Technical Information Service, Springfield, Virginia).

EFSTATHOPOULOS, E.P., KATRITSIS, D.G., KOTTOU, S., KALIVAS, N., TZANALARIDOU, E., GIAZITZOGLOU, E., KOROVESIS, S. and FAULKER, K. (2006). "Patient and staff radiation dosimetry during cardiac electrophysiology studies and catheter ablation procedures: A comprehensive analysis," Europace **8**(6), 443–448.

EHRLICH, P.J., DOHOO, I.R. and O'CALLAGHAN, M.W. (1999). "Results of bone scintigraphy in racing standardbred horses: 64 cases (1992–1994)," J. Am. Vet. Med. Assoc. **215**(7), 982–991.

EMSLEY, J. (2003). *Nature's Building Blocks, An A – Z Guide to the Elements* (Oxford University Press, New York).

EPA (1983). U.S. Environmental Protection Agency. "40 CFR Part 249 –Guideline for federal procurement of cement and concrete containing fly ash," 48 FR 4230–4253 (U.S. Government Printing Office, Washington).

EPA (1990). U.S. Environmental Protection Agency. *Idaho Radionuclide Study-Pocatello and Soda Springs, Idaho*, EPA/520/6-90/008. (U.S. Environmental Protection Agency, Las Vegas, Nevada).

EPA (1992). U.S. Environmental Protection Agency. *National Residential Radon Survey: Summary Report*, EPA 402-R-92-011 (U.S. Government Printing Office, Washington).

EPA (1993a). U.S. Environmental Protection Agency. *Radon Measurement in Schools,* EPA 402-R-92-014 (U.S. Government Printing Office, Washington).

EPA (1993b). U.S. Environmental Protection Agency. *Diffuse NORM Wastes. Waste Characterization and Preliminary Risk Assessment,* EPA 68-D20-155 (U.S. Environmental Protection Agency, Washington).

EPA (1997). U.S. Environmental Protection Agency. *Exposure Factors Handbook, Volume 3: Activity Factors,* EPA 600/P-95/002FC (National Technical Information Service, Springfield, Virginia).

EPA (1999). U.S. Environmental Protection Agency. *Biosolids Generation, Use, and Disposal in the United States,* EPA 530-R-99-009, http://www.biosolids.org/docs/18941.PDF (accessed February 3, 2009) (U.S. Environmental Protection Agency, Washington).

EPA (2000a). U.S. Environmental Protection Agency. *Evaluation of EPA's Guidelines for Technologically Enhanced Naturally Occurring Radioactive Materials (TENORM), Report to Congress,* EPA 402-R-00-01, http://www.epa.gov/radiation/docs/tenorm/402-r-00-001.pdf (accessed February 3, 2009) (U.S. Environmental Protection Agency, Washington).

EPA (2000b). U.S. Environmental Protection Agency. *Estimated Per Capita Water Ingestion in the United States, Based on Data Collected by the United States Department of Agriculture's 1994-96 Continuing Survey of Food Intakes by Individuals,* EPA-822-R-00-008 (National Technical Information Service, Springfield, Virginia).

EPA (2003a). U.S. Environmental Protection Agency. *EPA Assessment of Risks from Radon in Home,* EPA 402-R-03-003, http://www.epa.gov/radon/pdfs/402-r-03-003.pdf (accessed February 3, 2009) (National Technical Information Service, Springfield, Virginia).

EPA (2003b). U.S. Environmental Protection Agency. *Clean Watersheds Needs Survey 2000,* EPA-832-R-03-001, http://www.epa.gov/owm/mtb/cwns/2000rtc/toc.htm (accessed February 3, 2009) (U.S. Environmental Protection Agency, Washington).

EPA (2006). U.S. Environmental Protection Agency. *Building Assessment Survey and Evaluation (BASE) Study,* http://www.epa.gov/iaq/base (accessed February 3, 2009) (U.S. Environmental Protection Agency, Washington).

EPA (2007a). U.S. Environmental Protection Agency. *EPA Map of Radon Zones,* http://www.epa.gov/radon/zonemap.html (accessed February 3, 2009) (U.S. Environmental Protection Agency, Washington).

EPA (2007b). U.S. Environmental Protection Agency. *Technologically Enhanced Naturally Occurring Radioactive Materials from Uranium Mining, Vol. 1, Mining and Reclamation Background,* EPA 402-R-05-007, rev., http://www.epa.gov/radiation/docs/tenorm/402-r-08-005-voli/402-r-08-005-v1.pdf (accessed February 3, 2009) (U.S. Environmental Protection Agency, Washington).

EPA (2007c). U.S. Environmental Protection Agency. "Environmental radiation protection standards, Subpart B – Environmental standards for the uranium fuel cycle, Standards for normal operations," 40 CFR Part 190.10 (revised July 1) (U.S. Government Printing Office, Washington).

EPA (2008). U.S. Environmental Protection Agency. *Who Can Test or Fix Your Home?*, http://epa.gov/radon/radontest.html (accessed February 3, 2009) U.S. Environmental Protection Agency, Washington).

EVANS, R.D. (1980). "Engineers' guide to the elementary behavior of radon daughters," Health Phys. **38**(6), 1173–1197.

FAA (2004). Federal Aviation Administration. *CARI-6,* http://www.faa. gov/education_research/research/med_humanfacs/aeromedical/radio-biology/cari6 (accessed February 3, 2009) (National Technical Information Service, Springfield, Virginia).

FAULKNER, K., JAMES, H.V., CHAPPEL, C.L. and RAWLINGS, D.J. (1996). "Assessment of effective dose to staff in brachytherapy," Health Phys. **71**(5), 727–732.

FDA (1994). U.S. Food and Drug Administration. *Public Health Advisory: Avoidance of Serious X-Ray-Induced Skin Injuries to Patients During Fluoroscopically-Guided Procedures,* http://www.fda.gov/cdrh/fluor. html (accessed February 3, 2009) (U.S. Food and Drug Administration, Rockville, Maryland).

FDA (2003). U.S. Food and Drug Administration. *Nationwide Evaluation of X-Ray Trends (NEXT),* http://www.fda.gov/cdrh/radhlth/next.html (accessed February 3, 2009) (U.S. Food and Drug Administration, Rockville, Maryland).

FDA (2006). U.S. Food and Drug Administration. *Dose and Image Quality in Mammography: Trends During the First Decade of MQSA,* http:// www.fda.gov/CDRH/MAMMOGRAPHY/scorecard-article5-update. html (accessed February 3, 2009) (U.S. Food and Drug Administration, Rockville, Maryland).

FDA (2007a). U.S. Food and Drug Administration. *MQSA Facility Score-card: MQSA National Statistics,* http://www.fda.gov/CDRH/MAM-MOGRAPHY/scorecard-statistics.html (accessed December 14, 2007) (U.S. Food and Drug Administration, Rockville, Maryland).

FDA (2007b). U.S. Food and Drug Administration. "Performance standards for ionizing radiation emitting products. Fluoroscopy equipment," 21 CFR Part 1020.32, (revised April 1), http://www.accessdata. fda.gov/scripts/cdrh/cfdocs/cfcfr/CFRSearch.cfm (accessed February 3, 2009) (U.S. Government Printing Office, Washington).

FDA (2007c). U.S. Food and Drug Administration. "Performance standards for ionizing radiation emitting products. Television receivers," 21 CFR Part 1020.10 (revised April 1), http://www.accessdata.fda.gov/ scripts/cdrh/cfdocs/cfcfr/CFRSearch.cfm (accessed February 3, 2009) (U.S. Government Printing Office, Washington).

FDA (2007d). U.S. Food and Drug Administration. "Performance standards for ionizing radiation emitting products. Cabinet x-ray systems," 21 CFR Part 1020.40 (revised April 1), http://www.accessdata.fda.gov/ scripts/cdrh/cfdocs/cfcfr/CFRSearch.cfm (accessed February 3, 2009) (U.S. Government Printing Office, Washington).

FDA (2008). U.S. Food and Drug Administration. *Mammography, Information for Mammography Facility Personnel, Inspectors, and Consumers About the Implementation of the Mammography Quality Standards*

Act of 1992 (MQSA), http://www.fda.gov/cdrh/mammography/score-card-statistics.html (accessed January 30, 2008) (U.S. Food and Drug Administration, Rockville, Maryland).

FERRARI, A., PELLICCIONI, M. and PILLON, M. (1996). "Fluence to effective dose and effective dose equivalent conversion coefficients for photons from 50 keV to 10 GeV," Radiat. Prot. Dosim. **67**(4), 245–251.

FERRARI, A., PELLICCIONI, M., and PILLON, M. (1997a). "Fluence to effective dose and effective dose equivalent conversion coefficients for electrons from 5 MeV to 10 GeV." Radiat. Prot. Dosim. **69**(2), 97–104.

FERRARI, A., PELLICCIONI, M., and PILLON, M. (1997b). "Fluence to effective dose conversion coefficients for protons from 5 MeV to 10 TeV," Radiat. Prot. Dosim. **71**(2), 85–91.

FERRARI, A., PELLICCIONI, M., and PILLON, M. (1997c). "Fluence to effective dose conversion coefficients for neutrons up to 10 TeV," Radiat. Prot. Dosim. **71**(3), 165–173.

FERRARI, A., PELLICCIONI, M., and PILLON, M. (1997d). "Fluence-to-effective dose conversion coefficients for muons," Radiat. Prot. Dosim. **74**(4), 227–233.

FERRARI, A., PELLICCIONI, M., and PILLON, M. (1998). "Fluence to effective dose conversion coefficients for negatively and positively charged pions," Radiat. Prot. Dosim. **80**(4), 361–370.

FINK, R.M. (1950). *Biological Studies with Polonium, Radium, and Plutonium*, National Nuclear Energy Series, Division VI, Volume 3 (McGraw-Hill, New York).

FINLEY, V.L. (2004). *Princeton Plasma Physics Laboratory Annual Site Environmental Report for Calendar Years 2003 and 2004*, PPPL-4039, http://www.pppl.gov/pub_report//2005/PPPL-4039.pdf (accessed February 3, 2009) (Princeton Plasma Physics Laboratory, Princeton, New Jersey).

FOCAZIO, M.J., TIPTON, D., SHAPIRO, S.D. and GEIGER, L.H. (2006). "The chemical quality of self-supplied domestic well water in the United States," Ground Water Monit. Remediat. **26**(3), 92–104.

FRAASS, B.A. and VAN DE GEIJN, J. (1983). "Peripheral dose from megavolt beams," Med Phys. **10**(6), 809–818.

FRAME, P. and KOLB, W. (2005). *Living With Radiation: The First Hundred Years*, 4th ed. (William Kolb, Edgewater, Maryland).

FRIEDBERG, W. and COPELAND, K. (2003). U.S. Department of Transportation. *What Aircrews Should Know About Their Occupational Exposure to Ionizing Radiation*, DOT/FAA/AM-03/16, http://www.faa.gov/library/reports/medical/oamtechreports/2000s/media/0316.pdf (accessed February 3, 2009) (National Technical Information Service, Springfield, Virginia).

FRIEDBERG, W., COPELAND, K., DUKE, F.E., O'BRIEN, K., III and DARDEN, E.B., JR. (2000). "Radiation exposure during air travel: Guidance provided by the Federal Aviation Administration for air carrier crews," Health Phys. **79**(5), 591–595.

GELEIJNS, J., BROERSE, J.J., SHAW, M.P., SCHULTZ, F.W., TEEUWISSE, W., VAN UNNIK J.G. and ZOETELIEF, J. (1997). "Patient dose due to colon examination: Dose assessment and results from a survey in The Netherlands," Radiology **204**(2), 553–559.

GEORGE, A.C. and BRESLIN, A.J. (1980). "The distribution of ambient radon and radon daughters in residential buildings in the New Jersey-New York area," pages 1272 to1292 in *Natural Radiation Environment III*, Gesell, T.F. and Lowder, W.M., Eds. (National Technical Information Service, Springfield, Virginia).

GERUSKY, T.M. (1996). *The Pennsylvania Radon Story*, http://www.dep.state.pa.us/dep/deputate/airwaste/rp/Radon_Division/PA_Radon_Story1.htm (accessed February 3, 2009) (Pennsylvania Department of Environmental Protection, Harrisburg, Pennsylvania).

GESELL, T.F. and PRICHARD, H.M. (1975). "The technologically enhanced natural radiation environment," Health Phys. **28**(4), 361–366.

GIBBS, S.J. (2000). "Effective dose equivalent and effective dose: Comparison for common projections in oral and maxillofacial radiology," Oral Surg. Oral Med. Oral Pathol. Oral Radiol. Endod. **90**(4), 538–545.

GODOY, J.M., GOUVEA, V.A., MELO, D.R. and AZEREDO, A.M.G. (1992). "^{226}Ra / ^{210}Pb / ^{210}Po equilibrium in tobacco leaves," Radiat. Prot. Dosim. **45**(1), 299–300.

GORDON, M.S., GOLDHAGEN, P., RODBELL, K.P., ZABEL, T.H., TANG, H.H.K., CLEM, J.M. and BAILEY, P. (2004). "Measurement of the flux and energy spectrum of cosmic-ray induced neutrons on the ground," IEEE Trans. Nucl. Sci. **51**(6) 3427–3434.

GRASTY, R.L. (2002). *The Annual Effective Dose from Natural Sources of Ionizing Radiation in Canada*, Gamma-Bob Report 02-6 (Gamma-Bob Inc., Ottawa, Canada).

GRASTY, R.L. and LAMARRE, J.R. (2004). "The annual effective dose from natural sources of ionizing radiation in Canada," Radiat. Prot. Dosim. **108**(3), 215–226.

GUILLET, B., QUENTIN, P., WAULTIER, S., BOURRELLY, M., PISANO, P. and MUNDLER, O. (2005). "Technologist radiation exposure in routine clinical practice with ^{18}F-FDG PET," J. Nucl. Med. Technol. **33**(3), 175–179.

GUNNING, C. and SCOTT, A.G. (1982). "Radon and thoron daughters in housing," Health Phys. **42**(4), 527–528.

HARLEY, N.H. and PASTERNACK, B.S. (1972). "Alpha absorption measurements applied to lung dose from radon daughters," Health Phys. **23**(6), 771–782.

HARLEY, N.H. and PASTERNACK, B.S. (1982). "Environmental radon daughter alpha dose factors in a five-lobed human lung," Health Phys. **42**(6), 789–799.

HARLEY, N.H. and ROBBINS, E.S. (1992). "^{222}Rn alpha dose to organs other than the lung," Radiat. Prot. Dosim. **45**(1), 619-622.

HARLEY, N.H. and TERILLI, T.B. (1990). "Predicting annual average indoor ^{222}Rn concentration," Health Phys. **59**(2), 205–209.

HART, D. and WALL, B.F. (2002). *Radiation Exposure of the UK Population from Medical and Dental X-Ray Examinations*, Report NRPB-W4 (Health Protection Agency, London).

HART, D. and WALL, B.F. (2004). "UK population dose from medical x-ray examinations," Eur. J. Radiol. **50**(3), 285–291.

HAUSLEITER, J., MEYER, T., HERMANN, F., HADAMITZKY, M., KREBS, M., GERBER, T.C., MCCOLLOUGH, C., MARTINOFF, S., KASTRATI, A., SCHOMIG, A. and ACHENBACH, S. (2009). "Estimated radiation dose associated with cardiac CT angiography," JAMA **301**(5), 500–507.

HAWKINSON, J., TIMINS, J., ANGELO, D., SHAW, M., TAKATA, R. and HARSHAW, F. (2006). *Technical White Paper: Bone Densitometry*, CRCPD Publication E-06-5, http://crcpd.org/Pubs/BoneDensitometry-WhitePaper.pdf (accessed February 3, 2009) (Conference of Radiation Control Program Directors, Inc., Frankfort, Kentucky).

HEGGIE, J.C. and WILKINSON, L.E. (2000). "Radiation doses from common radiographic procedures: A ten year perspective," Australas. Phys. Eng. Sci. Med. **23**(4), 124–134.

HESS, C.T., MICHEL, J., HORTON, T.R., PRICHARD, H.M. and CONIGLIO, W.A. (1985). "The occurrence of radioactivity in public water supplies in the United States," Health Phys. **48**(5), 553–586.

HILL, C.R. (1965). "Polonium-210 in man," Nature **208**(9), 423–428.

HOPKE, P.K., JENSEN, B., LI, C.S., MONTASSIER, N., WASIOLEK, P., CAVALLO, A.J., GATSBY, K., SOCOLOW, R.H. and JAMES, A.C. (1995). "Assessment of the exposure to and dose from radon decay products in normally occupied homes," Environ. Sci. Technol. **29**(5), 1359–1364.

HOPPER, R.D., LEVY, R.A., RANKIN, R.C. and BOYD, M.A. (1991). "National ambient outdoor radon study," pages 79 to 94 in *Proceedings of the 1991 International Symposium on Radon and Radon Reduction Technology*, Dyess, T.M., Conrath, S.M., Hardin, C.M. and Cohen, S., Eds., EPA-600/9-91-037d (National Technical Information Service, Springfield, Virginia).

HUDA, W. and GKANATSIOS, N.A. (1998). "Radiation dosimetry for extremity radiographs," Health Phys. **75**(5), 492–499.

HUDA, W., ATHERTON, J.V., WARE, D.E. and CUMMING, W.A. (1997). "An approach for the estimation of effective radiation dose at CT in pediatric patients," Radiology **203**(2), 417–422.

HUDA, W., CHAMBERLAIN, C.C., ROSENBAUM, A.E. and GARRISI, W. (2001). "Radiation doses to infants and adults undergoing head CT examinations," Med. Phys. **28**(3), 393–399.

HUNOLD, P., VOGT, F.M., SCHMERMUND, A., DEBATIN, J.F., KERKHOFF, G., BUDDE, T., ERBEL, R., EWEN, K. and BARKHAUSEN, J. (2003). "Radiation exposure during cardiac CT: Effective doses at multi-detector row CT and electron-beam CT," Radiology **226**(1), 145–152.

HURWITZ, L.M., REIMAN, R.E., YOSHIZUMI, T.T., GOODMAN, P.C., TONCHEVA, G., NGUYEN, G. and LOWRY, C. (2007). "Radiation dose from contemporary cardiothoracic multidetector CT protocols with an anthropomorphic female phantom: Implications for cancer induction," Radiology **245**(3), 742–750.

HUTSON, S.S., BARBER, N.L., KENNY, J.F., LINSEY, K.S., LUMIA, D.S. and MAUPIN, M.A. (2005). *Estimated Use of Water in the United States in 2000*, (rev) USGS Circular 1268, http://pubs.usgs.gov/circ/2004/circ1268 (accessed February 4, 2009) (U.S. Geological Survey, Reston, Virginia).

IAEA (1996). International Atomic Energy Agency. *International Basic Safety Standards for Protection Against Ionizing Radiation and for the Safety of Radiation Sources*, Safety Series No. 115, STI/PUB/996 (International Atomic Energy Agency, Vienna, Austria).

IAEA (2004). International Atomic Energy Agency. *Extent of Environmental Contamination by Naturally Occurring Radioactive Material (NORM) and Technological Options for Mitigation,* Technical Report Series No. 419, STI/PUB/010/419 (International Atomic Energy Agency, Vienna).

ICRP (1977). International Commission on Radiological Protection. *Recommendations of the International Commission on Radiological Protection*, ICRP Publication 26, Ann. ICRP **1**(3) (Elsevier, New York).

ICRP (1991). International Commission on Radiological Protection. *1990 Recommendations of the International Commission on Radiological Protection*, ICRP Publication 60, Ann. ICRP **21**(1–3) (Elsevier, New York).

ICRP (1993). International Commission on Radiological Protection. *Protection Against Radon-222 at Home and at Work*, ICRP Publication 65, Ann. ICRP **23**(2) (Elsevier, New York).

ICRP (1994). International Commission on Radiological Protection. *Human Respiratory Tract Model for Radiological Protection*, ICRP Publication 66, Ann. ICRP **24**(1–3) (Elsevier, New York).

ICRP (1995). International Commission on Radiological Protection. *Age-Dependent Doses to Members of the Public from Intake of Radionuclides: Part 4, Inhalation Dose Coefficients,* ICRP Publication 71, Ann. ICRP **25**(3–4) (Elsevier, New York).

ICRP (1996). International Commission on Radiological Protection. *Age-Dependent Doses to the Members of the Public from Intake of Radionuclides: Part 5, Compilation of Ingestion and Inhalation Coefficients,* ICRP Publication 72, Ann. ICRP **26**(1) (Elsevier, New York).

ICRP (1998). International Commission on Radiological Protection. *Radiation Doses to Patients from Radiopharmaceuticals*, ICRP Publication 80, Ann. ICRP **28**(3) (Elsevier, New York).

ICRP (2000). International Commission on Radiological Protection. *Avoidance of Radiation Injuries from Medical Interventional Procedures,* ICRP Publication 85, Ann. ICRP **30**(2) (Elsevier, New York).

ICRP (2003). International Commission on Radiological Protection. *Relative Biological Effectiveness (RBE), Quality Factor (Q), and Radiation Weighting Factor (w_R),* ICRP Publication 92, Ann. ICRP **33**(4) (Elsevier, New York).

ICRP (2007a). International Commission on Radiological Protection. *The 2007 Recommendations of the International Commission on Radiological Protection*, ICRP Publication 103, Ann. ICRP **37**(2–4) (Elsevier, New York).

ICRP (2007b). International Commission on Radiological Protection. *Radiological Protection in Medicine*, ICRP Publication 105, Ann. ICRP **37**(6) (Elsevier, New York).

IEC (2002). International Electrotechnical Commission. *Medical Electrical Equipment–Part 2-44: Particular Requirements for the Safety of X-Ray Equipment for Computed Tomography*, International Standard IEC 60601-2-44, 2.1 ed., http://webstore.iec.ch/preview/info_iec60601-2-44%7Bed2.1%7Den.pdf (accessed February 3, 2009) (International Electrotechnical Commission, Geneva).

IMV (2004). IMV Medical Information Division. *Benchmark Report, Cardiac Cath Labs, 2003* (IMV Medical Information Division, Des Plaines, Illinois).

IMV (2005a). IMV Medical Information Division. *Benchmark Report, CT 2004* (IMV Medical Information Division, Des Plaines, Illinois).

IMV (2005b). IMV Medical Information Division. *Benchmark Report, Radiation Oncology 2004* (IMV Medical Information Division, Des Plaines, Illinois).

IMV (2006a). IMV Medical Information Division. *Benchmark Report, CT 2006* (IMV Medical Information Division, Des Plaines, Illinois).

IMV (2006b). IMV Medical Information Division. *Benchmark Report, Mammography 2005* (IMV Medical Information Division, Des Plaines, Illinois).

IMV (2006c). IMV Medical Information Division. *Benchmark Report, Nuclear Medicine 2005* (IMV Medical Information Division, Des Plaines, Illinois).

IMV (2006d). IMV Medical Information Division. *Benchmark Report, PET 2005/06* (IMV Medical Information Division, Des Plaines, Illinois).

IMV (2006e). IMV Medical Information Division. *Benchmark Report, Radiographic Fluoroscopy 2004/05* (IMV Medical Information Division, Des Plaines, Illinois).

IMV (2006f). IMV Medical Information Division. *Benchmark Report, Interventional Angiography 2004/05* (IMV Medical Information Division, Des Plaines, Illinois).

ISCORS (2003). Interagency Steering Committee on Radiation Standards. *Final Report. ISCORS Assessment of Radioactivity in Sewage Sludge: Radiological Survey Results and Analysis*, ISCORS Technical Report 2003-02, NUREG-1775 (National Technical Information Service, Springfield, Virginia).

ISCORS (2005a). Interagency Steering Committee on Radiation Standards. *Final Report. ISCORS Assessment of Radioactivity in Sewage Sludge: Modeling to Assess Radiation Doses*, ISCORS Technical Report 2004-03, NUREG-1783 (National Technical Information Service, Springfield, Virginia).

ISCORS (2005b). Interagency Steering Committee on Radiation Standards. *Final Report. ISCORS Assessment of Radioactivity in Sewage Sludge: Recommendations on Management of Radioactive Materials in Sewage Sludge and Ash at Publicly Owned Treatment Works*, ISCORS Technical Report 2004-04, DOE/EH-0668 (National Technical Information Service, Springfield, Virginia).

ISRAELI, M. (1985). "Deposition rates of Rn progeny in houses," Health Phys. **49**(6), 1069–1083.

JACOBI, W. and EISFELD, K. (1980). *Dose to Tissues and Effective Dose Equivalent by Inhalation of Radon-222, Radon 220 and Their Short-Lived Daughters,* GSF Report S-626 (National Research Center for Environment and Health, Neuherberg).

JAMES, A.C., BIRCHALL, A. and AKABANI, G. (2004). "Comparative dosimetry of BEIR VI revisited," Radiat. Prot. Dosim. **108**(1), 3–26.

JAVADI, M., MAHESH, M., MCBRIDE, G., VOICU, C., EPLEY, W., MERRILL, J. and BENGEL, F.M. (2008). "Lowering radiation dose for integrated assessment of coronary morphology and physiology: First experience with step-and-shoot CT angiography in a rubidium 82 PET-CT protocol," J. Nucl. Cardiol. **15**(6), 783–790.

JEDEC (2006). Joint Electron Device Engineering Council (JEDEC) Solid State Technology Association. "Annex A - Determination of terrestrial neutron flux (normative)" pages 55 to 69 in *JEDEC Standard: Measurement and Reporting of Alpha Particle and Terrestrial Cosmic Ray-Induced Soft Errors in Semiconductor Devices*, http://www.jedec. org/download/search/JESD89A.pdf (accessed February 3, 2009) (JEDEC Solid State Technology Association, Arlington, Virginia).

JESSEN, K.A., SHRIMPTON, P.C., GELEIJNS, J., PANZER, W. and TOSI, G. (1999). "Dosimetry for optimisation of patient protection in computed tomography," Appl. Radiat. Isotopes **50**(1), 165–172.

JESSEN, K.A., PANZER, W., SHRIMPTON, P.C., BONGARTZM, G., GELEIJNS, J., GOLDING, S.J., JURIK, A.G., LEONAR, M. and TOSI, G. (2000). *European Guidelines on Quality Criteria for Computed Tomography*, EUR 16262, http://www.drs.dk/guidelines/ct/quality/index.htm (accessed January 23, 2008) (European Commission, Luxembourg).

JOHNSON, R.H., JR., GEIGER, E. and ROSARIO, A., JR. (1990). "Cigarette smoking increases radon working level exposures to all occupants of the smoker's home," pages 1 to 19 in *Proceedings of the Fourth Annual Radon Conference* (American Association of Radon Scientists and Technologists, Fletcher, North Carolina).

JOHNSON, R.H., KLINE, R.S., GEIGER, E. and ROSARIO, A. (1991). "The effect of passive cigarette smoke on working level exposure in homes," pages 1 to 19 in *Proceedings of the 1991 International Symposium on Radon and Radon Reduction Technology*, Dyess, T.M., Conrath, S.M., Hardin, C.M. and Cohen, S., Eds., EPA-600/9-91-037d (National Technical Information Service, Springfield, Virginia).

KEMERINK, G.J., DE HAAN, M.W., VASBINDER, G.B.G, FRANTZEN, M.J., SCHULTZ, F.W., ZOETELIEF, J., JANSEN, J.T.M. and VAN

ENGELSHOVEN, J.M.A. (2003). "The effect of equipment set up on patient radiation dose in conventional and CT angiography of the renal arteries," Br. J. Radiol. **76**(909), 625–630.

KENDALL, G.M. and SMITH, T.J. (2002). "Doses to organs and tissues from radon and its decay products," J. Radiol. Prot. **22**(4), 389–406.

KHAN, S.M., NICHOLAS, P.E. and TERPILAK, M.S. (2004). "Radiation dose equivalent to stowaways in vehicles," Health Phys. **86**(5), 483–492.

KHATER, A.E.M. (2004). "Polonium-210 budget in cigarettes," J. Environ. Radioact. **71**(1), 33–41.

KHATER, A.E.M. and AL-SEWAIDAN, H.A.I. (2006). "Polonium-210 in cigarette tobacco," Int. J. Low Radiat. **3**(2/3), 224–233.

KHURSHEED, A. (2000). "Doses to systemic tissues from radon gas," Radiat. Prot. Dosim. **88**(2), 171–181.

KIM, K.P., MILLER, D.L., BALTER, S., KLEINERMAN, R.A., LINET, M.S., KWON, D. and SIMON, S.L. (2008). "Occupational radiation doses to operators performing cardiac catheterization procedures," Health Phys. **94**(3), 211–227.

KIRISITS, C., HEFNER, A., WEXBERG, P., POKRAJAC, B., GLOGAR, D., POTTER, R. and GEORG, D. (2004). "Estimation of doses to personnel and patients during endovascular brachytherapy applications," Radiat. Prot. Dosim. **108**(3), 237–245.

KNUTSON, E.O. and GEORGE, A.C. (1992). "Reanalysis of data on particle size distribution of radon progeny in uranium mines," pages 149 to 164 in *Indoor Radon and Lung Cancer: Reality or Myth*. Cross, F.T., Ed. (Battelle Press, Columbus, Ohio).

KOBLIK, P.D., HORNOF, W.J. and SEEHERMAN, H.J. (1988). "Scintigraphic appearance of stress-induced trauma of the dorsal cortex of the third metacarpal bone in racing thoroughbred horses: 121 cases (1978–1986)," J. Am. Vet. Med. Assoc. **192**(3), 390–395.

KOCHER, D.C. and ECKERMAN, K.F. (1988). "On inclusion of the dose to skin in the effective dose equivalent," Health Phys. **55**(5), 813–815.

KOENIG, T.R., WOLFF, D., METTLER, F.A. and WAGNER, L.K. (2001a). "Skin injuries from fluoroscopically guided procedures: Part 1, Characteristics of radiation injury," Am. J. Roentgenol. **177**, 3–11.

KOENIG, T.R., METTLER, F.A. and WAGNER, L.K. (2001b). "Skin injuries from fluoroscopically guided procedures: Part 2, Review of 73 cases and recommendations for minimizing dose delivered to patient," Am. J. Roentgenol. **177**, 13–20.

KUMAZAWA, S., NELSON, D.R. and RICHARDSON, A.C.B. (1984). *Occupational Exposure to Ionizing Radiation in the United States: A Comprehensive Review for the Year 1980 and a Summary of Trends for the Years 1960–1985,* EPA/520/1-84-005 (National Technical Information Service, Springfield, Virginia).

LANDA, E.R. and COUNCELL, T.B. (1992). "Leaching of uranium from glass and ceramic foodware and decorative items," Health Phys. **63**(3), 343–348.

LARIVIERE, D., PACKER, A.P., MARRO, L., LI, C., CHEN, J. and COR-
NETT, R.J. (2007). "Age dependence of natural uranium and thorium
concentrations in bone." Health Phys. **92**(2), 119–126.
LINDSAY, B.D., EICHLING, J.O., AMBOS, H.D, and CAIN, M.E. (1992).
"Radiation exposure to patients and medical personnel during radio-
frequency catheter ablation for supraventricular tachycardia," Am. J.
Cardiol. **70**(2), 218–223.
LIPOTI, J.A. (2008). "Exposure reduction through quality assurance for
diagnostic x-ray procedures," Health Phys. **95**(5), 577–585.
LMC (2003). Lockheed Martin Corporation. *Chart of the Nuclides and Iso-
topes*, 16th ed., http://www.ChartOfTheNuclides.com (accessed Febru-
ary 4, 2009) (Lockheed Martin Corporation, Cincinnati, Ohio).
LONGTIN, J.P. (1988). "Occurrence of radon, radium, and uranium in
groundwater," J. Am. Water Works Assoc. **80**(7), 84–93.
LUDLOW, J.B., DAVIES-LUDLOW, L.E., and WHITE, S.C. (2008).
"Patient risk related to common dental radiographic examinations:
The impact of 2007 International Commission on Radiological Protection recommendations regarding dose calculation," J. Am. Dent. Assoc.
139(19), 1237–1243.
MAHESH, M. and CODY, D.D. (2007). "Physics of cardiac imaging with
multiple-row detector CT," Radiographics **27**(5), 1495–1509.
MARCINOWSKI, F., LUCAS, R.M. and YEAGER, W.M. (1994). "National
and regional distributions of airborne radon concentrations in U.S.
homes," Health Phys. **66**(6), 699–706.
MARSH, J.W. and BIRCHALL, A. (2000). "Sensitivity analysis of the
weighted equivalent lung dose per unit exposure from radon progeny,"
Radiat. Prot. Dosim. **87**(3), 167–178.
MARSH, J.W., BIRCHALL, A., BUTTERWECK, G., DORRIAN, M.D.,
HUET, C., ORTEGA, X., REINEKING, A., TYMEN, G., SCHULER, C.,
VARGAS, A., VESSU, G. and WENDT, J. (2002). "Uncertainty analysis
of the weighted equivalent lung dose per unit exposure to radon prog-
eny in the home," Radiat. Prot. Dosim. **102**(3), 229–248.
MARSH, J.W., BIRCHALL, A. and DAVIS, K. (2005). "Comparative
dosimetry in homes and mines: estimation of K-factors," pages 290 to
298 in *The Natural Radiation Environment VII. Seventh International
Symposium on the Natural Radiation Environment*, McLaughlin, J.P.,
Simopoulos, E.S. and Steinhausler, F., Eds. (Elsevier, New York).
MARSHALL, N.W., CHAPPLE, C.L. and KOTRE, C.J. (2000). "Diagnostic
reference levels in interventional radiology," Phys. Med. Biol. **45**(12),
3833–3846.
MARTELL, E.A. (1974). "Radioactivity of tobacco trichromes and insolu-
ble cigarette smoke particles," Nature **249**, 215–217.
MARTIN, C.J. (2007). "Effective dose: How should it be applied to medical
exposures?" Br. J. Radiol. **80**, 639–647.
MARTONEN, T.B., HOFMANN, W. and LOWE, J.E. (1987). "Cigarette
smoke and lung cancer," Health Phys. **52**(2), 213–217.
MAURICE, E., TROSCLAIR, A., MERRITT, R., CARABALLO, R., MAL-
AR-CHER, A., HUSTEN, C. and PECHACEK, T. (2005). "Cigarette

smoking among adults — United States, 2004," Mortality Morbidity Weekly Rep. **54**(44), 1121–1124.

MCCOLLOUGH, C.H. (2003). "Patient dose in cardiac computed tomography," Herz. **28**(1), 1–6.

MCCOLLOUGH, C.H. and SCHUELER, B.A. (2000). "Calculation of effective dose," Med. Phys. **27**(5), 828–837.

MCCOLLOUGH, C., CODY, D., EDYVEAN, S., GEISE, R., GOULD, B., KEAT, N., HUDA, W., JUDY, P., KALENDER, W., MCNITT-GRAY, M., MORIN, R., PAYNE, T., STERN, S., ROTHENBERG, L., SHRIMPTON, P., TIMMER, J. and WILSON, C. (2008). *The Measurement, Reporting, and Management of Radiation Dose in CT*, AAPM Report 96, http://www.aapm.org/pubs/reports/RPT_96.pdf (accessed February 4, 2009) (American Association of Physicists in Medicine, College Park, Maryland).

MCCORMICK, L. (1992). "More consumer radiation sources," Health Phys. News **XX**(2), 5.

MCFADDEN, S.L., MOONEY, R.B. and SHEPHERD, H. (2002). "X-ray dose and associated risks from radiofrequency catheter ablation procedures," Br. J. Radiol. **75**, 253–265.

MCPARLAND, B.J. (1998). "A study of patient radiation doses in interventional radiological procedures," Br. J. Radiol. **71**(842), 175–185.

MDCH (2007). Michigan Department of Community Health. *Patient Radiation Exposure Information*, http://www.michigan.gov/mdch/0, 1607,7-132-27417_35791-46650--,00.html (accessed January 21, 2007) (Michigan Department of Community Health, Lansing, Michigan).

MDCH (2008). Michigan Department of Community Health. *Dental Intraoral Patient Exposures*, http://www.michigan.gov/mdch/0,1607,7-132-27417_35791_35798-46657--,00.html (accessed November 18, 2008) (Michigan Department of Community Health, Lansing, Michigan).

MEINHOLD, C.B. (1989). "Use of effective dose equivalent for external radiation exposures," Health Phys. **56**(4), 570.

METTLER, F.A., JR., WILLIAMS, A.G., CHRISTIE, J.H., MOSELEY, R.D. and KELSEY, C.A. (1985). "Trends and utilization of nuclear medicine in the United States: 1972–1982," J. Nucl. Med. **26**(2), 201–205.

METTLER, F.A., JR., WIEST, P.W., LOCKEN, J.A. and KELSEY, C.A. (2000). "CT scanning: Patterns of use and dose," J. Radiol. Prot. **20**, 353–359.

METTLER, F.A. JR, HUDA, W., YOSHIZUMI, T.T. and MAHESH, M. (2008a). "Effective doses in radiology and diagnostic nuclear medicine: A catalog." Radiology **248**(1), 254–263.

METTLER, F.A., JR., THOMADSEN, B.R., BHARGAVAN, M., GILLEY, D.B., GRAY, J.E., LIPOTI, J.A., MCCROHAN, J., YOSHIZUMI, T.T. and MAHESH, M. (2008b). "Medical radiation exposure in the U.S. in 2006: Preliminary results," Health Phys. **95**(5), 502–507.

MILLER, K.M. (1992). "Measurements of external radiation in United States dwellings," Radiat. Prot. Dosim. **45**(1), 535–539.

MILLER, D.L., BALTER, S., COLE, P.E., LU, H.T., BERENSTEIN, A., ALBERT, R., SCHUELER, B.A., GEORGIA, J.D., NOONAN, P.T., RUSSELL, E.J., MALISCH, T.W., VOGELZANG, R.L., GEISINGER, M., CARDELLA, J.F., ST. GEORGE. J., MILLER, G.L. and ANDERSON, J. (2003). "Radiation dose in interventional radiology procedures: The RAD-IR study," J. Vasc. Interv. Radiol. **14**, 977–990.

MOGHISSI, A.A., PARAS, P., CARTER, M.W. and BARKER, R.F., Eds. (1978). *Radioactivity in Consumer Products*, NUREG/CP-001 (National Technical Information Service, Springfield, Virginia).

MORIN, R.L., GERBER, T.C. and MCCOLLOUGH, C.H. (2003). "Radiation dose in computed tomography of the heart," Circulation **107**, 917–922.

MOROZ, B.B. and PARFENOV, Y.D. (1972). "Metabolism and biological effects of ^{210}Po," Atomic Energy Rev. **10**(2), 175–232.

MOYAL, A.E., SPOHRER, M.A., FARRIS, K., FREIER, W., GANTT, A., MATKOVICH, B., NAKASONE, J. and SCOTT, B. (2006). *Nationwide Evaluation of X-Ray Trends (NEXT), Tabulation and Graphical Summary of 2002 Abdomen/Lumbosacral Spine Survey*, CRCPD Publication E-06-2b, http://www.crcpd.org/Pubs/NEXT_docs/NEXT2002-Ab-LS_Spine.pdf (accessed February 3, 2009) (Conference of Radiation Control Program Directors, Inc., Frankfort, Kentucky).

MOYAL, A.E., FERRUOLO, J., CROSBY, J., KLOKEID, G., PLUS-QUELLIC, L. and SPOHRER, M.A. (2007). Conference of Radiation Control Program Directors, Inc. *Nationwide Evaluation of X-Ray Trends (NEXT): Tabulation and Graphical Summary of the 1999 Dental Radiographic Survey*, CRCPD Publication E-03-6-a, http://crcpd.org/Pubs/NEXT_docs/NEXT99Dental.pdf (accessed February 3, 2009) (Conference of Radiation Control Program Directors, Inc., Frankfort, Kentucky).

MQSA (2005). *Mammography Quality Standards Act (MQSA) of 1992* (as amended by MQSRA of 1998 and 2004), http://www.fda.gov/CDRH/MAMMOGRAPHY/mqsa-act.html (accessed February 4, 2009) (U.S. Food and Drug Administration, Rockville, Maryland).

MUELLER, T.J., LENTZ, F.L., BRANN, J.A. and MCLANE, B.P. (2007). *Occupational Radiation Exposure from U.S. Naval Nuclear Propulsion Plants and their Support Facilities, 2006*, Report NT-07-2 (U.S. Department of the Navy, Washington).

MYRICK, T.E., BERVEN, B.A. and HAYWOOD, F.F. (1983). "Determination of concentrations of selected radionuclides in surface soil in the U.S.," Health Phys. **45**(3), 631–642.

NAS/NRC (1972). National Academy of Sciences/National Research Council. *The Effects on Populations of Exposure to Low Levels of Ionizing Radiation, BEIR I*, Committee on the Biological Effects of Ionizing Radiations (National Academies Press, Washington).

NAS/NRC (1980). National Academy of Sciences/National Research Council. *The Effects on Populations of Exposure to Low Levels of Ionizing Radiation, BEIR III*, Committee on the Biological Effects of Ionizing Radiations (National Academies Press, Washington).

NAS/NRC (1999a). National Academy of Sciences/National Research Council. *Risk Assessment of Radon in Drinking Water*, Committee on Risk Assessment of Exposure to Radon in Drinking Water (National Academies Press, Washington).

NAS/NRC (1999b). National Academy of Sciences/National Research Council. *Health Effects of Exposure to Radon, BEIR VI*, Committee on the Biological Effects of Ionizing Radiations (National Academies Press, Washington).

NAS/NRC (2006). National Academy of Sciences/National Research Council. *Health Risks from Exposure to Low Levels of Ionizing Radiation: Phase 2, BEIR VII*, Board on Radiation Effects Research (National Academies Press, Washington).

NCHS (2006). National Center for Health Statistics. *Health, United States, 2006 with Chartbook on Trends in the Health of Americans* (U.S. Government Printing Office, Washington).

NCRP (1975). National Council on Radiation Protection and Measurements. *Natural Background Radiation in the United States*, NCRP Report No. 45 (National Council on Radiation Protection and Measurements, Bethesda, Maryland).

NCRP (1984a). National Council on Radiation Protection and Measurements. *Exposures from the Uranium Series with Emphasis on Radon and Its Daughters*. NCRP Report No. 77 (National Council on Radiation Protection and Measurements, Bethesda, Maryland).

NCRP (1984b). National Council on Radiation Protection and Measurements. *Evaluation of Occupational and Environmental Exposures to Radon and Radon Daughters in the United States,* NCRP Report No. 78 (National Council on Radiation Protection and Measurements, Bethesda, Maryland).

NCRP (1987a). National Council on Radiation Protection and Measurements. *Ionizing Radiation Exposure of the Population of the United States*, NCRP Report No. 93 (National Council on Radiation Protection and Measurements, Bethesda, Maryland).

NCRP (1987b). National Council on Radiation Protection and Measurements, *Exposure of the Population in the United States and Canada from Natural Background Radiation*, NCRP Report No. 94 (National Council on Radiation Protection and Measurements, Bethesda, Maryland).

NCRP (1987c). National Council on Radiation Protection and Measurements. *Public Radiation Exposure from Nuclear Power Generation in the United States*, NCRP Report No. 92 (National Council on Radiation Protection and Measurements, Bethesda, Maryland).

NCRP (1987d). National Council on Radiation Protection and Measurements. *Radiation Exposure of the U.S. Population from Consumer Products and Miscellaneous Sources*, NCRP Report No. 95 (National Council on Radiation Protection and Measurements, Bethesda, Maryland).

NCRP (1987e). National Council on Radiation Protection and Measurements. *Recommendations on Limits for Exposure to Ionizing*

Radiation, NCRP Report No. 91 (National Council on Radiation Protection and Measurements, Bethesda, Maryland).

NCRP (1989a). National Council on Radiation Protection and Measurements. *Exposure of the U.S. Population from Diagnostic Medical Radiation*, NCRP Report No. 100 (National Council on Radiation Protection and Measurements, Bethesda, Maryland).

NCRP (1989b). National Council on Radiation Protection and Measurements. *Exposure of the U.S. Population from Occupational Radiation*, NCRP Report No. 101 (National Council on Radiation Protection and Measurements, Bethesda, Maryland).

NCRP (1991). National Council on Radiation Protection and Measurements. *Misadministration of Radioactive Material in Medicine — Scientific Background*, NCRP Commentary No. 7 (National Council on Radiation Protection and Measurements, Bethesda, Maryland).

NCRP (1993a). National Council of Radiation Protection and Measurements, *Limitation of Exposure to Ionizing Radiation*, NCRP Report No. 116 (National Council of Radiation Protection and Measurements, Bethesda, Maryland).

NCRP (1993b). National Council on Radiation Protection and Measurements. *Radiation Protection in the Mineral Extraction Industry*, NCRP Report No. 118 (National Council on Radiation Protection and Measurements, Bethesda, Maryland).

NCRP (1995a). National Council on Radiation Protection and Measurements. *Principles and Application of Collective Dose in Radiation Protection*, NCRP Report No. 121 (National Council on Radiation Protection and Measurements, Bethesda, Maryland).

NCRP (1995b). National Council on Radiation Protection and Measurements. *Use of Personal Monitors to Estimate Effective Dose Equivalent and Effective Dose to Workers for External Exposure to Low-LET Radiation*, NCRP Report No. 122 (National Council on Radiation Protection and Measurements, Bethesda, Maryland)

NCRP (1995c). National Council on Radiation Protection and Measurements. *Radiation Exposure and High-Altitude Flights*, NCRP Commentary No. 12 (National Council on Radiation Protection and Measurements, Bethesda, Maryland)

NCRP (1996). National Council on Radiation Protection and Measurements. *Sources and Magnitude of Occupational and Public Exposures from Nuclear Medicine Procedures*, NCRP Report No. 124 (National Council on Radiation Protection and Measurements, Bethesda, Maryland).

NCRP (2003a). National Council on Radiation Protection and Measurements. *Pulsed Fast Neutron Analysis System Used in Security Surveillance*, NCRP Commentary No. 17 (National Council on Radiation Protection and Measurements, Bethesda, Maryland).

NCRP (2003b). National Council on Radiation Protection and Measurements. *Screening of Humans for Security Purposes Using Ionizing Radiation Scanning Systems*, NCRP Commentary No. 16 (National Council on Radiation Protection and Measurements, Bethesda, Maryland).

NCRP (2004a). National Council on Radiation Protection and Measurements. *A Guide to Mammography and Other Breast Imaging Procedures*, NCRP Report No. 149 (National Council on Radiation Protection and Measurements, Bethesda, Maryland).

NCRP (2004b). National Council on Radiation Protection and Measurements. *Radiation Protection in Veterinary Medicine*, NCRP Report No. 148 (National Council on Radiation Protection and Measurements, Bethesda, Maryland).

NCRP (2007). National Council on Radiation Protection and Measurements. *Radiation Protection and Measurement Issues Related to Cargo Scanning with Accelerator-Produced High-Energy X Rays*, NCRP Commentary No. 20 (National Council on Radiation Protection and Measurements, Bethesda, Maryland).

NEA (1983). Nuclear Energy Agency. *Dosimetric Aspects of Exposure to Radon and Thoron Daughter Products* (Organisation for Economic Co-operation and Development Publications and Information Center, Washington).

NEI (2007). Nuclear Energy Institute. *U.S. Nuclear Generating Statistics (1971–2007)*, http://nei.org/resourcesandstats/documentlibrary/reliableandaffordableenergy/graphicsandcharts/usnucleargenerating statistics (accessed February 4, 2009) (Nuclear Energy Institute, Washington).

NEOFOTISTOU, V., KAROUSSOU, A., LOBOTESI, H. and HOURDAKIS, K. (1998). "Patient dosimetry during interventional cardiology procedures," Radiat. Prot. Dosim. **80**(1), 151–154.

NICKOLOFF, E.L., KHANDJI, A. and DUTTA, A. (2000). "Radiation doses during CT fluoroscopy," Health Phys. **79**(6), 675–681.

NIKLASON, L.T., MARX, M.V. and CHAN, H.P. (1994). "The estimation of occupational effective dose in diagnostic radiology with two dosimeters," Health Phys. **67**(6), 611–615.

NISHIZAWA, K., MARUYAMA, T., TAKAYAMA, M., OKADA, M., HACHIYA, J. and FURUYA, Y. (1991). "Determinations of organ doses and effective dose equivalents from computed tomographic examination," Br. J. Radiol. **64**(757), 20–28.

NIST (2008). National Institute of Standards and Technology. *About the National Voluntary Laboratory Accreditation Program (NVLAP)*, http://ts.nist.gov/standards/accreditation/index.cfm (accessed February 4, 2009) (National Institute of Standards and Technology, Gaithersburg, Maryland).

NJDEP (1989). New Jersey Department of Environmental Protection. *Highlights of the Statewide Scientific Study of Radon* (New Jersey Department of Environmental Protection, Trenton, New Jersey).

NJDEP (2006a). New Jersey Department of Environmental Protection. *A Study of Technologically Enhanced Naturally Occurring Radioactive Material (TENORM) in Municipal Sludge Landis Sewage Authority* (New Jersey Department of Environmental Protection, Trenton, New Jersey).

NJDEP (2006b). New Jersey Department of Environmental Protection. *A Study of Technologically Enhanced Naturally Occurring Radioactive Material (TENORM) Municipal Sludge Cumberland County Utilities Authority* (New Jersey Department of Environmental Protection, Trenton, New Jersey).

NNDC (2008a). National Nuclear Data Center. *NuDat 2.4*, http://www.nndc.bnl.gov/nudat2 (accessed February 4, 2009) (Brookhaven National Laboratory, Upton, New York).

NNDC (2008b). National Nuclear Data Center. *Search Parameters,* ^{40}K, http://www.nndc.bnl.gov/chart/decaysearchdirect.jsp?nuc=40K&unc= nds (accessed February 4, 2009) (Brookhaven National Laboratory, Upton, New York).

NNDC (2008c). National Nuclear Data Center. *Chart of Nuclides*, http://www.nndc.bnl.gov/chart/reCenter.jsp?z=19&n=21 (accessed February 4, 2009) (Brookhaven National Laboratory, Upton, New York).

NRC (1988). U.S. Nuclear Regulatory Commission. *Final Generic Environmental Impact Statement on Decommissioning of Nuclear Facilities*, NUREG-0586, http://www.nrc.gov/reading-rm/doc-collections/ nuregs/staff/sr0586/sr0586.pdf (accessed February 4, 2009) (National Technical Information Service, Springfield, Virginia).

NRC (2007a). U.S. Nuclear Regulatory Commission. "Standards for protection against radiation. Definitions," 10 CFR Part 20.1003, http://www.nrc.gov/reading-rm/doc-collections/cfr/part020/part020-1003.html (accessed February 4, 2009) (U.S. Nuclear Regulatory Commission, Washington).

NRC (2007b). U.S. Nuclear Regulatory Commission. *Nuclear Material Events Database*, https://nmed.inl.gov (accessed February 4, 2009) (U.S. Nuclear Regulatory Commission, Washington).

NRC (2007c). U.S. Nuclear Regulatory Commission. *Unimportant Quantities of Source Material*, 10 CFR Part 40.13(c)(2)(i) and (iii), http://www. nrc.gov/reading-rm/doc-collections/cfr/part040/part040-0013.html (accessed February 4, 2009) (U.S. Nuclear Regulatory Commission, Washington).

NRC (2007d). U.S. Nuclear Regulatory Commission. "Radiological criteria for unrestricted use," 10 CFR Part 20.1402, http://www.nrc.gov/reading-rm/doc-collections/cfr/part020/part020-1402.html (accessed February 4, 2009) (U.S. Nuclear Regulatory Commission, Washington).

NRC (2007e). U.S. Nuclear Regulatory Commission. "Protection of the general population from releases of radioactivity," 10 CFR Part 61.41, http://www.nrc.gov/reading-rm/doc-collections/cfr/part061/part061-0041.html (accessed February 4, 2009) (U.S. Nuclear Regulatory Commission, Washington).

NRC (2008). U.S. Nuclear Regulatory Commission. *Generic Environmental Impact Statement for In-Situ Leach Uranium Milling Facilities –Draft Report for Comment*, NUREG-1910, http://www.nrc.gov/reading-rm/doc-collections/nuregs/staff/sr1910 (accessed February 4, 2009) (U.S. Nuclear Regulatory Commission, Washington).

OAKLEY, D.T. (1972). *Natural Radiation Exposure in the United States*, ORP/SID 72-1 (U.S. Environmental Protection Agency, Washington).

O'BRIEN, K. (2005). "The theory of cosmic-ray and high-energy solar-particle transport in the atmosphere," pages 29 to 44 in *The Natural Radiation Environment VII. Seventh International Symposium on the Natural Radiation Environment*, McLaughlin, J.P., Simopoulos, E.S. and Steinhausler, F., Eds. (Elsevier, New York).

O'BRIEN, K. and FRIEDBERG, W. (1994). "Atmospheric cosmic rays at aircraft altitudes," Environ. Intl. **20**(5), 645–663.

OTT, W.R. (1995). *Environmental Statistics and Data Analysis* (CRC Press, Boca Raton, Florida).

PAPASTEFANOU, C. (2007). "Radiation dose from cigarette tobacco," Radiat. Prot. Dosim. **123**(1), 68–73.

PDEP (2005). Pennsylvania Department of Environmental Protection. *Radiological Investigation Results for Pennsylvania Landfill Leachate*, http://www.dep.state.pa.us/brp/Radiation_Control_Division/SolidWaste Monitoring/LF%20Leachate%20Final%2010_03_051_web.pdf (accessed February 4, 2009) (Pennsylvania Department of Environmental Protection, Harrisburg, Pennsylvania).

PDEP (2006). Pennsylvania Department of Environmental Protection. *Radiological Investigation Results for Pennsylvania Landfill Leachate Fall 2005 Tritium Update*, http://www.dep.state.pa.us/brp/Radiation_Control_Division/SolidWasteMonitoring/Fall%2005%20LF%20 Leachate%20Tritium%20PRE%20FINAL_slw032906_8.pdf (accessed February 4, 2009) (Pennsylvania Department of Environmental Protection, Harrisburg, Pennsylvania).

PERES, A.C. and HIROMOTO, G. (2002). "Evaluation of ^{210}Pb and ^{210}Po in cigarette tobacco produced in Brazil," J. Environ. Radioact. **62**(1), 115–119.

PIESCH, E., BURGKHARDT, B. and ANTON, R. (1986). "Dose rate measurements in the beta-photon radiation field from UO_2 pellets and glazed ceramics containing uranium," Radiat. Prot. Dosim. **14**(2), 109–112.

PRICE, P.N., NERO, A., REVZAN, K., APTE, M., GELMAN, A. and BOSCARDIN, W.J. (2007). *High-Radon Project Home Page*, http://eetd.lbl.gov/IEP/high-radon (accessed February 4, 2009) (Lawrence Berkeley National Laboratory, Berkeley, California).

PSI (2003). Product Stewardship Institute. *Radioactive Materials Product Stewardship. A Background Report for the National Dialogue on Radioactive Materials Product Stewardship*, http://www.epa.gov/radiation/docs/source-management/psi-radmat-bkgrd-rpt.pdf (accessed February 4, 2009) (U.S. Environmental Protection Agency, Washington).

PUKKILA, O and KARILA, K. (1990). *Interventional Radiology – A Challenge for Radiation Protection* (Nordic Society for Radiation Protection, Ronneby, Sweden).

RADAR (2008). Radiation Dose Assessment Resource. *RADAR - Available Phantoms*, http://www.doseinfo-radar.com/RADARphan.html (accessed

February 4, 2009) (Radiation Dose Assessment Resource, Nashville, Tennessee).

RAMME, B. and THARANIYIL, M. (2004). *Coal Combustion Products Utilization Handbook,* http://wwwstg.we-energies.com/environmental/recycle_coalash.htm (accessed February 4, 2009) (Wisconsin Electric Power Company and Wisconsin Gas LLC, Milwaukee, Wisconsin).

RANNOU, A. (1987). *Contribution a l'etude du risque lie a la presence du radon 220 et du radon 222 dans 1'atmosphere des habitations,* Rapport CEA-R-5378 (Commissariat à l'Energie Atomique, Saclay, France).

REGULLA, D.F. and EDER, H. (2005). "Patient exposure in medical x-ray imaging in Europe," Radiat. Prot. Dosim. **114**(1–3), 11–25.

ROBINSON, J.P. and THOMAS, J. (1991). *Time Spent in Activities, Locations, and Microenvironments: A California-National Comparison. Project Report,* EPA-68-01-7325 (National Technical Information Service, Springfield, Virginia).

ROBINSON, C.M., YOUNG, J.G., WALLACE, A.B. and IBBETSON, V.J. (2005). "A study of the personal radiation dose received by nuclear medicine technologists working in a dedicated PET center," Health Phys. **88**(2)(Suppl. 1), S17–S21.

ROESSLER, G. and GUILMETTE, R. (2007). "Why ^{210}Po?," Health Phys. News **XXXV**(2), 1–9.

ROESSLER, C.E., SMITH, Z.A., BOLCH, W.E. and PRINCE, R.J. (1979). "Uranium and radium-226 in Florida phosphate materials," Health Phys. **37**(3), 269–277.

ROGERS, G.O., HUMMON, N.P. and STROM, D.J. (1990). "A preliminary model of radon exposure," in *New Risks: Issues and Management,* Cox, L.A. Jr. and Ricci, P.F., Eds. (Plenum Press, New York).

ROSENSTEIN, M. and WEBSTER, E.W. (1994). "Effective dose to personnel wearing protective aprons during fluoroscopy and interventional radiology," Health Phys. **67**(1), 88–89.

ROSENTHAL, L.S., MAHESH, M., BECK, T.J., SAUL, J.P., MILLER, J.M., KAY, N., KLEIN, L.S., HUANG, S., GILLETTE, P., PRYSTOWSKY, E., CARLSON, M., BERGER, R.D., LAWRENCE, J.H., YONG, P. and CALKINS, H. (1998). "Predictors of fluoroscopy time and estimated radiation exposure during radiofrequency catheter ablation procedures," Am. J. Cardiol. **82**(4), 451–458.

RSNA (2008). Radiological Society of North America. *Myelography,* http://www.radiologyinfo.org/en/pdf/myelography.pdf (accessed February 4, 2009) (Radiological Society of North America, Oak Brook, Illinois).

SAITO, K. and JACOB, P. (1995). "Gamma ray fields in the air due to sources in the ground," Radiat. Prot. Dosim. **58**(1), 29–45.

SAITO, K., PETOUSSI-HENSS, N. and ZANKL, M. (1998) "Calculation of effective dose and its variation from environmental gamma ray sources," Health Phys. **74**(6), 698–706.

SATO, T., TSUDA, S., SAKAMOTO, Y., YAMAGUCHI, Y. and NIITA, K. (2003). "Conversion coefficients from fluence to effective dose for heavy ions with energies up to 3 GeV/A," Radiat. Prot. Dosim. **106**(2), 137–144.

SAVIDOU, A., KEHAGIA, K. and ELEFTHERIADIS, K. (2006). "Concentration levels of ^{210}Pb and ^{210}Po in dry tobacco leaves in Greece," J. Environ Radioact. **85**(1), 94–102.

SCHERY, S.D. and GRUMM, D.M. (1992). "Thoron and its progeny in the atmospheric environment," pages 423 to 459 in *Gaseous Pollutants: Characterization and Cycling*, Nriagu, J.O., Ed. (John Wiley and Sons, Inc., Hoboken, New Jersey).

SCHLEIPMAN, A.R., CASTRONOVO, F.P., JR., DI CARLI, M.F. and DORBALA, S. (2006). "Occupational radiation dose associated with Rb-82 myocardial perfusion positron emission tomography imaging," J. Nucl. Cardiol. **13**(3), 378–384.

SCHNEIDER, S., KOCHER, D.C., KERR, G.D., SCOFIELD, P.A., O'DONNELL, F.R., MATTSEN, C.R., COTTER, S.J., BOGARD, J.S., BLAND, J.S. and WIBLIN, C. (2001). *Systematic Radiological Assessment of Exemptions for Source and Byproduct Materials*, NUREG 1717, http://www.nrc.gov/reading-rm/doc-collections/nuregs/staff/sr1717/nureg-1717.pdf (accessed February 4, 2009) (U.S. Nuclear Regulatory Commission, Washington).

SCHULTZ, F.W. and ZOETELIEF, J. (2005). "Dose conversion coefficients for interventional procedures," Radiat. Prot. Dosim. **117**(1–3), 225–230.

SCHWARTZ, D.J., DAVIS, B.J., VETTER, R.J., PISANSKY, T.M., HERMAN, M.G., WILSON, T.M., LAJOIE, W.N. and OBERG, A.L. (2003). "Radiation exposure to operating room personnel during transperineal interstitial permanent prostate brachytherapy," Brachytherapy **2**(1), 98–102.

SEIERSTAD, T., STRANDEN, E., BJERING, K., EVENSEN, M., HOLT, A., MICHALSEN, H.M. and WETTELAND, O. (2007). "Doses to nuclear technicians in a dedicated PET/CT centre utilising 18F fluorodeoxyglucose (FDG)," Radiat. Prot. Dosim. **123**(2), 246–249.

SHERBINI, S. and DECICCO, J. (2002) "Estimation of the effective dose when protective aprons are used in medical procedures: A theoretical evaluation of several methods," Health Phys. **83**(6), 861–870.

SHOPE, T.B. (1996). "Radiation-induced skin injuries from fluoroscopy," RadioGraphics **16**, 1195–1199.

SHOPE, T.B., GAGNE, R.M. and JOHNSON, G.C. (1981). "A method for describing the doses delivered by transmission x-ray computed tomography," Med. Phys. **8**(4), 488–495.

SHRIMPTON, P.C. and WALL, B.F. (2000) "Reference doses for paediatric computed tomography," Radiat. Prot. Dosim. **90**(1), 249–252.

SHRIMPTON, P.C., HILLIER, M.C., LEWIS, M.A and DUNN, M. (2006). "National survey of doses from CT in the UK: 2003," Br. J. Radiol. **79**(948), 968–980.

SKWARZEC, B., ULATOWSKI, J., STRUMINSKA, D.I. and BORYLO, A. (2001). "Inhalation of ^{210}Po and ^{210}Pb from cigarette smoking in Poland," J. Environ. Radioact. **57**(3), 221–230.

SMITH, K.R., CROCKETT, G.M., OATWAY, W.B., HARVEY, M.P., PENFORLD, J.S.S. and MOBBS, S.F. (2001). *Radiological Impact on the*

UK Population of Industries Which Use or Produce Materials Containing Enhanced Levels of Naturally Occurring Radionuclides, Part I: Coal-Fired Electricity Generation, NRPB-R327 (Health Protection Agency, London).

SMITH, T.B., BANOVAC, K.L., MCCANN, G.M., PARROTT, J.D., SHEPHERD, J.C. and SOBEL, P.A. (2003). *Consolidated NMSS Decommissioning Guidance,* NUREG 1757, Vol. 1, rev. 1 (National Technical Information Service, Springfield, Virginia).

SNM (2008). Society of Nuclear Medicine. *Practice Management* http://interactive.snm.org/index.cfm?PageID=772&RPID=18 (accessed February 4, 2009) (Society of Nuclear Medicine, Reston, Virginia).

SNYDER, W.S., FORD, M.R., WARNER, G.G. and WATSON, S.B. (1975). *"S," Absorbed Dose per Unit Cumulated Activity for Selected Radionuclides and Organs,* MIRD Pamphlet No. 11, http://interactive.snm.org/docs/MIRD%20Pamphlet%2011.1-69.pdf (accessed February 4, 2009) (Society of Nuclear Medicine, Reston, Virginia).

STABIN, M.G. and SIEGEL, J.A. (2003). "Physical models and dose factors for use in internal dose assessment," Health Phys. **85**(3), 294–310.

STANNARD, J.N. (1988). *Radioactivity and Health: A History* (National Technical Information Service, Springfield, Virginia).

STEINHAUSLER, F. (1996). "Environmental ^{220}Rn: A review," Environ. Int. **22**(Suppl. 1), S1111–S1123.

STERN, S.H., FREIER, W., FARRIS, K., GANTT, A., MATKOVICH, B., NAKASONE, J., NEAL, J., SCOTT, R. and SPOHRER, M.A. (2007). *Nationwide Evaluation of X-Ray Trends (NEXT): Tabulation and Graphical Summary of 2000 Survey of Computed Tomography,* CRCPD Publication E-07-2, http://www.crcpd.org/Pubs/NEXT_docs/NEXT2000-CT.pdf (accessed February 3, 2009) (Conference of Radiation Control Program Directors, Inc., Frankfort, Kentucky).

STOVALL, M., BLACKWELL, C.R., CUNDIFF, J., NOVACK, D.H., PALTA, J.R., WAGNER, L.K., WEBSTER, E.W. and SHALEK, R.J. (1995). "Fetal dose from radiotherapy with photon beams: Report of AAPM Radiation Therapy Committee Task Group No. 36," Med. Phys. **22**(1), 63–82.

STROM, D.J. (2007). *Default Assumptions and Methods for Atomic Weapons Employer Dose Reconstruction,* Battelle TIB-5000, http://www.cdc.gov/niosh/ocas/pdfs/tibs/b-t5000-r0.pdf (accessed February 4, 2009) (National Institute for Occupational Safety and Health, Cincinnati, Ohio).

STROM, D.J. and STANSBURY, P.S. (2000). "Determining parameters of lognormal distributions from minimal information," PNNL-SA-32215. Am. Ind. Hyg. Assoc. J. **61**, 877–880.

STROM, D.J., LYNCH, T.P. and WEIER, D.R. (2009). *Radiation Doses to Hanford Workers from Natural Potassium-40,* PNNL-18240 (Pacific Northwest National Laboratory, Richland, Washington).

SULEIMAN, O.H., SPELIC, D.C., CONWAY, B., HART, J.C., BOYCE, P.R. and ANTONSEN, R.G. (1999). "Radiographic trends of dental offices and dental schools," J. Am. Dental Assoc. **130**(7), 1104–1110.

SWANN, C., MATTHEWS, J. ERICKSEN, R. and KUSZMAUL, J. (2004). *Evaluations of Radionuclides of Uranium, Thorium, and Radium Associated with Produced Fluids, Precipitates, and Sludges from Oil, Gas, and Oilfield Brine Injections Wells in Mississippi, Final Report,* http://www.olemiss.edu/depts/mmri/programs/norm_final.pdf (accessed February 4, 2009) (University of Mississippi, University, Mississippi).

SZABO, Z. and DEPAUL, V. (1998). *Radium-226 and Radium-228 in Shallow Ground Water, Southern New Jersey,* Fact Sheet FS-062-98 (U.S. Geological Survey, West Trenton, New Jersey).

SZENDRO, G., AXELSSON, B. and LEITZ, W. (1995). "Computed tomography practice in Sweden. Quality control, techniques and patient dose," Radiat. Prot. Dosim. **57**(1–4), 469–473.

TEEUWISSE, W.M., GELEIJNS, J., BROERSE, J.J., OBERMANN, W.R. and VAN PERSIJN VAN MEERTEN, E.L. (2001). "Patient and staff dose during CT guided biopsy, drainage and coagulation," Br. J. Radiol. **74**(884), 720–726.

THWAITES, J. H., RAFFERTY, M.W., GRAY, N., BLACK, J. and STOCK, B. (1996). "A patient dose survey for femoral arterogram diagnostic radiographic examinations using a dose-area product meter," Phys. Med. Biol. **41**(5), 899–907.

TIMMER, S.G., ECCLES, J. and O'BRIEN, K. (1985). "How children use time," pages 353 to 380 in *Time, Goods, and Well-Being,* Juster, F.T. and Stafford, F.P., Eds. (University of Michigan, Ann Arbor, Michigan).

TOKONAMI, S., YANG, M. and SANADA, T. (2001). "Contribution from thoron on the response of passive radon detectors," Health Phys. **80**(6), 612–615.

TOMASEK, L., ROGEL, A., LAURIER, D. and TIRMARCHE, M. (2008). "Dose conversion of radon exposure according to new epidemiological findings," Radiat. Prot. Dosim. **130**(1), 98–100.

TSANG, A.M. and KLEPEIS, N.E. (1996). *Results Tables from a Detailed Analysis of the National Human Activity Pattern Survey (NHAPS) Response* (U.S. Environmental Protection Agency, Washington).

TSCHIERSCH, J., LI, W.B. and MEISENBERG, O. (2007). "Increased indoor thoron concentrations and implication to inhalation dosimetry," Radiat. Prot. Dosim. **127**(1–4), 73–78.

TSO, T.C., HALLDEN, N.A. and ALEXANDER, L.T. (1964). "Radium-226 and polonium-210 in leaf tobacco and tobacco soil," Science **146**(3647), 1043–1045.

TSO, T.C., HARLEY, N. and ALEXANDER, L.T. (1966). "Source of lead-210 and polonium-210 in tobacco," Science **153**(3738), 880–882.

TU, K.W., GEORGE, A.C., LOWDER, W.M. and GOGOLAK, C.V. (1992). "Indoor thoron and radon progeny measurements," Radiat. Prot. Dosim. **45**(1), 557–560.

UMTRCA (1978). Uranium Mill Tailings Radiation Control Act. Public Law 95-604 (November 8), 92 Stat. 3021, as amended (U.S. Government Printing Office, Washington).

UNSCEAR (1966). United Nations Scientific Committee on the Effects of Atomic Radiation. *Report of the United Nations Scientific Committee on the Effects of Atomic Radiation*, http://www.unscear.org/unscear/en/publications/1966.html (accessed February 4, 2009) (United Nations Publications, New York).

UNSCEAR (1972). United Nations Scientific Committee on the Effects of Atomic Radiation. *Ionizing Radiation: Levels and Effects. A Report of the United Nations Scientific Committee on the Effects of Atomic Radiation to the General Assembly, with Annexes*, http://www.unscear.org/unscear/en/publications/1972.html (accessed February 4, 2009) (United Nations Publications, New York).

UNSCEAR (1977). United Nations Scientific Committee on the Effects of Atomic Radiation. *Sources and Effects of Ionizing Radiation. United Nations Scientific Committee on the Effects of Atomic Radiation 1977 Report to the General Assembly, with Annexes*, http://www.unscear.org/unscear/en/publications/1977.html (accessed February 4, 2009) (United Nations Publications, New York).

UNSCEAR (1982). United Nations Scientific Committee on the Effects of Atomic Radiation. *Ionizing Radiation: Sources and Biological Effects. United Nations Scientific Committee on the Effects of Atomic Radiation 1982 Report to the General Assembly, with Annexes*, http://www.unscear.org/unscear/en/publications/1982.html (accessed February 4, 2009) (United Nations Publications, New York).

UNSCEAR (1988). United Nations Scientific Committee on the Effects of Atomic Radiation. *Sources, Effects and Risks of Ionizing Radiation, United Nations Scientific Committee on the Effects of Atomic Radiation 1988 Report to the General Assembly, with Scientific Annexes*, http://www.unscear.org/unscear/en/publications/1988.html (accessed February 4, 2009) (United Nations Publications, New York).

UNSCEAR (1993). United Nations Scientific Committee on the Effects of Atomic Radiation. *Sources and Effects of Ionizing Radiation, United Nations Scientific Committee on the Effects of Atomic Radiation 1993 Report to the General Assembly, with Scientific Annexes*, http://www.unscear.org/unscear/en/publications/1993.html (accessed February 4, 2009) (United Nations Publications, New York).

UNSCEAR (2000). United Nations Scientific Committee on the Effects of Atomic Radiation. *Sources and Effects of Ionizing Radiation, Volume I: Sources, United Nations Scientific Committee on the Effects of Atomic Radiation 2000 Report to the General Assembly, with Scientific Annexes*, http://www.unscear.org/unscear/en/publications/2000_1.html (accessed February 4, 2009) (United Nations Publications, New York).

USCB (2005). U.S. Census Bureau. *American Housing Survey for the United States: 2003*, http://www.census.gov/hhes/www/housing/ahs/ahs03/tab29.htm (accessed February 9, 2009) (U.S. Census Bureau, Washington).

USCB (2006a). U.S. Census Bureau. *National and State Population Estimates, Annual Population Estimates 2000 to 2006*, http://www.census.

gov/popest/states/NST-annest.html (accessed December 22, 2006) (U.S. Census Bureau, Washington).

USCB (2006b). U.S. Census Bureau. *National Population Estimates-Characteristics, National Sex and Age, Annual Estimates of the Population by Sex and Five-Year Age Groups for the United States: April 1, 2000 to July 1, 2005*, NC-EST2005-01, http://www.census.gov/popest/national/asrh/NC-EST2005-sa.html (accessed February 4, 2009) (U.S. Census Bureau, Washington).

USCB (2006c). U.S. Census Bureau. *Data Table, Estimates for 12.2006*, www.census.gov/popest/national/asrh/files/NC-EST2006-ALLDATA-R-File14.dat (accessed February 4, 2009) (U.S. Census Bureau, Washington).

USCB (2007a). U.S. Census Bureau. *U.S. Statistics in Brief—Resident Population of States and DC*, http://www.census.gov/compendia/statab/files/statepop.html (accessed March 7, 2008) (U.S. Census Bureau, Washington).

USCB (2007b). U.S. Census Bureau. *Construction and Housing: Housing Units and Characteristics*, http://www.census.gov/compendia/statab/cats/construction_housing/housing_units_and_characteristics.html (accessed March 7, 2008) (U.S. Census Bureau, Washington).

USCB (2008). U.S. Census Bureau. *United States Census 2000*, http://www.census.gov/main/www/cen2000.html (accessed February 4, 2009) (U.S. Census Bureau, Washington).

USDA (2001a). U.S. Department of Agriculture. *Acres of Small Built-Up Areas, by Year*, http://www.nrcs.usda.gov/technical/NRI/maps/mappdfs/m5793.pdf (accessed February 4, 2009) (U.S. Department of Agriculture, Washington).

USDA (2001b). U.S. Department of Agriculture. *Acres of Large Urban Built-Up Land, by Year*, http://www.nrcs.usda.gov/technical/NRI/maps/mappdfs/m5792.pdf (accessed February 4, 2009) (U.S. Department of Agriculture, Washington).

USDA (2003). U.S. Department of Agriculture. *National Resources Inventory 2001 Annual NRI, Urbanization and Development of Rural Land*, http://www.nrcs.usda.gov/technical/NRI/2001/urban.pdf (accessed February 4, 2009) (U.S. Department of Agriculture, Washington).

USDA (2006). U.S. Department of Agriculture. *Farms, Land in Farms, and Livestock Operations: 2005 Summary*, http://usda.mannlib.cornell.edu/usda/nass/FarmLandIn//2000s/2006/FarmLandIn-01-31-2006.pdf (accessed February 4, 2009) (U.S. Department of Agriculture, Washington).

USGS (1997). U.S. Geological Survey. *Radioactive Elements in Coal and Fly Ash: Abundance, Forms, and Environmental Significance*, Fact Sheet FS-163-97, http://pubs.usgs.gov/fs/1997/fs163-97/FS-163-97.html (accessed February 4, 2009) (U.S. Geological Survey, Denver).

USGS (1999). U.S. Geological Survey. *Naturally Occurring Radioactive Materials (NORM) in Produced Water and Oil-Field Equipment-An Issue for the Energy Industry*, Fact Sheet FS-142-99, http://pubs.usgs.

gov/fs/fs-0142-99/index.html (accessed February 4, 2009) (U.S. Geological Survey, Denver).

USGS (2005a). U.S. Geological Survey. *Map of Potassium Concentrations*, http://pubs.usgs.gov/of/2005/1413/namkmap.htm (accessed February 4, 2009) (U.S. Geological Survey, Reston, Virginia).

USGS (2005b). U.S. Geological Survey. *Map of Uranium Concentrations*, http://pubs.usgs.gov/of/2005/1413/namumap.htm (accessed February 4, 2009) (U.S. Geological Survey, Reston, Virginia).

USGS (2005c). U.S. Geological Survey. *Map of Thorium Concentrations*, http://pubs.usgs.gov/of/2005/1413/namthmap.htm (accessed February 4, 2009) (U.S. Geological Survey, Reston, Virginia).

USGS (2005d). U.S. Geological Survey. *Ternary Map of Gamma-Ray Data*, http://pubs.usgs.gov/of/2005/1413/namccmcmy.htm (accessed February 4, 2009) (U.S. Geological Survey, Reston, Virginia).

USGS (2005e). U.S. Geological Survey. *Map of Cosmic-Ray Exposure*, http://pubs.usgs.gov/of/2005/1413/cosmicmap.htm (accessed February 4, 2009) (U.S. Geological Survey, Reston, Virginia).

VAN UNNIK, J.G., BROERSE, J.J., GELEIJNS, J., JANSEN, J.T., ZOE-TELIEF, J. and ZWEERS, D. (1997). "Survey of CT techniques and absorbed dose in various Dutch hospitals," Br. J. Radiol. **70**(832), 367–371.

VLIETSTRA, R.E., WAGNER, L.K., KOENIG, T. and METTLER, F. (2004). "Radiation burns as a severe complication of fluoroscopically guided cardiological interventions," J. Intervent. Cardiol. **17**(3), 131–142.

WARE, D.E., HUDA, W., MERGO, P.J. and LITWILLER, A.L. (1999). "Radiation effective doses to patients undergoing abdominal CT examinations," Radiology **210**, 645–650.

WATERS, M., BLOOM, T.F. and GRAJEWSKI, B. (2000). "The NIOSH/FAA Working Women's Health Study: Evaluation of the cosmic-radiation exposures of flight attendants," Health Phys. **79**(5), 553–559.

WEBSTER, E.W. (1989). "EDE for exposure with protective aprons," Health Phys. **56**(4), 568–569.

WILLIAMS, J.R. (1997). "The interdependence of staff and patient doses in interventional radiology," Br. J. Radiol. **70**(833), 498–503.

WILSON, A.J. and SCOTT, L.M. (1992). "Characterization of radioactive petroleum piping scale with an evaluation of subsequent land contamination," Health Phys. **63**(6), 681–685.

WINKLER-HEIL, R., HOFMANN, W., MARSH, J.W. and BIRCHALL, A. (2007). "Comparison of radon lung dosimetry models for the estimation of dose uncertainties," Radiat. Prot. Dosim. **127**(1–4), 27–30.

WOLBARST, A.B., CHIU, W.A., YU, C., AIELLO, K., BACHMAIER, J.T., BASTIAN, R.K., CHENG, J-J., GOODMAN, J., HOGAN, R., JONES A.R., KAMBOJ, S., LENHARTT, T., OTT, W.R., RUBIN, A., SALOMON, S.N., SCHMIDT, D.W. and SETLOW, L.W. (2006). "Radioactive materials in biosolids: Dose modeling," Health Phys. **90**(1), 16–30.

ZIELINSKI, R.A. and BUDAHN, J.R. (1998). "Radionuclides in fly ash and bottom ash: Improved characterization based on radiography and low energy gamma-ray spectrometry," Fuel **77**(4), 259–267.

ZWEERS, D., GELEIJNS, J., AARTS, N.J., HARDAM, L.J., LAMERIS, J.S., SCHULTZ, F.W. and SCHULTZ-KOOL, L.J. (1998). "Patient and staff radiation dose in fluoroscopy-guided TIPS procedures and dose reduction, using dedicated fluoroscopy exposure settings," Br. J. Radiol. **71**(846), 672–676.

The NCRP

The National Council on Radiation Protection and Measurements is a non-profit corporation chartered by Congress in 1964 to:

1. Collect, analyze, develop and disseminate in the public interest information and recommendations about (a) protection against radiation and (b) radiation measurements, quantities and units, particularly those concerned with radiation protection.
2. Provide a means by which organizations concerned with the scientific and related aspects of radiation protection and of radiation quantities, units and measurements may cooperate for effective utilization of their combined resources, and to stimulate the work of such organizations.
3. Develop basic concepts about radiation quantities, units and measurements, about the application of these concepts, and about radiation protection.
4. Cooperate with the International Commission on Radiological Protection, the International Commission on Radiation Units and Measurements, and other national and international organizations, governmental and private, concerned with radiation quantities, units and measurements and with radiation protection.

The Council is the successor to the unincorporated association of scientists known as the National Committee on Radiation Protection and Measurements and was formed to carry on the work begun by the Committee in 1929.

The participants in the Council's work are the Council members and members of scientific and administrative committees. Council members are selected solely on the basis of their scientific expertise and serve as individuals, not as representatives of any particular organization. The scientific committees, composed of experts having detailed knowledge and competence in the particular area of the committee's interest, draft proposed recommendations. These are then submitted to the full membership of the Council for careful review and approval before being published.

The following comprise the current officers and membership of the Council:

Officers

President	Thomas S. Tenforde
Senior Vice President	Kenneth R. Kase
Secretary and Treasurer	David A. Schauer

357

Members

John F. Ahearne
Edward S. Amis, Jr.
Sally A. Amundson
Kimberly E. Applegate
Benjamin R. Archer
Stephen Balter
Steven M. Becker
Joel S. Bedford
Mythreyi Bhargavan
Eleanor A. Blakely
William F. Blakely
Wesley E. Bolch
Thomas B. Borak
Andre Bouville
Leslie A. Braby
David J. Brenner
James A. Brink
Brooke R. Buddemeier
Jerrold T. Bushberg
John F. Cardella
Charles E. Chambers
Polly Y. Chang
S.Y. Chen
Mary E. Clark
Michael L. Corradini
Allen G. Croff
Paul M. DeLuca
Christine A. Donahue
David A. Eastmond
Stephen A. Feig
Alan J. Fischman
Patricia A. Fleming
John R. Frazier

Donald P. Frush
Ronald E. Goans
Robert L. Goldberg
Raymond A. Guilmette
Roger W. Harms
Kathryn Held
F. Owen Hoffman
Roger W. Howell
Timothy J. Jorgensen
Kenneth R. Kase
Ann R. Kennedy
William E. Kennedy, Jr.
David C. Kocher
Ritsuko Komaki
Amy Kronenberg
Susan M. Langhorst
Edwin M. Leidholdt
Howard L. Liber
James C. Lin
Jill A. Lipoti
Paul A. Locke
Jay H. Lubin
C. Douglas Maynard
Debra McBaugh
Ruth E. McBurney
Fred A. Mettler, Jr.
Charles W. Miller
Donald L. Miller
William H. Miller
William F. Morgan
Stephen V. Musolino
David S. Myers
Bruce A. Napier
Gregory A. Nelson

Andrea K. Ng
Carl J. Paperiello
Terry C. Pellmar
R. Julian Preston
Jerome C. Puskin
Abram Recht
Michael T. Ryan
Adela Salame-Alfie
Beth A. Schueler
Thomas M. Seed
J. Anthony Seibert
Stephen M. Seltzer
Edward A. Sickles
Steven L. Simon
Paul Slovic
Christopher G. Soares
Daniel J. Strom
Thomas S. Tenforde
Julie E.K. Timins
Richard E. Toohey
Lawrence W. Townsend
Elizabeth L. Travis
Fong Y. Tsai
Richard J. Vetter
Chris G. Whipple
Robert C. Whitcomb, Jr.
Stuart C. White
Gayle E. Woloschak
Shiao Y. Woo
Andrew J. Wyrobek
X. George Xu
R. Craig Yoder
Marco A. Zaider

Distinguished Emeritus Members

Warren K. Sinclair, *President Emeritus;* Charles B. Meinhold, *President Emeritus*
S. James Adelstein, *Honorary Vice President*
W. Roger Ney, *Executive Director Emeritus*
William M. Beckner, *Executive Director Emeritus*

Seymour Abrahamson
Lynn R. Anspaugh
John A. Auxier
William J. Bair
Harold L. Beck
Bruce B. Boecker
John D. Boice, Jr.
Robert L. Brent
Antone L. Brooks
Randall S. Caswell
J. Donald Cossairt
James F. Crow
Gerald D. Dodd
Sarah S. Donaldson
William P. Dornsife
Keith F. Eckerman
Thomas S. Ely

R.J. Michael Fry
Thomas F. Gesell
Ethel S. Gilbert
Robert O. Gorson
Joel E. Gray
Arthur W. Guy
Eric J. Hall
Naomi H. Harley
William R. Hendee
Donald G. Jacobs
Bernd Kahn
Charles E. Land
John B. Little
Roger O. McClellan
Barbara J. McNeil
Kenneth L. Miller

Dade W. Moeller
A. Alan Moghissi
Wesley L. Nyborg
John W. Poston, Sr.
Andrew K. Poznanski
Genevieve S. Roessler
Marvin Rosenstein
Lawrence N. Rothenberg
Henry D. Royal
William J. Schull
Roy E. Shore
John E. Till
Robert L. Ullrich
Arthur C. Upton
F. Ward Whicker
Susan D. Wiltshire
Marvin C. Ziskin

Lauriston S. Taylor Lecturers

John D. Boice, Jr. (2009) *Radiation Epidemiology: The Golden Age and Remaining Challenges*

Dade W. Moeller (2008) *Radiation Standards, Dose / Risk Assessments, Public Interactions, and Yucca Mountain: Thinking Outside the Box*

Patricia W. Durbin (2007) *The Quest for Therapeutic Actinide Chelators*

Robert L. Brent (2006) *Fifty Years of Scientific Research: The Importance of Scholarship and the Influence of Politics and Controversy*

John B. Little (2005) *Nontargeted Effects of Radiation: Implications for Low-Dose Exposures*

Abel J. Gonzalez (2004) *Radiation Protection in the Aftermath of a Terrorist Attack Involving Exposure to Ionizing Radiation*

Charles B. Meinhold (2003) *The Evolution of Radiation Protection: From Erythema to Genetic Risks to Risks of Cancer to ?*

R. Julian Preston (2002) *Developing Mechanistic Data for Incorporation into Cancer Risk Assessment: Old Problems and New Approaches*

Wesley L. Nyborg (2001) *Assuring the Safety of Medical Diagnostic Ultrasound*

S. James Adelstein (2000) *Administered Radioactivity: Unde Venimus Quoque Imus*

Naomi H. Harley (1999) *Back to Background*

Eric J. Hall (1998) *From Chimney Sweeps to Astronauts: Cancer Risks in the Workplace*

William J. Bair (1997) *Radionuclides in the Body: Meeting the Challenge!*

Seymour Abrahamson (1996) *70 Years of Radiation Genetics: Fruit Flies, Mice and Humans*

Albrecht Kellerer (1995) *Certainty and Uncertainty in Radiation Protection*

R.J. Michael Fry (1994) *Mice, Myths and Men*

Warren K. Sinclair (1993) *Science, Radiation Protection and the NCRP*

Edward W. Webster (1992) *Dose and Risk in Diagnostic Radiology: How Big? How Little?*

Victor P. Bond (1991) *When is a Dose Not a Dose?*

J. Newell Stannard (1990) *Radiation Protection and the Internal Emitter Saga*

Arthur C. Upton (1989) *Radiobiology and Radiation Protection: The Past Century and Prospects for the Future*

Bo Lindell (1988) *How Safe is Safe Enough?*

Seymour Jablon (1987) *How to be Quantitative about Radiation Risk Estimates*

Herman P. Schwan (1986) *Biological Effects of Non-ionizing Radiations: Cellular Properties and Interactions*

John H. Harley (1985) *Truth (and Beauty) in Radiation Measurement*

Harald H. Rossi (1984) *Limitation and Assessment in Radiation Protection*

Merril Eisenbud (1983) *The Human Environment—Past, Present and Future*

Eugene L. Saenger (1982) *Ethics, Trade-Offs and Medical Radiation*

James F. Crow (1981) *How Well Can We Assess Genetic Risk? Not Very*

Harold O. Wyckoff (1980) *From "Quantity of Radiation" and "Dose" to "Exposure" and "Absorbed Dose"—An Historical Review*

Hymer L. Friedell (1979) *Radiation Protection—Concepts and Trade Offs*

Sir Edward Pochin (1978) *Why be Quantitative about Radiation Risk Estimates?*

Herbert M. Parker (1977) *The Squares of the Natural Numbers in Radiation Protection*

Currently, the following committees are actively engaged in formulating recommendations:

Program Area Committee 1: Basic Criteria, Epidemiology, Radiobiology, and Risk

SC 1-13 Impact of Individual Susceptibility and Previous Radiation Exposure on Radiation Risk for Astronauts
SC 1-15 Radiation Safety in NASA Lunar Missions'
SC 1-16 Uncertainties in the Estimation of Radiation Risks and Probability of Disease Causation
SC 1-17 Second Cancers and Cardiopulmonary Effects After Radiotherapy
SC 85 Risk of Lung Cancer from Radon

Program Area Committee 2: Operational Radiation Safety

SC 2-2 Key Decision Points and Information Needed by Decision Makers in the Aftermath of a Nuclear or Radiological Terrorism Incident
SC 2-3 Radiation Safety Issues for Image-Guided Interventional Medical Procedures
SC 2-4 Self Assessment of Radiation Safety Programs

Program Area Committee 3: Nuclear and Radiological Security and Safety

Program Area Committee 4: Radiation Protection in Medicine

SC 4-1 Management of Persons Contaminated with Radionuclides
SC 4-2 Population Monitoring and Decontamination Following a Nuclear/ Radiological Incident
SC 4-3 Diagnostic Reference Levels in Medical Imaging: Recommendations for Application in the United States
SC 4-4 Risks of Ionizing Radiation to the Developing Embryo, Fetus and Nursing Infant

Program Area Committee 5: Environmental Radiation and Radioactive Waste Issues

SC 64-22 Design of Effective Effluent and Environmental Monitoring Programs

Program Area Committee 6: Radiation Measurements and Dosimetry

SC 6-3 Uncertainties in Internal Radiation Dosimetry
SC 6-4 Fundamental Principles of Dose Reconstruction

In recognition of its responsibility to facilitate and stimulate cooperation among organizations concerned with the scientific and related aspects of radiation protection and measurement, the Council has created a category of NCRP Collaborating Organizations. Organizations or groups of organizations that are national or international in scope and are concerned with scientific problems involving radiation quantities, units, measurements and effects, or radiation protection may be admitted to collaborating status by the Council. Collaborating Organizations provide a means by which NCRP can gain input into its activities from a wider segment of society. At the same time, the relationships with the Collaborating Organizations facilitate wider dissemination of information about the Council's activities, interests and concerns. Collaborating Organizations have the opportunity to comment on draft reports (at the time that these are submitted to the members of the Council). This is intended to capitalize on the fact that Collaborating Organizations are in an excellent position to both contribute to the identification of what needs to be treated in NCRP reports and to identify problems that might result from proposed recommendations. The present Collaborating Organizations with which NCRP maintains liaison are as follows:

American Academy of Dermatology
American Academy of Environmental Engineers
American Academy of Health Physics
American Academy of Orthopaedic Surgeons
American Association of Physicists in Medicine
American Bracytherapy Society
American College of Cardiology
American College of Medical Physics
American College of Nuclear Physicians
American College of Occupational and Environmental Medicine
American College of Radiology
American Conference of Governmental Industrial Hygienists
American Dental Association
American Industrial Hygiene Association
American Institute of Ultrasound in Medicine
American Medical Association
American Nuclear Society
American Pharmaceutical Association
American Podiatric Medical Association
American Public Health Association
American Radium Society
American Roentgen Ray Society
American Society for Radiation Oncology
American Society of Emergency Radiology
American Society of Health-System Pharmacists
American Society of Nuclear Cardiology
American Society of Radiologic Technologists
Association of Educators in Imaging and Radiological Sciences
Association of University Radiologists
Bioelectromagnetics Society
Campus Radiation Safety Officers
College of American Pathologists
Conference of Radiation Control Program Directors, Inc.
Council on Radionuclides and Radiopharmaceuticals
Defense Threat Reduction Agency
Electric Power Research Institute
Federal Aviation Administration
Federal Communications Commission
Federal Emergency Management Agency
Genetics Society of America
Health Physics Society
Institute of Electrical and Electronics Engineers, Inc.
Institute of Nuclear Power Operations
International Brotherhood of Electrical Workers

National Aeronautics and Space Administration
National Association of Environmental Professionals
National Center for Environmental Health/Agency for Toxic Substances
National Electrical Manufacturers Association
National Institute for Occupational Safety and Health
National Institute of Standards and Technology
Nuclear Energy Institute
Office of Science and Technology Policy
Paper, Allied-Industrial, Chemical and Energy Workers International
    Union
Product Stewardship Institute
Radiation Research Society
Radiological Society of North America
Society for Cardiovascular Angiography and Interventions
Society for Pediatric Radiology
Society for Risk Analysis
Society of Cardiovascular Computed Tomography
Society of Chairmen of Academic Radiology Departments
Society of Interventional Radiology
Society of Nuclear Medicine
Society of Radiologists in Ultrasound
Society of Skeletal Radiology
U.S. Air Force
U.S. Army
U.S. Coast Guard
U.S. Department of Energy
U.S. Department of Housing and Urban Development
U.S. Department of Labor
U.S. Department of Transportation
U.S. Environmental Protection Agency
U.S. Navy
U.S. Nuclear Regulatory Commission
U.S. Public Health Service
Utility Workers Union of America

NCRP has found its relationships with these organizations to be extremely valuable to continued progress in its program.

Another aspect of the cooperative efforts of NCRP relates to the Special Liaison relationships established with various governmental organizations that have an interest in radiation protection and measurements. This liaison relationship provides: (1) an opportunity for participating organizations to designate an individual to provide liaison between the organization and NCRP; (2) that the individual designated will receive copies of draft NCRP reports (at the time that these are submitted to the members of the Council) with an invitation to comment, but not vote; and (3) that new NCRP efforts might be discussed with liaison individuals as appropriate, so that they might have an opportunity to make suggestions on new studies and related matters. The following organizations participate in the Special Liaison Program:

Australian Radiation Laboratory
Bundesamt fur Strahlenschutz (Germany)

Canadian Nuclear Safety Commission
Central Laboratory for Radiological Protection (Poland)
China Institute for Radiation Protection
Commissariat a l'Energie Atomique (France)
Commonwealth Scientific Instrumentation Research Organization
    (Australia)
European Commission
Health Council of the Netherlands
Health Protection Agency
International Commission on Non-ionizing Radiation Protection
International Commission on Radiation Units and Measurements
International Radiation Protection Association
Japanese Nuclear Safety Commission
Japan Radiation Council
Korea Institute of Nuclear Safety
Russian Scientific Commission on Radiation Protection
South African Forum for Radiation Protection
World Association of Nuclear Operators
World Health Organization, Radiation and Environmental Health

NCRP values highly the participation of these organizations in the Special Liaison Program.

The Council also benefits significantly from the relationships established pursuant to the Corporate Sponsor's Program. The program facilitates the interchange of information and ideas and corporate sponsors provide valuable fiscal support for the Council's program. This developing program currently includes the following Corporate Sponsors:

Duke Energy Corporation
GE Healthcare
Global Dosimetry Solutions, Inc.
Landauer, Inc.
Nuclear Energy Institute

The Council's activities have been made possible by the voluntary contribution of time and effort by its members and participants and the generous support of the following organizations:

3M
3M Health Physics Services
Agfa Corporation
Alfred P. Sloan Foundation
Alliance of American Insurers
American Academy of Dermatology
American Academy of Health Physics
American Academy of Oral and Maxillofacial Radiology
American Association of Physicists in Medicine
American Cancer Society
American College of Medical Physics
American College of Nuclear Physicians
American College of Occupational and Environmental Medicine

American College of Radiology
American College of Radiology Foundation
American Dental Association
American Healthcare Radiology Administrators
American Industrial Hygiene Association
American Insurance Services Group
American Medical Association
American Nuclear Society
American Osteopathic College of Radiology
American Podiatric Medical Association
American Public Health Association
American Radium Society
American Roentgen Ray Society
American Society for Radiation Oncology
American Society for Therapeutic Radiology and Oncology
American Society of Radiologic Technologists
American Veterinary Medical Association
American Veterinary Radiology Society
Association of Educators in Radiological Sciences, Inc.
Association of University Radiologists
Battelle Memorial Institute
Canberra Industries, Inc.
Chem Nuclear Systems
Center for Devices and Radiological Health
College of American Pathologists
Committee on Interagency Radiation Research and Policy Coordination
Commonwealth Edison
Commonwealth of Pennsylvania
Consolidated Edison
Consumers Power Company
Council on Radionuclides and Radiopharmaceuticals
Defense Nuclear Agency
Defense Threat Reduction Agency
Eastman Kodak Company
Edison Electric Institute
Edward Mallinckrodt, Jr. Foundation
EG&G Idaho, Inc.
Electric Power Research Institute
Electromagnetic Energy Association
Federal Emergency Management Agency
Florida Institute of Phosphate Research
Florida Power Corporation
Fuji Medical Systems, U.S.A., Inc.
Genetics Society of America
Global Dosimetry Solutions
Health Effects Research Foundation (Japan)
Health Physics Society
ICN Biomedicals, Inc.
Institute of Nuclear Power Operations
James Picker Foundation

Martin Marietta Corporation
Motorola Foundation
National Aeronautics and Space Administration
National Association of Photographic Manufacturers
National Cancer Institute
National Electrical Manufacturers Association
National Institute of Standards and Technology
New York Power Authority
Philips Medical Systems
Picker International
Public Service Electric and Gas Company
Radiation Research Society
Radiological Society of North America
Richard Lounsbery Foundation
Sandia National Laboratory
Siemens Medical Systems, Inc.
Society of Nuclear Medicine
Society of Pediatric Radiology
Southern California Edison Company
U.S. Department of Energy
U.S. Department of Labor
U.S. Environmental Protection Agency
U.S. Navy
U.S. Nuclear Regulatory Commission
Victoreen, Inc.
Westinghouse Electric Corporation

Initial funds for publication of NCRP reports were provided by a grant from the James Picker Foundation.

NCRP seeks to promulgate information and recommendations based on leading scientific judgment on matters of radiation protection and measurement and to foster cooperation among organizations concerned with these matters. These efforts are intended to serve the public interest and the Council welcomes comments and suggestions on its reports or activities.

NCRP Publications

NCRP publications can be obtained online in both hard- and soft-copy (downloadable PDF) formats at http://NCRPpublications.org. Professional societies can arrange for discounts for their members by contacting NCRP. Additional information on NCRP publications may be obtained from the NCRP website (http://NCRPonline.org) or by telephone (800-229-2652, ext. 25) and fax (301-907-8768). The mailing address is:

NCRP Publications
7910 Woodmont Avenue
Suite 400
Bethesda, MD 20814-3095

Abstracts of NCRP reports published since 1980, abstracts of all NCRP commentaries, and the text of all NCRP statements are available at the NCRP website. Currently available publications are listed below.

NCRP Reports

No.   Title

8   *Control and Removal of Radioactive Contamination in Laboratories* (1951)

22   *Maximum Permissible Body Burdens and Maximum Permissible Concentrations of Radionuclides in Air and in Water for Occupational Exposure* (1959) [includes Addendum 1 issued in August 1963]

25   *Measurement of Absorbed Dose of Neutrons, and of Mixtures of Neutrons and Gamma Rays* (1961)

27   *Stopping Powers for Use with Cavity Chambers* (1961)

30   *Safe Handling of Radioactive Materials* (1964)

32   *Radiation Protection in Educational Institutions* (1966)

35   *Dental X-Ray Protection* (1970)

36   *Radiation Protection in Veterinary Medicine* (1970)

37   *Precautions in the Management of Patients Who Have Received Therapeutic Amounts of Radionuclides* (1970)

38   *Protection Against Neutron Radiation* (1971)

40   *Protection Against Radiation from Brachytherapy Sources* (1972)

41   *Specification of Gamma-Ray Brachytherapy Sources* (1974)

42   *Radiological Factors Affecting Decision-Making in a Nuclear Attack* (1974)

44   *Krypton-85 in the Atmosphere—Accumulation, Biological Significance, and Control Technology* (1975)

46   *Alpha-Emitting Particles in Lungs* (1975)

366

146 *Approaches to Risk Management in Remediation of Radioactively Contaminated Sites* (2004)

147 *Structural Shielding Design for Medical X-Ray Imaging Facilities* (2004)

148 *Radiation Protection in Veterinary Medicine* (2004)

149 *A Guide to Mammography and Other Breast Imaging Procedures* (2004)

150 *Extrapolation of Radiation-Induced Cancer Risks from Nonhuman Experimental Systems to Humans* (2005)

151 *Structural Shielding Design and Evaluation for Megavoltage X- and Gamma-Ray Radiotherapy Facilities* (2005)

152 *Performance Assessment of Near-Surface Facilities for Disposal of Low-Level Radioactive Waste* (2005)

153 *Information Needed to Make Radiation Protection Recommendations for Space Missions Beyond Low-Earth Orbit* (2006)

154 *Cesium-137 in the Environment: Radioecology and Approaches to Assessment and Management* (2006)

155 *Management of Radionuclide Therapy Patients* (2006)

156 *Development of a Biokinetic Model for Radionuclide-Contaminated Wounds and Procedures for Their Assessment, Dosimetry and Treatment* (2006)

157 *Radiation Protection in Educational Institutions* (2007)

158 *Uncertainties in the Measurement and Dosimetry of External Radiation* (2007)

159 *Risk to the Thyroid from Ionizing Radiation* (2008)

160 *Ionizing Radiation Exposure of the Population of the United States* (2009)

Binders for NCRP reports are available. Two sizes make it possible to collect into small binders the "old series" of reports (NCRP Reports Nos. 8–30) and into large binders the more recent publications (NCRP Reports Nos. 32–160). Each binder will accommodate from five to seven reports. The binders carry the identification "NCRP Reports" and come with label holders which permit the user to attach labels showing the reports contained in each binder.

The following bound sets of NCRP reports are also available:

Volume I. NCRP Reports Nos. 8, 22
Volume II. NCRP Reports Nos. 23, 25, 27, 30
Volume III. NCRP Reports Nos. 32, 35, 36, 37
Volume IV. NCRP Reports Nos. 38, 40, 41
Volume V. NCRP Reports Nos. 42, 44, 46
Volume VI. NCRP Reports Nos. 47, 49, 50, 51
Volume VII. NCRP Reports Nos. 52, 53, 54, 55, 57
Volume VIII. NCRP Report No. 58
Volume IX. NCRP Reports Nos. 59, 60, 61, 62, 63
Volume X. NCRP Reports Nos. 64, 65, 66, 67
Volume XI. NCRP Reports Nos. 68, 69, 70, 71, 72
Volume XII. NCRP Reports Nos. 73, 74, 75, 76
Volume XIII. NCRP Reports Nos. 77, 78, 79, 80
Volume XIV. NCRP Reports Nos. 81, 82, 83, 84, 85

Volume XV. NCRP Reports Nos. 86, 87, 88, 89
Volume XVI. NCRP Reports Nos. 90, 91, 92, 93
Volume XVII. NCRP Reports Nos. 94, 95, 96, 97
Volume XVIII. NCRP Reports Nos. 98, 99, 100
Volume XIX. NCRP Reports Nos. 101, 102, 103, 104
Volume XX. NCRP Reports Nos. 105, 106, 107, 108
Volume XXI. NCRP Reports Nos. 109, 110, 111
Volume XXII. NCRP Reports Nos. 112, 113, 114
Volume XXIII. NCRP Reports Nos. 115, 116, 117, 118
Volume XXIV. NCRP Reports Nos. 119, 120, 121, 122
Volume XXV. NCRP Report No. 123I and 123II
Volume XXVI. NCRP Reports Nos. 124, 125, 126, 127
Volume XXVII. NCRP Reports Nos. 128, 129, 130
Volume XXVIII. NCRP Reports Nos. 131, 132, 133
Volume XXIX. NCRP Reports Nos. 134, 135, 136, 137
Volume XXX. NCRP Reports Nos. 138, 139
Volume XXXI. NCRP Report No. 140
Volume XXXII. NCRP Reports Nos. 141, 142, 143
Volume XXXIII. NCRP Report No. 144
Volume XXXIV. NCRP Reports Nos. 145, 146, 147
Volume XXXV. NCRP Reports Nos. 148, 149
Volume XXXVI. NCRP Reports Nos. 150, 151, 152
Volume XXXVII, NCRP Reports Nos. 153, 154, 155
Volume XXXVIII, NCRP Reports Nos. 156, 157, 158

(Titles of the individual reports contained in each volume are given previously.)

NCRP Commentaries

No.   Title

1   *Krypton-85 in the Atmosphere—With Specific Reference to the Public Health Significance of the Proposed Controlled Release at Three Mile Island* (1980)

4   *Guidelines for the Release of Waste Water from Nuclear Facilities with Special Reference to the Public Health Significance of the Proposed Release of Treated Waste Waters at Three Mile Island* (1987)

5   *Review of the Publication, Living Without Landfills* (1989)

6   *Radon Exposure of the U.S. Population—Status of the Problem (1991)*

7   *Misadministration of Radioactive Material in Medicine—Scientific Background* (1991)

8   *Uncertainty in NCRP Screening Models Relating to Atmospheric Transport, Deposition and Uptake by Humans* (1993)

9   *Considerations Regarding the Unintended Radiation Exposure of the Embryo, Fetus or Nursing Child* (1994)

10   *Advising the Public about Radiation Emergencies: A Document for Public Comment* (1994)

11   *Dose Limits for Individuals Who Receive Exposure from Radionuclide Therapy Patients* (1995)

12   *Radiation Exposure and High-Altitude Flight* (1995)

Proceedings of the Annual Meeting

13 *Genes, Cancer and Radiation Protection,* Proceedings of the Twenty-seventh Annual Meeting held on April 3-4, 1991 (including Taylor Lecture No. 15) (1992)

14 *Radiation Protection in Medicine,* Proceedings of the Twenty-eighth Annual Meeting held on April 1-2, 1992 (including Taylor Lecture No. 16) (1993)

15 *Radiation Science and Societal Decision Making,* Proceedings of the Twenty-ninth Annual Meeting held on April 7-8, 1993 (including Taylor Lecture No. 17) (1994)

16 *Extremely-Low-Frequency Electromagnetic Fields: Issues in Biological Effects and Public Health,* Proceedings of the Thirtieth Annual Meeting held on April 6-7, 1994 (not published).

17 *Environmental Dose Reconstruction and Risk Implications,* Proceedings of the Thirty-first Annual Meeting held on April 12-13, 1995 (including Taylor Lecture No. 19) (1996)

18 *Implications of New Data on Radiation Cancer Risk,* Proceedings of the Thirty-second Annual Meeting held on April 3-4, 1996 (including Taylor Lecture No. 20) (1997)

19 *The Effects of Pre- and Postconception Exposure to Radiation,* Proceedings of the Thirty-third Annual Meeting held on April 2-3, 1997, Teratology **59**, 181–317 (1999)

20 *Cosmic Radiation Exposure of Airline Crews, Passengers and Astronauts,* Proceedings of the Thirty-fourth Annual Meeting held on April 1-2, 1998, Health Phys. **79**, 466–613 (2000)

21 *Radiation Protection in Medicine: Contemporary Issues,* Proceedings of the Thirty-fifth Annual Meeting held on April 7-8, 1999 (including Taylor Lecture No. 23) (1999)

22 *Ionizing Radiation Science and Protection in the 21st Century,* Proceedings of the Thirty-sixth Annual Meeting held on April 5-6, 2000, Health Phys. **80**, 317–402 (2001)

23 *Fallout from Atmospheric Nuclear Tests—Impact on Science and Society,* Proceedings of the Thirty-seventh Annual Meeting held on April 4-5, 2001, Health Phys. **82**, 573–748 (2002)

24 *Where the New Biology Meets Epidemiology: Impact on Radiation Risk Estimates,* Proceedings of the Thirty-eighth Annual Meeting held on April 10-11, 2002, Health Phys. **85**, 1–108 (2003)

25 *Radiation Protection at the Beginning of the 21st Century–A Look Forward,* Proceedings of the Thirty-ninth Annual Meeting held on April 9–10, 2003, Health Phys. **87**, 237–319 (2004)

26 *Advances in Consequence Management for Radiological Terrorism Events,* Proceedings of the Fortieth Annual Meeting held on April 14–15, 2004, Health Phys. **89**, 415–588 (2005)

27 *Managing the Disposition of Low-Activity Radioactive Materials,* Proceedings of the Forty-first Annual Meeting held on March 30–31, 2005, Health Phys. **91**, 413–536 (2006)

28 *Chernobyl at Twenty,* Proceedings of the Forty-second Annual Meeting held on April 3–4, 2006, Health Phys. **93**, 345–595 (2007)

29 *Advances in Radiation Protection in Medicine,* Proceedings of the Forty-third Annual Meeting held on April 16-17, 2007, Health Phys. **95**, 461–686 (2008)

Lauriston S. Taylor Lectures

Symposium Proceedings

NCRP Statements

No.   Title

1   "Blood Counts, Statement of the National Committee on Radiation
    Protection," Radiology **63**, 428 (1954)
2   "Statements on Maximum Permissible Dose from Television
    Receivers and Maximum Permissible Dose to the Skin of the Whole
    Body," Am. J. Roentgenol., Radium Ther. and Nucl. Med. **84**, 152
    (1960) and Radiology **75**, 122 (1960)
3   *X-Ray Protection Standards for Home Television Receivers, Interim
    Statement of the National Council on Radiation Protection and
    Measurements* (1968)
4   *Specification of Units of Natural Uranium and Natural Thorium,
    Statement of the National Council on Radiation Protection and
    Measurements* (1973)
5   *NCRP Statement on Dose Limit for Neutrons* (1980)
6   *Control of Air Emissions of Radionuclides* (1984)
7   *The Probability That a Particular Malignancy May Have Been Caused
    by a Specified Irradiation* (1992)
8   *The Application of ALARA for Occupational Exposures* (1999)
9   *Extension of the Skin Dose Limit for Hot Particles to Other External
    Sources of Skin Irradiation* (2001)
10 *Recent Applications of the NCRP Public Dose Limit Recommendation
    for Ionizing Radiation* (2004)

Other Documents

The following documents were published outside of the NCRP report, commentary and statement series:

Somatic Radiation Dose for the General Population, Report of the Ad Hoc
    Committee of the National Council on Radiation Protection and
    Measurements, 6 May 1959, Science **131** (3399), February 19,
    482–486 (1960)
Dose Effect Modifying Factors in Radiation Protection, Report of
    Subcommittee M-4 (Relative Biological Effectiveness) of the National
    Council on Radiation Protection and Measurements, Report BNL
    50073 (T-471) (1967) Brookhaven National Laboratory (National
    Technical Information Service, Springfield, Virginia)
*Residential Radon Exposure and Lung Cancer Risk: Commentary on
    Cohen's County-Based Study*, Health Phys. **87**(6), 656–658 (2004)

Index